09

Integrating Healthcare with Information and Communications Technology

Integrating Healthcare with Information and Communications Technology

Edited by

WENDY CURRIE

Professor and Head
Information Systems and Management Group
Warwick Business School

and

DAVID FINNEGAN

Associate Professor
Information Systems and Management Group
Warwick Business School

Radcliffe Publishing
Oxford • New York

Radcliffe Publishing Ltd
18 Marcham Road
Abingdon
Oxon OX14 1AA
United Kingdom

www.radcliffe-oxford.com

Electronic catalogue and worldwide online ordering facility.

ISBN-13: 978 184619 300 2

The paper used for the text pages of this book is FSC certified. FSC (The Forest Stewardship Council) is an international network to promote responsible management of the world's forests.

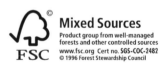

Mixed Sources
Product group from well-managed forests and other controlled sources
www.fsc.org Cert no. SGS-COC-2482
© 1996 Forest Stewardship Council

Typeset by Pindar NZ, Auckland, New Zealand
Printed and bound by TJI Digital, Padstow, Cornwall, UK

Contents

About the editors   vii
Contributors   ix

PART ONE Transforming Healthcare Services using ICT   1

1 Integrating healthcare   3
   Wendy Currie

2 Information systems (IS) integration approaches
   in healthcare: a critical review   35
   David Finnegan and Khairil Azhar Abdul Hamid

3 Modernising healthcare: really connecting for health?   65
   Annabelle Mark

4 Integrating healthcare with ICT   85
   John Powell

5 The National Programme for IT (NPfIT): is there a better way?   95
   Sean Brennan

PART TWO Electronic Health Records   111

6 Electronic health records for patient-centred healthcare   113
   Nick Gaunt

7 Integrating electronic health records   135
   Wendy Currie, David Finnegan and Khairil Azhar Abdul Hamid

8 The NHS National Programme for Information Technology:
   a socio-technical systems perspective   183
   Ken Eason

PART THREE Global ICT Adoption and Implementation in Healthcare   205

  9 New IT and the Kaiser Chiefs: EMR integration in the Aloha State   207
    Tim Scott

10 Some insights into the national healthcare systems of the
    United Kingdom and the Netherlands   241
    Matthew Waritay Guah

11 Customer value and lean operations in a self-care setting   255
    Jannis Angelis, Cameron Watt and Mairi Macintyre

    Index   267

About the editors

Wendy Currie is Professor and Head of the Information Systems and Management Group at Warwick Business School. She holds a PhD in Management and a BSc in Sociology. Her research focuses on the information and communications technology and change in private and public sector organisations with particular interest in governance, compliance, audit and evaluation. She has obtained research funding from the European Union, EPSRC, ESRC and from industry. Recent projects have included a longitudinal study on the National Programme for IT, managing ICT in healthcare organisations, implementing compliance systems in financial services firms, and cross-national policy and practice on security, identity and management systems. In 2005, she set up the MSc Information Systems and Management course at Warwick Business School, which aims to promote the 'university apprentice' scheme by placing students in organisations for their dissertation work. The course is now a leader in this market and is currently expanding each year. Wendy is on the editorial board of seven academic journals and regularly publishes her research work. She currently serves as Hon Treasurer with an education charity, the Fellowship of Postgraduate Medicine. She is co-founder (with David Finnegan) of the Business, Technology, Leadership and Management research unit at Warwick and regularly consults with organisations on ICT strategy, change management, audit and evaluation.

Dr David Finnegan gained a PhD in Information Systems from Warwick Business School, focusing on business systems integration and customer relationship management. With 20 years of senior management experience, he specialises in business systems integration. His PhD in this area was sponsored by IBM. With an international background in management and IT consultancy, he combines research and experiential learning where students apply theory to practice. For the MSc in Information Systems and Management, he partnered with Deloitte to give students a working experience of the management consultancy life cycle with a close coupling between theory and practice. This fulfils the vision of this course and his ambition to provide business school students with practically based work placements (a university apprenticeship model). Previous roles have included working for the Swedish Home Office and working in the e-business environment in strategic leadership, mentoring and auditing roles. David moved into academia where he carries out research into ICT business, management and leadership. He recently published a book on customer relationship management and is currently working on a research study comparing integrated healthcare in Sweden and the UK.

Contributors

Dr Jannis Angelis is an Assistant Professor of Operations Management at Warwick Business School, where he teaches operations management and strategy, and an associated researcher with the Centre for Technology, Policy and Industrial Development at MIT. Following a doctorate on numerical flexibility and productivity in FMCGs at Cambridge, Dr Angelis worked in venture capital in London. Prior roles also include work on competitiveness at Harvard, flexibility and productivity at Stanford and Berkeley, lean and behavioural operations at Cambridge, high performance practices in aerospace at Oxford, and Asian export processing zones at the UN.

Sean Brennan had a long career in the NHS, initially in Pathology then as a General Manager and Information Manager responsible for the (then) Resource Management Initiative, Medical Audit and IT staff. In the mid-1990s Sean was seconded to the Department of Health as Clinical Audit Advisor and then appointed Project Manager for the national Electronic Patient Record Project in England. In 2000, Sean joined Northgate Information Solutions (formerly MDIS) as Head of Healthcare Strategy, experiencing life in the commercial sector. Two years later he launched Clinical Matrix Limited, a network of consultants engaged in strategy development, business cases, clinical change management and general healthcare informatics projects for the NHS and commercial customers. His bestselling book *The NHS IT Project: The Biggest Computer Programme in the World . . . Ever!* was published in April 2005 by Radcliffe Publishing and considers the National Programme for IT (NPfIT), as being delivered by Connecting for Health (CfH), in the context of the last 20 years of health IT.

Ken Eason is Professor Emeritus in the Department of Human Sciences at Loughborough University and Senior Consultant in the Bayswater Institute in London. For 40 years Ken has researched the impact of IT on organisations using socio-technical systems theory as an explanatory framework and has published widely on the challenges of integrating technical developments with changing organisational reality. As an action researcher he has worked with IT suppliers and user organisations to develop user-centred design methods by which human and organisational issues can be treated in systems development. This work was conducted in organisations including publishers and libraries developing digital libraries, military organisations procuring new systems and banks, utilities, city firms and government departments upgrading their electronic systems. A continuous thread since 1978, however, has been work with healthcare organisations on the implementation of successive waves of e-health systems. His book *Information Technology and Organisational Change* became a standard text in the teaching of socio-technical approaches on information system courses. After 30 years at Loughborough University, Ken became the Director of the Bayswater Institute in 2002 to focus on action research work with organisations. From 2004 to 2009 he worked extensively with NHS trusts on the implementation issues of the NHS National Programme for IT.

Dr Nick Gaunt is Specialist Associate in Technology and Product Innovation NHS Institute for Innovation and Improvement, based at the University of Warwick. Following a first career as a senior hospital doctor in the UK NHS and a career-long interest and professional involvement in health informatics and information security, Nick spent several years leading local Health Informatics Services in Devon. During that time he was responsible for developing an electronic health record demonstrator that aggregated clinical records into a patient-centred and controlled web environment. It was an early example of how e-health systems might support the end-to-end patient journey, integrated care pathways and healthcare business processes focused around the patient rather than the clinician. Sadly, the lessons were not transferred into the subsequent National Programme for IT. His current role as a Specialist Associate in the NHS Institute for Innovation and Improvement draws together this experience and the theory and practice of improvement and large-scale change, to foster healthcare transformation through the innovative application of technologies. Professional interests include approaches to influencing the adoption of disruptive technologies, the application of complexity science to healthcare improvement, and the modelling and simulation of healthcare processes to support business change.

Dr Matthew Waritay Guah is Assistant Professor at Erasmus School of Economics, Erasmus University, Rotterdam. His research focus is organisational issues surrounding emerging technologies in the healthcare and financial industries. Other research interests include neo-institutional theory, socioeconomic impacts of IS on government services delivery, resistance to IS, organisational reform, IS infrastructure, strategic planning for IS – with a more general interest in the cognitive, material and social relationships between science, technology and business as well as their implications for present-day understandings of creativity and innovation. He holds a PhD in Information Systems and Management Controls from Warwick Business School, MSc in Technology Management from University of Manchester, and BSc (Honours) from Salford University, UK. He came into academia with a wealth of industrial experience spanning over 10 years (Merrill Lynch, CITI Bank, HSBC, British Airways, and United Nations). He has authored *Managing Very Large IT Projects* and

Internet Strategy: The Road to Web Services (with Wendy Currie). He has published widely in the information systems and management journals and is editor-in-chief for the *International Journal of Healthcare Delivery Reform Initiatives*. He has been track chair for major IS conferences (ICIS, ECIS, AMCIS, etc.). He is a member of ERIM, AIS, UKAIS and BMiS.

Khairil Azhar Abdul Hamid is an IT professional with over nine years' experience in technical implementation and support, technical account management and technology consultancy in mission-critical computing environments. He has held various roles during a seven-year tenure at Hewlett Packard Malaysia as a systems engineer, account support manager and technology consultant prior to earning an MSc in Information Systems and Management from the University of Warwick. He also holds a BEng in Electrical and Electronic Engineering from the University of Nottingham. Khairil has been involved in numerous IT infrastructure deployment and integration projects for large multinational corporations ranging from the telecommunications to manufacturing industries, to financial services and commercial enterprises, as well as public sector organisations. Khairil is currently an Information Systems Architect attached to Hewlett Packard's Solution Infrastructure Practice within the Technology Solutions Group. He specialises in IT solution consulting and technical service delivery for enterprise customers that enable these large organisations to best utilise and integrate cutting-edge infrastructure technologies to achieve their business goals. His primary areas of expertise include enterprise data storage, systems virtualisation and high availability solutions. Khairil's information systems subjects of interest include IT governance and information systems strategy.

Mairi Macintyre is currently leading work on a major project for the WIMRC Next Generation Healthcare Processes theme at WMG of the University of Warwick, which combines systems thinking with operations management and psychology. She has a breadth of sector experience from manufacturing and service, public and private. The research is both multidisciplinary and multi-sector. With a mathematical and engineering background, Mairi has worked extensively with organisations that have undergone or intend to undergo lean or other process transformations.

Annabelle Mark is Professor of Healthcare Organisation at Middlesex University and Director of the NHS Human Resource Management Training Scheme which is, for the third year running, top of the Times Graduate Schemes HR programmes across all sectors of the economy in the UK. An Honorary Professor at Glasgow University and Eminent Research Visitor 2009–11 at the University of Western Sydney, Australia, she had a 10-year career in the NHS before becoming an academic in the 1980s. A Fellow of both the Institute of Healthcare Management and the Royal Society of Medicine, she is the first elected Chair of the Society for Studies in Organising Healthcare (SHOC) affiliated to the Academy of Social Sciences and founding academic of the international biennial conference Organisational Behaviour in Healthcare. Her publications and research focus on the development of professionals and technology in organising and changing healthcare, demarketing and managing demand, including research on NHS Direct in the UK, the role of emotion in healthcare organisation, including an award-winning special edition of the *Journal of Health Organisation & Management*, and international health development including pan-European research on the quality of working life.

Dr John Powell is Associate Clinical Professor in Epidemiology and Public Health at the University of Warwick and an Honorary NHS Consultant. He undertakes research in the area of e-health. His interests include the social aspects of connected health, the use of the internet as a tool for delivering health services, and e-research methods. His current projects include an investigation of consumer use of the NHS Direct website; a study of an Internet-based cardiac rehabilitation programme; development of a virtual reality treatment of anxiety; a study of knowledge management in the NHS; and a study of networked technologies and carers of people with dementia. He has worked at the Department of Health and for independent health information websites.

Dr Tim Scott is Senior Lecturer in Organisation at St Andrews University School of Management. After trying jobs as varied as roof-tiler and trawlerman, he started a British Rail career as a signalman in 1979, resigning from the post of Senior Industrial Relations Officer in 2000. During his early career, he began to read for a first degree in the humanities with the Open University. This was abandoned after two years to read for an MA in Organisational Analysis and Behaviour at the University of Lancaster. After a brief return to BR, he resigned to take up a scholarship-funded PhD at the University of Hull. He then entered health services research and was awarded a Harkness Fellowship in 2002–3. He has also worked at The University of York, and UC Berkeley. Tim has published a wide range of articles, including studies of improving communication with patients about their cancer or heart disease, organisational culture, health information technology, and ethnography. He has published books on healthcare performance and organisational culture; an account of implementing new information technology in Kaiser Permanente; and, most recently, a post-structural revision of organisation studies. His current teaching and research focus is on the history and interpretation of advertising as social communication.

Dr Cameron Watt has worked in the creative industry for over 20 years. After completing an MBA in 1994 he continued in the industry in brand development. His PhD focused on the role of trust and stakeholder relationships in facilitating creativity in organisations. He has lectured widely on the subject of creativity, innovation and branding at a number of universities and design schools, including Warwick Manufacturing Group, Kingston Business School and the University for the Creative Arts. He has been working with the National Health Service investigating the implementation and diffusion of Lean to improve service provision. In a consultancy role he acts as a creativity, change and innovation diffusion consultant for a number of organisations.

PART ONE

Transforming Healthcare Services using ICT

CHAPTER 1

Integrating healthcare

Wendy Currie

ABOUT THIS BOOK

The challenge to provide a nationwide integrated healthcare service continues unabated in the 21st century as politicians and managers drive through policies to modernise the UK National Health Service (NHS). Government policy to 'modernise' the NHS for the past four decades has produced a series of white papers and reports (e.g. Patients First, 1969, The Griffiths Report, 1983, Working for Patients, 1989, The New NHS, 1997, The NHS Plan, 2000, Delivering 21st Century IT Support for the NHS, 2002, High Quality Care for All, 2008). While the overriding theme of these contributions has been the introduction of private-sector-style practices and procedures into the UK NHS, the consequences have often led to confusion and chaos as continuous change initiatives have produced unintended outcomes such as process and service fragmentation rather than integration (Currie and Guah 2007). The key research question addressed in this edited volume is: How can ICT be used to develop market-driven healthcare (more variety and choice of service providers for patients) against the current background of relative stability and persistence in healthcare practices (institutionalised practices) while simultaneously moving from a fragmented (disparate healthcare services) to an integrated (seamless services) healthcare industry?

To answer this question, contributions were sought from a team of academic and practitioner experts, with many years' experience of researching and/or working in healthcare. This book is divided into three parts. Part One considers the broad issue of transforming healthcare using ICTs. It focuses upon market, organisational, managerial and technical aspects of ICT-enabled transformation of healthcare. Part Two considers the topic of electronic health records (EHRs), which is a broader agenda than electronic medical or patient records. International governments are currently introducing policies to develop and implement EHRs to move healthcare away from a supplier-driven to a consumer-driven approach. The chapters focus on theoretical and practical issues. Part Three considers the global healthcare integration challenge featuring research studies from different countries. Empirical work includes studies from Scandinavia, the US, UK and the Netherlands to provide a basis for comparison of different clinical and non-clinical healthcare systems. While cross-national comparisons need to recognise socio-political, cultural and economic diversity, they provide some valuable lessons on different policies and practices of ICTs in healthcare, some of which may be transferable across geographical and organisational boundaries.

INTEGRATING HEALTHCARE: A 21ST-CENTURY CHALLENGE

The academic and practitioner communities recognise the challenge of integrating healthcare to improve service delivery to patients, yet few studies exist which identify the broad range of themes and issues necessary to achieve this goal. Our lengthy review of the literature points to multiple silos where clinicians are unlikely to read studies on ICT and healthcare published in management and IT journals, and academics and practitioners interested in business, management and IT issues are also unlikely to refer to clinical and health informatics journals. Such a narrow scholarly and practitioner focus inevitably leads to poor understanding of the broader clinical and non-clinical challenges of introducing large-scale ICT change in healthcare organisations. Figure 1.1 identifies four broad disciplines or fields of investigation that publish studies on ICT in healthcare. From a clinical perspective, studies commonly focus on issues such as ICT for clinical decision making and support and related issues of patient safety and medical error. Studies from the more general business and management literature tend to emphasise issues of organisational transformation and change. Whereas some of these studies focus on the macro level of analysis, including the political impetus for driving through changes in healthcare, other studies consider how managers and healthcare professionals may impose or become the recipients of change in healthcare organisations. Many of these contributions include case study scenarios on the adoption, implementation and evaluation of ICT change.

Alongside clinical and managerial studies, we identify two further technology-focused areas that overlap. Each area draws academics and practitioners from a variety of disciplines and backgrounds. Within the field of information systems and technology, a range of studies look at the 'engineering' problems of introducing large-scale ICT into healthcare organisations. Many of these studies stem from the field of computer science and engineering and often consider the technical imperative to be the most important and challenging issue. Studies in this field highlight the technical changes which take place, such as how hospitals have moved from the early radiology systems of the 1960s, through to the patient administrative systems in the 1970s, to the personal computers of the 1980s, the Internet of the 1990s, and more recently, the issue of software as a service and the networked society of the 21st century (Carter 2008). Recently, the information systems and technology domain has considered the technical challenges of data security and protection, particularly as electronic data storage of patient records carries additional risks over paper records (Johns 2008). Coupled with the work in this area, the field of health informatics

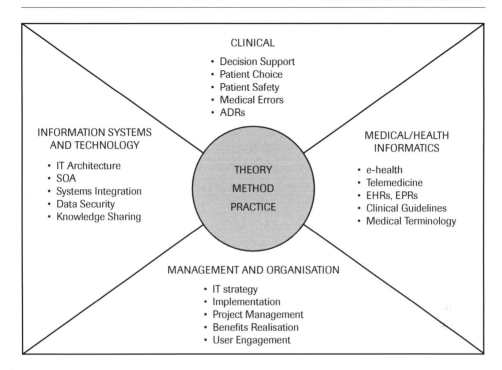

FIGURE 1.1 Integrating healthcare

fully embraces the link between healthcare and information technology. Health or medical informatics is defined as the intersection of information science, computer science and healthcare. The subject considers the 'resources, devices, and methods required to optimise the acquisition, storage, retrieval, and use of information in health and biomedicine. Health informatics tools include not only computers but also clinical guidelines, formal medical terminologies, and information and communication systems'.

Since the literature on ICT and healthcare is spread across several disciplines, with academics and practitioners tending to restrict their participation to their own professional groups and subject areas, it is not surprising that our review of the literature reveals a tendency among writers to revisit issues and debates that are well rehearsed in some areas but not in others. For example, within the management and organisation literature, the notion that IT is not simply about the technical imperative, but also about policies, people, processes and practices, is a perennial issue. However, in the field of medical/health informatics, which has commonly produced studies that identify the engineering and technical challenges of introducing ICT into healthcare, authors welcome studies on the socio-technical approach to evaluation (de Lusignan and Aarts 2008). Spanning different disciplines is a fruitful exercise since it reveals a rich source of material on different, yet related, themes and issues on the deployment and use of ICT in healthcare organisations. We would therefore encourage an interdisciplinary focus, particularly to avoid reinventing the wheel.

The next three sections present an overview of some of the literature from various disciplinary areas organised around specific themes and issues. This is not an exhaustive list of the literature, but an attempt to isolate studies which embrace ICT as a driver for change or more broadly discuss issues around innovation and transformation. One of our observations from reading the range of papers is that the more general business and management literature tends to 'black box' technology, whereby technology is peripheral to the wider managerial and organisational issues. While this perspective offers an interesting and insightful contribution to managing change within healthcare settings, it often underplays the role of technology, and, more importantly, specific technical applications which may be integral to the change process. Equally, the health informatics and IT literature often underplays the importance of 'people' issues, often aggregating this critical element under the term 'human factors'. In this regard, human behaviour is often seen as 'rational' and amenable to performance measurement if not management. From our analysis of the literature, we delineate three broad interdisciplinary themes which we consider integral to the relationship between ICT and healthcare. They are: institutional and organisational change and ICT; ICT architecture, applications, process and systems integration; and performance measurement, risk assessment and benefits realisation.

INSTITUTIONAL/ORGANISATIONAL CHANGE AND ICT

The fields of business management and health informatics are replete with studies on institutional/organisational change and ICT. The former offers a broad range of studies which focus on policy and economic issues relating to value creation in public services and redefining the healthcare industry. These contributions consider how publicly funded healthcare organisations may adopt methods and practices used in the private sector to create a 'New Public Management' (Moore 1995) which better serves the public interest. More specifically, the global healthcare industry is perceived to be in a parlous state as budgets soar without a commensurate increase in service levels to patients and citizens (Porter and Teisberg 2006). While these studies do not identify ICT as a leading contender to improve healthcare services, other writers more specifically consider the role of innovation and technology in healthcare (Casebeer, Harrison and Mark 2006). An earlier study identified how the UK NHS introduced a Resource Management Initiative (RMI) to deploy information systems to connect medical activity to resource usage and to costs (Bloomfield 1991:701). This study showed how IT was used to improve 'greater communication, planning and control, and even to bring about changes in organisational cultures'.

Since the late 1980s, ICT has been increasingly linked with the performance management of healthcare organisations, together with studies on how management methods and practices developed in the private sector have been introduced into public services. These initiatives include total quality management techniques (Currie 1995), business process re-engineering (McNulty and Ferlie 2002, 2004; Willcocks and Currie 1997) knowledge management (Currie and Suhomlinova 2006) and, more recently, new variants on quality management and lean manufacturing (Boaden, Harvey, Moxham, *et al.* 2008).

While these practices may produce variable benefits across healthcare services, many writers caution that simply applying management tools and techniques from the private sector into healthcare is not a guarantee for success (Willcocks and Currie 1997), particularly as each sector is governed by different management philosophies, policies, practices and procedures. In conjunction with studies on policy and market drivers for ICT, others focus on technology-enabled improvement in service delivery in healthcare. This is partly fuelled by government policy to introduce ICT as a change agent in transforming the healthcare industry (*see* Department of Health reports 2000, 2002) and also ICT adoption and diffusion practices in specific clinical or non-clinical organisational settings, e.g. cardiology, renal dialysis, patient administration. An integral part of studying ICT in healthcare is the recognition that health professionals are governed by different management practices, embedded into organisational structures and cultures. The notion that new management practices can easily translate across private sector settings into healthcare is somewhat misguided. As writers have identified, it is important to understand the contextual nature of medical information and how it is used by professionals in their day-to-day activities (Berg 1999). Thus implementing an information system in banking or manufacturing will be very different from doing so in a hospital.

Empirical research into the design and implementation of ICTs in the UK NHS has found that poor user engagement is a significant barrier to adoption (Currie and Guah 2007). Despite the label of a national health service, ICTs have developed across a very fragmented system over the past 50 years, not helped by the constant structural and organisational changes in the service. So, whereas some healthcare organisations (e.g. the large hospitals) have invested more money into developing ICTs, albeit in specific clinical and non-clinical settings, other less well-resourced providers have not been able to embrace the full benefits from technical change (Brennan 2005). This is a significant factor in understanding the potential and actual adoption of ICTs, particularly as the level of IT maturity (i.e. the understanding, ability to use, propensity to use and perceived effectiveness of ICT) varies considerably across the landscape of healthcare providers. For example, a teaching hospital may be a world leader in renal dialysis and therefore invest considerable resources in developing ICT to retain its status. The same organisation, however, may be less inclined to invest in other forms of technology (devices or software), particularly where clinicians show little interest. Introducing technology is therefore closely related to the contextual situation, so quick-fix solutions are unlikely to produce satisfactory results (Doolin 2004; Currie 1995). The institutional/organisational change and ICT literature provides a useful multi-level analysis on the importance of understanding policy, organisational and managerial issues in the adoption and diffusion of ICTs. One observation is that the ICT or technical aspects are often underplayed as contributions highlight structural, cultural and ethical factors, thus ignoring the varying effects of different technology artefacts across organisations, departments and units.

TABLE 1.1 Institutional and organisational change and ICT

Policy and market drivers for ICT	Healthcare policy, ICT and transformation in healthcare, health economics and global challenges, the history and development of ICTs in healthcare, medical/professional bodies and their comments on government ICT policy, market-driven approaches to healthcare.	Bloomfield 1991, Brennan 2005, Burgoyne, Brown, Hindle, *et al.* 1997, British Computer Society 2006, British Medical Association 2007, Brown 2001, Currie and Guah 2007, de Lusignan and Aarts 2008, Ham 2004, Harrison 2004, Institute of Medicine 2002, Klein 2001, Mohan 2002, Payne and Rhia 2006, Pollock 2005, Scott, Ruef, Mendel, *et al.* 2000, Summers 2007.
ICT service delivery in healthcare	Primary care (GPs and practice team) are 'high maturity' in terms of provision of ICT hardware and software.	Luftman 2000, Majeed 2003, Ondo and Smith 2006.
	Secondary care (hospital doctors, nurses, administrators) are 'low maturity' users of ICT.	
	Supplier knowledge/capability of NHS/ healthcare industry.	
	'Best practice' scenarios of ICT adoption and implementation.	
Management practice	The role of management in changing healthcare practices.	Herzlinger 1989, Kyu Kim and Michelman 1990, Berry, Mirabito and Berwick 2004.
Structure/culture	Structural and cultural issues which inhibit introduction of ICT.	Lee 1971, Casebeer, Harrison and Mark 2006.
	Poor communication channels between clinical/non-clinical (managerial and administrative) staff.	
	Lack of clinical engagement.	
	Unclear key performance indicators for evaluating ICT.	
	Financial/cost constraints.	
	Lack of training.	
Medical information and informatics	Contextual nature of medical information.	Berg 1999, Brownbridge, Lilford and Tindle-Biscoe 1988, Friedman and Abbas 2003, Mandl and Lee 2002.

Design	Poor 'user engagement' between government, ICT suppliers, NHS staff and public at design stage.	Currie and Guah 2006, Jeffcott and Johnson 2002.
	Lack of consensus about data inputs for summary/detailed care record.	
	Records need to reflect the needs of all clinicians, not only GPs.	
	Confusion about mechanisms to keep parts of the record confidential (sealing).	
Ethics	Lack of agreement about assumed or explicit consent for information sharing.	Currie and Guah 2007, Carter 2008.
	Poor communication between government/NHS executives and public/patients about summary care record.	

ICT ARCHITECTURE, APPLICATIONS, PROCESS AND SYSTEMS INTEGRATION

The more technically focused literature, particularly from the health informatics or information systems and technology fields, is complementary to the former, more broader institutional and organisational approach, since it considers the technical and engineering challenges of introducing new hardware and software in healthcare settings. Whereas the health informatics literature looks at technologies designed and applied to healthcare, there is a wealth of literature from the information systems and technology area that considers these challenges across different geographical, industrial, organisational and operational contexts. Our observations from reading this literature give support to the view that many engineering and technical challenges faced by other sectors are similar to healthcare. However, these challenges may differ when professional, clinical and managerial factors are considered. For example, it is important to recognise that introducing manufacturing methods and practices, such as total quality management and just-in-time manufacturing, into healthcare may not produce the desired benefits as the engineering and technical challenges may be less significant compared with cultural and managerial issues (Currie 1995).

The literature which considers ICT architecture, design, process and systems integration is highly relevant to healthcare professionals, particularly as many change management initiatives are designed to implement new systems to improve service delivery in healthcare. Within the field of health informatics, there are many studies on how ICT can enhance clinical decision making, particularly as new technologies come on stream. Healthcare IT has been described as an 'alphabet soup' (Thomas 2006) as new acronyms are increasingly introduced. Confusion exists about the acronyms electronic health records (EHRs), electronic medical records (EMRs) and personal health records (PHRs). They are defined respectively as, 'EHRs provide clinicians with access to patient information and provide evidence-based decision support; EMRs are the electronic version of a legal health record; PHRs are digital health records that are owned, updated and controlled by the consumer' (Thomas

2006: 100). PHRs are also likely to be referred to as electronic patient records (EPRs). Whether these definitions are adopted or not, a common understanding is needed between politicians, healthcare providers, academics and the public more generally, particularly as each type of record implies different access, usage, accountability and responsibility levels, each of which relate to economic, social, professional, managerial and technical issues.

Many studies on electronic records consider the technical imperatives such as the content, structure, use and impacts. The challenge to develop electronic records (medical, patient or health) is a global one, with different countries pursuing a variety of policies for adoption and implementation. In the United States, electronic health records are seen as one solution to reducing the number of medical errors, which account for 44 000 to 98 000 people dying in hospitals every year (Kohn, Corrigan, Donaldson 1999). A national poll found that 4 out of 10 people believe that quality of care was declining across the health service despite rising healthcare budgets (Carter 2008). The US Congressional Budget Office predicts that total spending on healthcare will increase from 16% of the economy in 2007 to 25% in 2025 (Health Reform Summit Committee 2008). Electronic records, with functionality for automated error checking, clinical decision support, and reliable information flow and integration among different individuals and departments involved in patient care, are viewed as an integral part of making healthcare less error prone and more efficient for clinicians and patients.

A recent publication shows that, in spite of the potential of electronic records, less than 20% of US physicians are using these systems (DesRoches, Campbell, Rao 2008). Two challenges are identified. The first is to develop appropriate clinical and financial expectations, and to build or buy the skills needed for successful implementation (Carter 2008). While these studies are US-centric, the issues are transferable to other nations, as the challenge to develop electronic records is being confronted by politicians, professionals and public.

In the United Kingdom, the Labour Government embarked upon an ambitious programme in 2002 to develop a National Care Record System (NCRS) to provide all citizens in England with an electronic summary care record containing basic data such as name, address, GP, blood group, allergies, etc. (the National Programme for IT (NPfIT) is discussed by various authors in this volume). Research into the development of the NCRS reveals disappointing results. Two National Audit Office Reports (2006, 2008) focused on the slow progress, marked by a range of problems, i.e. poor user engagement among clinicians, software design problems, failure of suppliers to meet targets, budget problems at implementation sites, changes to the programming code to include additional features and functionality, low IT maturity (capabilities and skills) in healthcare organisations, failure to set and meet performance targets, poor understanding of risk assessment and benefits realisation. Academic research has also identified a range of issues and concerns about introducing electronic records, with some studies looking in-depth at the institutionalisation of professional, managerial and technical work (Currie and Guah 2007) and others focusing on the more practical barriers to implementation (Hendy, Reeves, Fulop, *et al.* 2005).

Alongside the engineering and technical challenges to design electronic records, it is noteworthy that different levels of IT maturity exist among healthcare providers. In the UK, primary care is provided by general practitioners (GPs) who are physicians/ doctors running their own practices or surgeries. More generally, these individuals are likely to be relatively knowledgeable about the latest ICT, having used patient administration systems for many years. Within secondary care providers, i.e. hospital consultants, nurses, junior doctors, managers and administrators, knowledge of software applications for both clinical and non-clinical use is highly variable. Secondary care is more likely to be a 'late mover' in ICT adoption, particularly in terms of hardware and software implementation compared with primary care (Brennan 2005). So even if the technology is well developed and capable of providing clinicians and patients with good data for decision making, healthcare organisations will need to develop the IT governance and management capabilities to successfully implement electronic records.

In Table 1.2, this issue is placed under our technical theme of ICT architecture, applications, process and systems integration. However, governance and compliance issues should not simply reside with technical departments within healthcare organisations, since these matters are the direct responsibility of senior executives and clinicians. In fact, one of the public criticisms about introducing electronic records concerns data security and protection, with some leading academics calling for a boycott in using the government-led initiative to develop the NCRS (www.thebigoptout. com). This website, which promotes the NHS Confidentiality Campaign, was

> set up to protect patient confidentiality and to provide a focus for patient-led opposition to the government's NHS Care Records System. This system is designed to be a huge national database of patient medical records and personal information (sometimes referred to as the NHS 'spine') with no opt-out mechanism for patients at all. . . . Your medical confidentiality is at risk from this new database, as over a million NHS employees and central government bureaucrats will have access to not only your medical records but also your demographic details, name, address, NHS Number, GP details, phone number (even if it's ex-directory) and mobile number.

Campaigns of this nature reflect a growing concern among people about the confidentiality of public data. Despite serious data losses by government departments, agencies and employees, there is greater concern about misplaced electronic data as opposed to data held on paper sources. The collection, storage, retrieval and manipulation of patient data within the healthcare system has often invited criticism about poor governance, especially where patient notes are misplaced as they pass from one health provider to another. Recognising the public concerns about data security of electronic records, a definition of information governance was given by Harry Clayton, National Director for Patients and the Public and Chair, Care Record Development Board: 'the structures, policies and practice of the DH, the NHS and its suppliers to ensure the confidentiality and security of all records, and especially patient records, and to enable the ethical use of them for the benefit of individual patients and the public good' (Cayton 2006, p. 2).

New technology offers the potential to integrate business processes using secure networks, although it is evident that more work needs to be done to convince various stakeholders about the merits of storing large amounts of sensitive data electronically.

TABLE 1.2 ICT architecture, applications, process and systems integration

Migration to new ICT platforms	Accelerated obsolescence of ICT. Maturity of new ICT platforms (i.e. service-oriented architecture). Standards (protocols).	Janz 2005, Cartwright 2000.
IT governance and management	Information management organisation (i.e. responsibility/reporting structures); project management and timescales for implementing ICTs; Systems integration across NHS organisations; data security and protection.	Carter 2008, Johns 2008.
Electronic health/ medical/patient records	Defining the content, structure, content, use and impact of EHRs, adoption of EPRs.	Carter 2008, DesRoches, Campbell, Rao, *et al.* 2008, Hampton 2008, Hayrinen, Saranto and Nykanen 2007, Hippisley-Cox, Pringle, Cater, *et al.* 2003, Kim and Johnson 2002, Makoul, Curry and Tang 2001, Rifkin 2001, Rigby, Budgen, Turner, *et al.* 2007, Scott, Rundall, Vogt, *et al.* 2007, Thomas 2006.
Customer relationship management and integration	Level at which ICT improves service delivery. Ability of ICT to generate data/ information/knowledge for clinical/ non-clinical decision making. Workflow of ICTs.	Finnegan and Willcocks 2006, 2007. Nerenz 1992.
Knowledge-based processes	Knowledge sharing, knowledge-based processes.	Currie and Suhomlinovar 2006 Currie 1989 2003.
Service-oriented architecture/web services	Value creation using web services.	Currie and Parikh 2006 Dogac, Laceci, Kirbas, *et al.* 2006.
Re-engineering business processes and transformation	Process innovation and transformation, re-engineering healthcare.	Davenport 1993, Hammer and Champy 1990, McNulty and Ferlie 2002, McNulty and Ferlie 2004, Willcocks and Currie 1997.

PERFORMANCE MEASUREMENT, RISK ASSESSMENT AND BENEFITS REALISATION

The academic field of information systems located in business and management departments has a significant track record in evaluating the benefits and risks of information technology. While much of this work stems from the management accounting field (Kaplan and Norton 1992), there are many studies within information systems that identify quantitative and qualitative key performance indicators (KPIs) to measure value creation or potential risk (Currie 1989, 1995, 2004). From our review of the literature, it is interesting to note that the concept of evaluation is used differently by the business and management and health informatics communities. The former community tends to perceive information systems as 'business' systems, which are amenable to some form of measurement and assessment. Investment in information systems, whether in banking, manufacturing or healthcare, should not be perceived as anything other than a means to improve the operations and performance of an organisation. Notwithstanding the limitations of quantitative measures such as return on investment and capital asset depreciation, it is important that ICTs used in healthcare are introduced as part of a sound business case as opposed to political rhetoric. The latter community of health informatics tends to emphasise the benefits from ICT to the user community, i.e. clinicians, nurses, administrators and patients as a decision-making tool (Brown and Warmington 2002; Gagnon and Scott 2005; Heathfield, Pitty and Hanka 1998), more than for its potential to reduce costs and transform business processes. More recently, the British Computer Society (2006) has highlighted the importance of perceiving ICT projects as 'business change projects' where informatics should consume around 4% of turnover and be 'business led' as opposed to technically led.

Performance measurement and risk assessment are critical factors in conducting a pragmatic evaluation into ICT in healthcare. Yet studies show that simply gathering quantitative data on isolated ICT systems without considering the wider organisational structural, cultural and managerial issues is seldom useful (Greenhalgh, MacFarlane, Bate, *et al.* 2005). Equally, measuring key performance indicators without acting on this information is an exercise in data collection rather than technology management. We therefore concur with the view that, 'As with medicine, management is and will likely always be a craft that can be learned only through practice and experience' (Pfeffer and Sutton, 2005). To evaluate ICT, it is important to understand how business processes may change as a result of introducing technology. Common tools and techniques include value chain analysis (Porter and Teisberg 2006), process mapping (Hunt 1996) and balanced scorecard (Kaplan and Norton 1992). Mixed data collection methods are useful to provide a rich picture of how clinical staff, non-clinical staff and patients interact with ICTs within healthcare organisations.

One of the issues relating to evaluation of ICT is, 'What is being evaluated?' Table 1.3 identifies a range of issues that encapsulate the beginning and end of the ICT project process. For example, many sponsored evaluations on ICT, such as the summary care record for the National Programme for IT (Greenhalgh, Wood, Bratan, *et al.* 2008) are ex-post evaluations, which seek to assess what has been achieved at the implementation stage. Even though the IT system may not be fully implemented, there is an expectation on the part of the sponsor that it will be fully adopted by users at some stage in the future. Prior research (Currie 1989) has identified the importance of understanding the ex-ante side of evaluation (before implementation), particularly in terms of comparing secondary source data (i.e. IT strategy documentation) about what is expected from the ICT, with primary data in the form of ex-post rationalisations from respondents about the outcome of the ICT (following implementation). This is a useful exercise as vast differences are usually unveiled between the two stages, e.g. ex-post and ex-ante. A common finding is that perceptions about what the ICT is intended to achieve vary considerably from an initial shopping list of potential benefits to significant changes in what is eventually introduced.

Rossi, Lipsey and Freeman (2004) identify a number of categories for a systematic evaluation. They include: needs assessment, programme theory, process analysis, impact analysis, cost-benefit and cost-effectiveness analysis. A needs assessment examines the nature of the problem the programme is designed to address. This involves identifying stakeholder groups affected by the programme and how/if their working practices are likely to change. The programme theory is the formal description of the concepts and design of the programme. Programme theory delineates the components of the programme and shows anticipated short and long-term effects. An analysis of the programme theory considers how an organisation will achieve desired outcomes as well as unforeseen consequences (both positive and negative). Programme theory drives the hypotheses to be tested in the evaluation. The development of a logic model may further build common understanding among stakeholders. Process analysis and modelling go beyond the theory of the formal aims and objectives of the programme and evaluate how the programme is being implemented. Evaluation and implementation are therefore separate focal areas. The impact analysis considers causal effects of the programme. Finally, cost-benefit or cost-effectiveness analysis assesses the efficiency, performance and risks of the programme. Evaluations occurring across sites may therefore identify 'best practice' scenarios.

We discuss the issue of evaluation in more detail in the next section which considers the development of the National Programme for Information Technology (NPfIT) in the UK National Health Service.

THE NATIONAL PROGRAMME FOR IT IN THE UK NHS

Following a period of relative underinvestment in ICT over three decades, in 2002 the government pledged to spend around £6.2 billion on the NPfIT to deliver four large-scale IT-enabled projects:

1   a National Care Records Service (NCRS) for capturing, storing, retrieving and modifying patient medical records on a national database;
2   an Electronic Appointments Booking system (later becoming Choose and Book), where GPs and patients can book hospital appointments using a computer system;

TABLE 1.3 Performance measurement, risk assessment and benefits realisation

Adoption/access	Clear guidelines on user access to record.	Greenhalgh, Wood, Bratan, *et al.* 2008.
	Availability of record (i.e. 24/7).	
	Usability, actual usage, functionality, impact of pilot and delivered systems and services.	
	'Early' and 'late' adopter issues/concerns.	
Implementation opportunities and barriers	Variable quality of data/information in GP systems.	Clement and McDonald 1997, Doolin 2004, Heathfield, Pitty and Hanka 1998, Hendy, Reeves, Fulop, *et al.* 2005, Wyatt 1998.
	Link between opt-in/opt-out and data quality, if patient is seen as key to ensuring quality and accuracy of the record.	
	Difficulty in uploading data that is currently free text.	
	Ensuring that the proposed levels of patient participation in information sharing are real and work.	
	Defining responsibility for maintaining the summary record.	
	Deciding access rights to the Personal Demographics Service (directory or integral part of system), role-based access.	
Data quality and management	Security and integrity of record.	Brown and Warmington 2002, Callaghan and Wistow 2006
	Accuracy, reliability, timeliness of data/information.	
	Disaster recovery (i.e. systems outages).	
	Clear distinction between confidential and non-confidential data.	
	Error (recording/correction).	
Quality of care	Using performance indicators to improve quality of care.	Majeed, Lester and Bindman 2007.

(continued)

Patient safety	Ongoing monitoring of data to avoid system/human error.	Amarasingham, Plantinga, Diener-West, *et al.* 2009, Bate and Robert 2006, Davidsen, *et al.* 1988, Kohn, Corrigan and Donaldson 1999.
	Reduction in adverse drug reactions (ADRs).	
	Patient data sharing across geographical areas between clinicians.	
	Variance among health professionals in use of ICT to detect abnormal reports and to log and confirm effectiveness of actions to address important test abnormalities.	
	Variance in effective use of pharmacy software for drug/disease/patient interaction alerts.	
	Variances in medication areas across 'early' and 'late' adopter sites.	
	Patient satisfaction levels in accessing/interpreting record.	
Benefits realisation	Costs and benefits of introducing ICTs.	Currie 2003, Goldzweig, Towfigh, Maglione *et al.* 2009.
IT audit, evaluation and risk assessment	Evaluating public sector ICT projects.	Currie 1995, Cross 2005, Gagnon and Scott 2005, Greenhalgh, Robert, MacFarlane, *et al.* 2005, Kaplan and Norton 1992, Greenhalgh, Wood, Bratan, *et al.* 2008, Majeed, Lester and Bindman 2007, Chapman, Zechel, Carter *et al.* 2004.

3 the Picture Archiving and Communications System (PACs) to capture and send digital images of X-rays and scans; and

4 an Electronic Prescription Service (EPS) to enable patients to collect their prescriptions from hospital and high-street pharmacies more efficiently. These systems would be supported by a new National Network (N3) to provide a 'rapid, secure, robust and reliable' network across the NHS with sufficient capacity to enable efficient communication between NHS organisations.

The NCRS was the most resource intensive in terms of time and money since it was designed to give all English citizens an electronic record in the form of three distinct services:

1 Summary Care Record
   — Essential elements of a person's electronic record, extracted from general practice notes.
   — Essential elements relating to that person from other organisations where they receive care.
2 Detailed Care Record
   — The person's electronic record for that organisation
   — Elements of all electronic records relating to that person from other organisations.
3 HealthSpace
   — A personal health organiser and protected link to their Summary Care Record for every person who chooses to have one.

The move to develop electronic health records for clinicians, NHS managers, administrators and patients has evolved from previous decades where electronic medical records were used primarily for clinical purposes. As a subset of the NPfIT, which aims to 'help deliver a better NHS that gives public and patients services that fit the twenty-first century' (Department of Health 2002) the NCRS emerged from a series of policy documents which identified key strands in government policy to introduce 'lifelong electronic records of patients' in a report called Information for Health (Department of Health 1998). This was followed by further government reports including the NHS Plan (Department of Health 2000) outlining an information strategy for the 'modern NHS' and Building the Information Core (Department of Health 2001) on how to implement the NHS plan. These publications contain policy recommendations that influenced the publication of the Wanless Report (Wanless 2002) that spearheaded the launch of the NPfIT.

Information management is a critical activity within the NHS. In 2003, there were around 650 million prescriptions dispensed in the community, and nearly 5.5 million people were admitted to hospital for planned treatment. In addition, there were 13.3 million outpatient consultations, and nearly 13.9 million people attended Accident and Emergency (A&E), of whom 4.3 million were emergency admissions (Connecting for Health 2004). Management and administration costs in the NHS were around £170 million, and a further £14 billion was spent on IT in

2006/7 (National Audit Office 2006). Notwithstanding the increase in the annual NHS IT budget, the pursuit of IT-enabled business change is challenging, not least because of the low maturity in IT (particularly in secondary care) compared with other industrial sectors, such as banking. From a period of virtually no computers in the 1960s and 70s, the NHS has developed a vast array of disparate IT systems (Brennan 2005). Primary care is relatively advanced compared with secondary care, as GPs have tended to invest in IT systems for patient administration and medical record keeping. Similarly, retail pharmacies have invested in IT to improve the efficiency and operations of their business. Among the first IT systems was the patient administration system (PAS) in the early 1960s. This was followed by laboratory and radiology systems in the 1970s, and hospital information support systems (HISS) and resource management in the 1980s. As computer technology proliferated during the 1980s and 1990s, the NHS began to implement ICTs for service improvement in healthcare. However, the accelerated obsolescence of ICT (from mainframes in the 1960s/70s, to PCs in the 1980s/90s, and now service-oriented architectures from 2000 onwards) imposes significant challenges for implementing the NCRS, particularly as clinical and non-clinical data is currently being migrated from legacy ICT architectures to remote (web-based) platforms. Constantly changing technologies pose significant challenges to introducing a NCRS across healthcare services, particularly as healthcare professionals will need to adapt to the inevitable changes to clinical and administrative working practices if the new systems are to succeed.

EVALUATING THE NCRS

The aim of the NCRS is to use electronic health records to deliver direct care to patients. How this will be achieved in practice remains to be seen, as the project timescales for developing and implementing the system have been delayed, from an initial 'go-live' plan for 2010 to a revised plan for 2014 (National Audit Office 2008). Healthcare professionals currently generate records for encounters or episodes of care. These records are accessible to and shared by the immediate team (primary and secondary care). This procedure will continue, although the introduction of the NCRS across the NHS is to be supplemented by key information from other organisations that provide care to patients. The combined patient record from one organisation (i.e. GP practice) with information from other healthcare providers (i.e. secondary care) will comprise the Detailed Care Record. However, where two providers share an integrated local record, a care professional at one provider will be unable to access the whole record held by another provider. Data capture, input, retrieval, manipulation and sharing are all relevant in the evaluation of the NCRS, particularly since a variety of NHS providers and clinical and non-clinical staff may have access to, and responsibility for, information management and governance.

In addition to NHS staff, a patient attending an NHS appointment at one provider (e.g. hypertension clinic) may expect that all health professionals who provide care will contribute to their record by inputting data. For example, a receptionist may record the date/time of an appointment. A clinician will upload clinical notes to the record. The record will be available to that organisation on a need-to-know basis (i.e. through role-based access and a legitimate relationship). When a patient is referred to another NHS provider, unless he or she chooses to limit participation, that provider will have access to all or part of their NHS Care Record. The organisation may choose only to access the Summary Care Record on the basis of 'implied consent'. However, when the patient is attending several NHS providers for more complex care, it may be necessary for all these organisations to access all or some parts of the aggregate contribution to the Detailed Care Record. This data will facilitate NHS staff to carry out clinical and non-clinical activities enabled by shared access to the Detailed Care Record (i.e. ordering tests/monitoring results). Wider access to the record will require 'explicit consent' of the patient, although in time this level of access may become implicit (the implied/explicit spectrum of patient consent to the record is currently a contentious issue in some areas within the media and healthcare organisations). The scope for allowing access to a patient's record would necessitate explicit consent from NHS providers such as opticians, family planning clinics and incontinence advice services. Members of the public are further given the scope to change their decisions about who should have access and contribute to their NHS Care Record.

The right of patients to have access to their records is now widely acknowledged in ethical, legal and policy frameworks. This is based on the principles of the individual's right to self-determination and to privacy, as laid down in the European Convention on Human Rights. In UK legislation, right to access is defined by the Data Protection Act 1998 and is reflected in NHS policy through the NHS Plan and Information for Health/Building the Core. There is also a growing desire by the public and health professionals to share the healthcare records as a part of the increasing participation of patients in their care. The advent of Internet-based services, increasing computer literacy within the health profession and general public, and robust information ICT, has given the public access to the vast wealth of material on health and illness, spawned an industry of online healthcare, and made possible the shift from the present-day fragmented medical record spread across, and controlled by, several healthcare organisations towards a unified, patient-controlled health record.

While patients have the right to view their records, they may not gain any real benefit other than being aware of what has been written about them, having the opportunity to correct errors and to seek clarification or explanation during subsequent consultations. In contrast, allowing interaction with their records offers patients considerable additional benefits: health and lifestyle advice tailored to their needs; opportunities to contribute to the record; ability to communicate with their carers, and to share their concerns with other patients through online support groups; being reminded of appointments or availability of new information in their record. Interaction also improves healthcare by improving patients' understanding of their care, helping them prepare for consultations (e.g. through pre-clinic online questionnaires), providing a framework through which patients can contribute to their record, and supporting telecare (Gaunt 2001).

The involvement of patients in accessing their records is part of a wider move towards developing electronic health records which are classified as 'a repository of patient data in digital form, stored and exchanged securely, and accessible by multiple authorised users' (where they contain) 'retrospective, concurrent, and prospective information. . . . to support continuing, efficient and quality integrated healthcare' (Hayrinen, Saranto, Nykanen 2007). In terms of the current development of electronic records for patients, we note the British Medical Association's comment that, 'Whilst the BMA supports the sharing of information to improve patient care, we are disappointed that the architecture of a system, which will have huge implications to the delivery of healthcare, was commissioned and built prior to stakeholder consultation' (www.BMA.org.uk). A similar note of caution is expressed by the Information Commissioner's Office who claimed to receive a number of enquiries from the public relating to the introduction of EPRs in England. Thus, 'Many of these individuals have expressed concern at the plans and are worried that their health records will be available to everyone across the NHS' (Information Commissioner's Office 2007).

In almost a decade since its launch in 2002, the NPfIT has been a regular news item in the media, often discussed in less than favourable terms, and occasionally described as a 'computer disaster'. As the largest, non-military, publicly funded IT programme worldwide, the NPfIT was always going to be contentious, particularly as politicians linked the programme with a wider policy agenda to transform healthcare services in England. From the start, the NPfIT was given stringent performance targets where external suppliers would be paid only when they had implemented working systems. The government agency Connecting for Health was set up to procure systems from preferred suppliers. Only a handful of suppliers were able to tender for the multi-million-pound contacts. From the outset, England was divided into a geographical patchwork of five clusters: (1) North West, West Midlands, (2) North East, (3) East of England, East Midlands, (4) Southern, and (5) London. The suppliers CSC Corporation, Accenture, Fujitsu and British Telecom were each given responsibility for one or more of the clusters. These local service providers (LSPs) would subcontract work to other suppliers.

The NCRS was the most ambitious programme of work under the NPfIT umbrella, with an initial phased deployment timetable running from June 2004 to December 2010. From its inception, the NPfIT was beset with political and practical problems. By 2006, a National Audit Office Report (2006) reported serious shortfalls in the progress of the NPfIT. Achieving the targets across the spectrum of the IT projects was delayed, as deployments across NHS organisations were patchy. The report reported that 9600 initial deployments of software to NHS entities had been made across the five clusters by April 2006. These included 7639 Choose and Book deployments, and 1153 Electronic Prescribing Service deployments. The NCRS was running into some serious problems as concerns were expressed about data security and integrity, particularly where millions of patient records were held on the Spine and potentially accessible to thousands of NHS staff. The report stressed that Connecting for Health placed considerable efforts on the procurement of IT systems as a response to previous problems where procurement had been 'haphazard' within the NHS. One of the aims of the NPfIT was 'to provide a strong central direction of IT development, and increase the rate of take up of advanced IT' (p. 1). Connecting for Health negotiated contracts with IT service suppliers, recognising that, once new systems were developed, additional work was needed to introduce them into the NHS. This involved integrating new systems with existing (legacy) IT systems and 'configuring them to meet local circumstances, training staff to use them, and adapting ways of working to make the best of the solutions' (p. 1).

Faced with serious delays, the report offered 10 recommendations to Connecting for Health. They included: ensuring that a robust engineering-based timetable for delivery is introduced and capable of being met by the suppliers; better communication with NHS staff about how these changes will affect them; stronger management of supplier performance, including imposing penalties for late delivery; better quantification of the benefits delivered by the programme; more understanding of how the NPfIT impacts on local NHS IT expenditure; a comparison of early adopter NHS organisations to use their experience to help identify and quantify the service and efficiency improvements of new systems; additional training and development programmes, e.g. project management; the creation of more National Clinical Leads to drive through the change programme; and building capabilities in NHS organisations through passing on best practices in areas such as contracts management.

The issues raised in the 2006 National Audit Office report were relevant and timely but did not go far enough in terms of unpacking some of the more serious structural, organisational, managerial and technical problems of the NPfIT. This was picked up in the media where continued criticism of the programme highlighted ongoing delays, lack of clinical buy-in to the programme, unmet targets, and security and patient safety issues.

In 2008, a second National Audit Office (2008) report was published which monitored progress since the previous report. It stressed that 'the context within which the Programme is being delivered is complex and constantly changing, with new requirements arising from policy and operational changes in the NHS' (p. 7). Since 2006, the structure governing NPfIT had changed from five clusters to only three: (1) London, (2) the North West & West Midlands and Southern England, (3) the North East and Eastern England. In addition, strategic health authorities were reduced from 28 to only 10, with further changes including the expansion of foundation trusts and new plans to introduce polyclinics outlined in the Darzi Report (Darzi 2008).

This report identified five management challenges to support the delivery of the programme: the importance of achieving strong leadership and governance; maintaining the confidence of patients that their records will be secure; securing the support and involvement of clinicians and other NHS staff; managing suppliers effectively; and deploying and using the systems effectively at local level. Six recommendations were offered to realise the vision of the programme. Among them were closer communication between the NHS Connecting for Health and the strategic health authorities with NHS organisations about the deployment plans of the NCRS. The lessons learned from the experiences of the three 'early adopter' sites should be better communicated to other NHS organisations, particularly as plans to develop the Lorenzo system for the North, Midlands and East areas have been considerably delayed.

Recognising the difficulty in precisely evaluating the 'state of play' of the various IT systems of the NPfIT, ongoing monitoring and reporting on system development, deployment, cost and performance was seen as important. This included communication with NHS staff and externally to Parliament, and not just between NHS executives and the local service providers. It was reported that some trusts were still to be convinced about the benefits of adopting the NCRS, so more work was needed to address trusts' concerns about potential benefits of the system. SHAs were advised to hire people with programme-management skills to work with trusts and LSPs. Greater attention to benefits realisation was recommended, particularly to increase the commitment to the programme by NHS staff. Improvements in security were further recommended to ensure that patients could be assured that their personal data would be secure at all times. More work on data protection and monitoring levels of public confidence in the programme was advised.

Recognising that the NHS is a 'late adopter' of ICT compared with other sectors, such as financial services and manufacturing, the IT maturity across the NHS is variable, so moving from under-utilisation of computers to integrated electronic records offers many challenges. As government reports from the last decade suggest, the NHS was expected to play 'catch up' with ICT strategy and implementation, and the centrist, top-down approach was seen by politicians as the best way to achieve this objective. Yet the perception that the NHS is a level playing field for ICT adoption is not the reality. Rather, ICT adoption and diffusion across NHS organisations continues to be fragmented, ad hoc and sporadic. A recent report funded by Connecting for Health, which looked at the early adopter programme for the Summary Care Record (Greenhalgh, Wood, Bratan, et al. 2008) highlighted considerable confusion about issues of data security and integrity among NHS staff and patients. These issues and concerns, however, need to be resolved at the functional and technical specification of an ICT project (e.g. before software development begins) rather than several years into the project. This raises important questions about whether ICT should be introduced as part of a top-down, centrist policy-making approach (e.g. government, strategic health authority), or as part of a localised, decentralised strategy (e.g. PCT, IT department, clinical/administrative unit).

CENTRALISATION OR DECENTRALISATION?

The choice between centralised and decentralised ICT adoption is a perennial issue in information systems strategy and management. Advantages for centralisation in the context of the NPfIT in the NHS are given as: more scope to reduce costs due to larger discounts awarded to high cost/value contracts; more technical standardisation of systems and applications across the NHS; ability to achieve systems integration with fewer suppliers working together; opportunity to raise IT maturity/capability in NHS from large-scale investment; backing of government to use ICT to transform healthcare service delivery to enable patients to actively seek 'choice'; buy-in from senior NHS executives.

Advantages for decentralisation focus on: importance of allowing individual NHS clinicians and managers to actively become engaged in ICT decision making at local level; encouraging a sense of 'ownership' of ICT solutions at the clinical and non-clinical levels; developing IT maturity/capability at the strategic (e.g. planning, programme management, benefits realisation, risk assessment, procurement, contracts negotiation and management) levels, as well as the operational (implementation, project management, training, IT support) levels.

A LOCAL SOLUTION

As late as August 2006, the Acting NHS Chief Executive, Sir Ian Carruthers, sent a letter to SHA Chief Executives. It stressed that SHA Chief Executives are appointed Senior Responsible Officers (SROs) for implementation and benefits realisation of the NPfIT, and should also put in place implementation programmes to identify benefits streams. NPfIT was repositioned within the NHS to incorporate the National Local Ownership Programme (NLOP). The NLOP objectives were designed to align governance arrangements with the new SRO roles; to clarify roles and responsibilities; strengthen local governance and ownership to achieve the right balance between national and local needs; establish structures and processes to ensure mutual accountability; reinforce the value from NPfIT; define and implement clinical engagement; and improve NHS Connecting for Health programme decision-making capability. The NLOP was thus a direct response to the realisation that centrist ICT initiatives usually result in a lack of 'buy-in' from managers and staff at local level. This has been witnessed in private and public sector settings, particularly in complex administrative structures, such as the NHS. The NLOP aimed to clarify the issues around accountability and responsibility for the NPfIT. More senior level NHS engagement in the programme was sought, yet Connecting for Health would continue to be responsible for the NPfIT commercial strategy and contractual negotiations. SHAs in three groups (London, South, North East and Midlands) would work together to achieve the strategy.

CLINICAL INVOLVEMENT AND IT MANAGEMENT

One of the concerns raised by the two National Audit Office reports (2006, 2008) is the need for greater clinical involvement in the NPfIT. While Connecting for Health regularly gives examples of how their various clinical leads hold events (e.g. workshops, meetings, on-site visits) with healthcare organisations and individuals to convey information about the NPfIT, concerns about lack of clinical involvement and how NPfIT is managed continue.

BENEFITS REALISATION AND RISK ASSESSMENT

The NPfIT is intended as a major policy initiative to transform healthcare services in England. It is a major change-management programme designed to transform the way healthcare services are offered in the 21st century. From an investment perspective, however, the NPfIT is consuming vast amounts of taxpayers' money and should therefore be evaluated as a business-change programme, using robust methods and tools to measure and assess benefits realisation and risk assessment. In the current economic environment where the 'credit crunch' is witnessing the demise of banks, the rising cost of living for the public and fears about job security, costs consumed by the NPfIT will be more closely scrutinised in the media. Financial budgets in healthcare are increasingly challenged, particularly as politicians and executives need to make uncomfortable choices about healthcare services, including whether new drugs and treatments are offered to NHS patients. While the final target for expenditure on the NPfIT is estimated in some quarters to be around £20 billion, a critical question is whether it offers value for money.

IT SUPPLIER CONTRACTS/CAPABILITY

The NPfIT represents an extensive outsourcing initiative where leading third-party IT suppliers develop and implement the various systems, including the National Care Records Service, Choose and Book, the Picture Archiving and Communications Systems, the Electronic Prescription Service and the N3 Network. Through national application service providers (NASPs) and local service providers (LSPs), major companies such as Accenture, Fujitsu, British Telecom and CSC would work with independent software vendors (ISVs) to introduce the applications. One of the major aims of the NPfIT was to enter into tough negotiations with IT suppliers to procure systems at a discounted rate. Payment would only be made once working systems were fully implemented. Unfortunately, the burden of meeting ambitious performance targets coupled with the fact that ICT adoption and implementation in healthcare is dependent upon many factors (e.g. organisational, cultural, economic and technical factors) proved too challenging for some IT suppliers. First Accenture then Fujitsu terminated their contracts with Connecting for Health, with the inevitable negative press coverage about the NPfIT as a whole.

Given the fact that healthcare is considered a 'follower' in ICT adoption, rather than a 'leader', the years of under-investment in software applications, particularly in secondary care, suggests that IT maturity (both at the supplier and customer levels) is low. This is also referred to as 'IT-readiness', although this term is used mostly to describe the purchaser of systems, rather than the provider. Assessing the maturity of the IT supplier and customer is critical as low maturity on both sides is likely to result in low adoption, resistance from staff and low morale. In addition, evaluating whether the IT supplier can deliver on promises is invaluable, particularly as the capabilities of technology systems and applications are routinely 'over-hyped' by suppliers to secure contracts. Respondents voiced mixed views about the capabilities of IT suppliers, especially during the implementation phase.

THE FUTURE OF NPfIT

So what is the future of the NPfIT? Will the various systems ever be fully implemented? Will it achieve tangible benefits for patients, NHS staff and the taxpayer? From the evidence, the answer to these questions is not simply 'yes' or 'no', given the complexity of the programme as a whole. But one thing is certain: unless more stringent measures are put in place to strategically manage and evaluate the NPfIT, it will not achieve anything like the range of benefits set out in earlier government reports.

What needs to be done? As the largest publicly funded healthcare ICT programme worldwide, the NPfIT has lacked three essential requirements for realising tangible benefits. They fall into three areas: (1) business and ICT strategic planning; (2) implementation and evaluation; and (3) risk assessment/benefits realisation. First, the 'big bang' approach to NPfIT was highly risky and guaranteed to put enormous financial pressure on NHS budgets. There are plenty of examples in financial services and manufacturing to show that large-scale IT-enabled change programmes need to be fully supported by a clear and convincing business case. The business case for NPfIT was obscured by political expediency where increased ICT expenditure was linked to policy objectives to achieve 'transformational change' in the NHS. Paradoxically, while we talk of a 'national' health service, the NHS has undergone excessive restructuring over the past two decades, where a centrist approach to ICT strategy and planning does not fit well with its decentralised structure. Primary and secondary healthcare providers have tended to develop localised strategies for ICT, so any business case needs to take into account the complex system integration issues relating to clinical and non-clinical technologies. This needs to be combined with a thorough mapping of the business (clinical and non-clinical) processes to understand what is needed in terms of functionality and how it will be achieved technically. Unfortunately, the documentation supporting the NPfIT has not provided detailed scenarios using business process mapping methods and techniques, as this task has apparently been left to NHS managers and suppliers. Understanding the current and planned business processes, however, is essential to reveal potential problems during the implementation phase.

Second, the implementation and evaluation of the NPfIT has lacked the stringent management approaches essential for large-scale ICT programmes. These include the application of both quantitative and qualitative techniques. The earlier choice to restrict ICT suppliers to a select few with responsibilities for subcontracting appeared sensible but it created 'regional monopolies', seemingly at odds with government rhetoric that advocates competition in the marketplace. An assessment of the global software market would have shown that, while the chosen few suppliers have good knowledge and understanding of management and ICT consultancy, their knowledge and capability to supply the NHS needed further maturity. Yet learning 'on the job' in such a high-profile and risky 'expedition' into ICT-driven healthcare is risky and time-consuming. Implementation of novel systems such as the NCRS and Choose and Book in particular needed to secure the 'buy-in' of clinicians and other stakeholders, rather than be based on the assumption that staff and patients will come to accept systems over time. There is plenty of research to show this rarely happens as resistance to ICTs often results in low adoption and diffusion.

Evidence shows that GP surgeries use established electronic patient records systems, so convincing them to take new systems at greater cost was never going to be easy. The task was made more difficult as Choose and Book was initially designed as an electronic appointments booking system and later morphed into as system where GPs would offer a patient four appointment options. The new system was less attractive to GPs as it extended their patient appointments and did not provide the seamless process it was designed to achieve. Also, to be effective, the system would require cultural and behavioural change, particularly as patients were required to become more active in choosing treatment options.

Poor implementation strategies were identified where clinical engagement was not fully developed by the programme. An essential component of all successful ICT implementations is to engage key decision makers and users of systems at an early stage. Clinicians were very keen to discuss ICT issues but felt disenfranchised from the NPfIT as very little information about the programme had penetrated to the grass roots level. Even some ICT departments at NHS organisations knew little about the NPfIT as they focused instead on implementing other ICTs. Poor clinical engagement continues to be a major issue generating much resistance to the programme.

Third, risk assessment and evaluation of NPfIT was largely confined to monitoring implementation targets and issuing penalties on suppliers if systems were late or not fully functional. While much of the emphasis by Connecting for Health was placed on procurement of ICT systems, little attention was given to developing stringent programme and project management methods and techniques. The 'big bang' approach of NPfIT further increased risks and costs, particularly as introducing new systems was seen as unnecessary and costly by many clinicians. With all large-scale ICT change, it is important to evaluate how new systems will integrate with older (legacy) systems. The 'one size fits all' philosophy was risky because much of the implementation focused on the functionality of new applications, and not on connectivity with existing applications. An example is where electronic patient records are retained locally but need to be accessed remotely for treating a patient. This requires a robust systems integration solution to seamlessly connect disparate ICTs across remotes sites. Working closely with local sites is therefore essential to resolve integration problems.

Despite earlier government reports advising that large-scale ICT programmes should be treated as business initiatives, the NPfIT has focused almost exclusively on technology procurement. Management, organisational and cultural issues have been underplayed. This has resulted in several own goals as the media has continuously reported missed deadlines and problems with suppliers, having now lost Accenture and Fujitsu from the programme. Recognising the need to expand the preferred supplier network, the National Local Ownership Programme now allows the NHS to work with additional suppliers to meet programme objectives. This creates opportunity and risk. On one hand, it is common business practice to issue requests for tenders (RFTs) from different suppliers to gain an understanding of market offerings.

Caution is needed, however, to ensure that Connecting for Health and the NHS have the appropriate skills to evaluate competing bids, and to continue to monitor and audit supplier performance, not just on site but in the marketplace. Integrating systems will become more important, so it will be essential to carefully demarcate responsibilities and deliverables between suppliers. With the present arrangements of using fewer suppliers, it is clear that costs have escalated due to 'contract add-ons', so using more suppliers may encourage competition and mitigate the risks of 'supplier lock-in'.

Currently, the programme has invested around £3.6 billion pursuing its original goals. Now that the NCRS is running some four years late with an expected completion date of between 2009/10, it is time to take stock of the programme. The PACs, EPS and N3 systems have produced some promising results, yet Choose and Book continues to be unpopular with many GPs. Although there are many calls to scrap the programme, clinicians are generally supportive and recognise the potential benefits of ICTs. However, government-led ICT change is unlikely to win hearts and minds, particularly as poorly developed software design and implementation strategies can result in unforeseen consequences where patient safety is compromised rather than improved. One solution is to scale down the timescales of introducing the NCRS and work towards redefining the business case for electronic health records. While this strategy is akin to reverse engineering, many NHS organisations have already delayed procurement and implementation of the NPfIT systems as they work towards meeting their other ICT priorities. While there are several success stories of how ICT can improve healthcare service delivery and practice, the scale and scope of the NPfIT needs to be supported at a root and branch level. The business case needs to be widely accepted throughout the NHS, as communicating potential and actual benefits through a public relations exercise will just extend the gap between rhetoric and reality. Finally, this research raises some serious issues about the vision and direction of the NPfIT, and suggests that focusing upon the dis-benefits and risks will achieve greater scope for improvement than offering a 'blue sky' strategy for the programme which is not shared among NHS staff and public alike. The following recommendations are based on the results of this research in addition to 25 years' experience of carrying out IT audits for private and public sector organisations.

CONCLUDING ISSUES

➤ Politicians should not determine national policy for ICT as evidence from prior research shows that large-scale public sector ICT projects are rarely completed within time and budget with the desired benefits. A cross-party group which works closely with IT suppliers, SHAs and NHS trusts is more likely to be impartial and detached in evaluating ICT solutions. The high financial investment in ICT to achieve ICT-enabled transformation in healthcare requires the input from a multi-political and disciplinary team (e.g. business leaders, academics, clinicians, NHS managers, patients, the public, community/ healthcare workers).

➤ Best practice examples in procurement of ICTs from other industries (e.g. financial services and manufacturing) should be considered, particularly where case studies show how legacy (existing) ICTs can be integrated with new systems. Research evidence shows that similar challenges of integration and workflow are found across different industries and business processes, so lessons can be learnt where appropriate and relevant.

➤ The business case for the NCRS needs to be revisited. The thorny issues about patient data security, integrity, confidentiality and access need to be resolved if the NCRS is to be fully rolled out across the NHS. The case for retaining patient records centrally as opposed to locally needs to be made more convincingly to clinicians and the wider public.

➤ The business processes for Choose and Book have not resulted in a seamless system for GPs, other healthcare professionals and for patients. C&B should be returned to an electronic booking system for hospital/outpatient appointments where patient choice is supported by the clinical knowledge and integrity of the healthcare professional. Patient choice should not be used to replace the role of the GP as this will lead to infringements in patient safety.

➤ Politicians need to address the issue that large-scale ICT implementation in a climate of constant change is highly challenging. ICTs in healthcare need to be properly evaluated using modern management techniques such as business process mapping and gap analysis. The procurement of the systems in the NPfIT is disjointed from their implementation and clinical/user engagement. ICT adoption and diffusion needs to be understood as a holistic activity with the involvement of relevant stakeholders. Introducing technology as an 'out-of-the-box' solution will not win the hearts and minds of individuals. More work needs to be done to show how ICT change will benefit patients, clinicians and the wider public.

➤ The initial creation of regional monopolies using only a few ICT suppliers has now been replaced with the National Local Ownership Programme. Extending the NLOP is essential to encourage more competition and choice to SHAs and NHS trusts to pilot and procure new ICTs for a range of clinical and non-clinical applications. More devolvement of decision making about specific ICT products and services needs to be given to SHAs and NHS trusts. In particular, pilot schemes need to be used to test and evaluate a range of ICTs, rather than adopting a technology solution from a limited choice of suppliers.

➤ Competition among ICT suppliers should be encouraged to generate a 'value for money' climate in the NHS. NHS management needs to gain capabilities and skills in negotiating contracts in the global software market. Lessons from 'best practice' can be learned from other industries. ICT suppliers need to be evaluated on their levels of knowledge and capability of healthcare. Low maturity of working in healthcare is a risk that should not be paid for solely by the English taxpayer.

➤ Large-scale ICT change is accompanied by cultural and behaviour change. Much more work needs to be done through training schemes and pilot projects to convince NHS staff of the benefits. More engagement of stakeholders is needed as many successful ICTs begin at the 'grass roots' level with a 'technical champion' (who may be a clinician) taking the lead. Poor clinical engagement continues to be a major issue generating much resistance to the NPfIT, so measures to involve all staff should be introduced.

➤ More rigorous risk assessment and evaluation of NPfIT is needed as imposing targets and issuing penalties to suppliers when systems are late or not fully functional is not conducive to building cooperative business relationships. The current investment in ICT in the NHS needs to be evaluated in conjunction with new expenditure, particularly as some of these systems are still working well. Given the devolved structure of the NHS, the 'one size fits all' approach is risky and so more attention should now be on the functionality of new applications and their connectivity with existing applications.

REFERENCES

Amarasingham R, Plantinga L, Diener-West M, *et al*. Clinical information technologies and inpatient outcomes. *Arch Intern Med*. 2009; 169(2): 108–14.

Bate P, Robert G. Experience-based design: from redesigning the system around the patient to co-designing services with the patient. 2006; 15: 307–10. Available at: www.qshc.bjm.com

Berg M. The contextual nature of medical information. *Int J Med Inform*. 1999; 56: 51–60.

Berry LL, Mirabito AM, Berick DM. A health care agenda for business. *Sloan Manage Rev*. 2004; 45(4): 56–64.

Bloomfield BP. The role of information systems in the UK National Health Service: action at a distance and the fetish of calculation. *Soc Stud Sci*. 1991; 21: 701–34.

Boaden R, Harvey G, Moxham C, *et al*. *Quality Improvement: theory and practice in healthcare*. Warwick: NHS Institute for Innovation and Improvement; 2008.

Brennan S. *The NHS IT Project*. Oxford: Radcliffe Publishing; 2005.

British Computer Society. *The Way Forward for NHS Health Informatics. A report on behalf of the British Computer Society (BCS) by the BCS Health Informatics Forum Strategic Panel*; 15 December 2006.

British Medical Association. BMA response to clinical development of the NHS care records service. 2007. Available at: www.bma.org.uk/ap.nsf/Content/ncrsresponse

Brown PJB, Warmington V. Data quality probes: exploiting and improving the quality of electronic patient record data and patient care. *Int J Med Inform*. 2002; 68: 91–8.

Brown T. Modernization or failure? IT development projects in the UK public sector. *Finan Account Manage*. 2001; 17(4): 363–81.

Brownbridge G, Lilford RJ, Tindle-Biscoe S. Use of a computer to take booking histories in a hospital antenatal clinic. *Med Care*. 1988; 26(5): 474–87.

Burgoyne JG, Brown DH, Hindle A, *et al*. A multidisciplinary identification of issues associated with 'contracting' in market-orientated health service reforms. *Br J Manage*. 1997; 3(39): 39–49.

Cabinet Office. *Transformational Government, Enabled by Technology*. Cm 6683. London: HMSO; 2005.

Callaghan GD, Wistow G. Publics, patients, citizens, consumers? Power and decision making in primary health care. *Public Admin.* 2006; 84(3): 583–601.

Carter JH. What is the electronic health record? In: Carter JH, editor. *Electronic Health Records.* Philadelphia: ACP Publishing; 2008. pp. 3–18.

Cartwright L. Reach out and heal someone: telemedicine and the globalization of healthcare. *Health.* 2000; 4(3): 347–77.

Casebeer AL, Harrison A, Mark AL, editors. *Innovations in Health Care.* Basingstoke: Palgrave MacMillan; 2006.

Cayton H. *Information Governance in the Department of Health and the NHS.* Department of Health, London; 2006.

Chapman JL, Zechel A, Carter YH, *et al.* Systematic review of recent innovations in service provision to improve access to primary care. *Br J Gen Pract.* 2004; May: 374–81.

Clement J, McDonald MD. The barriers to electronic medical record systems and how to overcome them. *J Am Med Inform Assoc.* 1997; 4(3): 213–21.

Collins T. Doctors attacks health IT codes. *Computer Weekly,* 6 February 2003, p. 4.

Connecting for Health. Business Plan, 2004. Available at: www.connectingforhealth. nhs.uk

Cross M. Special report: public sector IT failures. *Prospect.* October 2005, pp. 48–52.

Currie G, Suhomlinova O. The impact of institutional forces upon knowledge sharing in the UK NHS: the triumph of professional power and the inconsistency of policy. *Public Admin.* 2006; 84(1): 1–30.

Currie WL. The art of justifying new technology to top management. *Omega.* 1989; 17(5): 409–18.

Currie WL. *Management Strategy for IT.* London: Pitman; 1995.

Currie W. Computerising the Stock Exchange: a comparison of two information systems. *New Technology, Work and Employment.* 1997; 12(2): 75–83.

Currie W. A knowledge-based risk assessment system for evaluating web-enabled application outsourcing projects. *Int J Proj Manage.* 2003; 21(3): 207–17.

Currie WL. *Value Creation from E-Business.* London: Butterworth-Heinemann; 2004.

Currie WL. The organizing vision of application service provision: a process-oriented analysis. *Information and Organization.* 2004; 14: 237–67.

Currie WL, Guah MW. IT-enabled healthcare delivery: the UK National Health Service. *Inf Syst Manage.* 2006; Spring: 7–22.

Currie WL, Guah MW. A national program for IT in the organizational field of healthcare: an example of conflicting institutional logics. *J Inf Technol.* 2007; 22: 235–48.

Currie W, Parikh M. Value creation in web services: an integrative model. *J Strat Inf Syst.* 2006; 15(2): 153–74.

Darzi, Professor the Lord (Darzi) of Denham. *High Quality Care for All: NHS next stage review final report.* Department of Health, 2008.

Davenport TH. *Process Innovation: reengineering work through information technology.* Cambridge, MA: Harvard Business School Press; 1993.

Davidsen F, *et al.* Adverse drug reactions and drug non-compliance. *Eur J Clin Pharmacol.* 1988; 34: 83–6.

de Lusignan S, Aarts J. UK's national programme for IT welcomes recommendations for a more socio-technical approach to evaluation: a commentary on the Greenhalgh evaluation of the summary care record. *Inform Prim Care.* 2008; 16: 75–7.

Department of Health. *Information for Health: an information strategy for the modern NHS 1998–2005*. Department of Health; 1998.

Department of Health. *Building the Information Core: implementing the NHS Plan*. London, Department of Health; 2001.

Department of Health. *Delivering 21st Century IT Support for the NHS*. London: Department of Health; 2002.

Department of Health. *The NHS in England: the operating framework for 2007/8*. London: Department of Health; 2007.

Department of Health. *Health Informatics Review: 10104*. London: Department of Health; 2008.

Department of Health. *High Quality Care for All: NHS next stage review final report*. London: Department of Health; 2008.

DesRoches CM, Campbell EG, Rao SR, *et al.* Electronic health records in ambulatory care: a national survey. *N Engl J Med.* 2008; 359(1): 50–60.

Dogac A, Laceci GB, Kirbas S, *et al.* Artemis: deploying semantically enriched web services in the healthcare domain. *Inf Syst.* 2005; Special Issue: 321–339.

Doolin B. Power and resistance in the implementation of a medical management information system. *Inf Syst.* 2004; 14: 343–62.

Finnegan D, Willcocks L. Knowledge management in the introduction of CRM Systems: tacit/non-codified knowledge transfer, subcultures and impacts. *Proceedings of the International Management Technology Conference*; Orlando, FL; 2004.

Finnegan D, Willcocks L. Knowledge issues in the introduction of CRM systems: tacit knowledge, psychological contracts, subcultures and impacts. *Proceedings of the European Conference in Information Systems*; Regensburg, MA; 2005.

Finnegan D, Willcocks L. Knowledge sharing issues in the introduction of a new technology. *J Enter Inf Manage.* 2006; 19(6): 568–90.

Finnegan DJ, Willcocks LP. *Implementing CRM*. Chichester: Wiley; 2007.

Friedman CP, Abbas UL. Is medical informatics a mature science? A review of measurement practice in outcome studies of clinical systems. *Int J Med Inform.* 2003; 69: 261–72.

Gagnon M-P and Scott RE. Striving for evidence in e-health evaluation: lessons from health technology assessment. *J Telemed Telecare.* 2005; (Suppl. 2): S34–6.

Gaunt N. *Initial Evaluation of Patient Interaction with Electronic Health Record*. South and West Devon Community ERDIP; 2001.

Goldzweig CL, Towfigh A, Maglione M, *et al.* Costs and benefits of health information technology: new trends from the literature. *Health Aff.* 2009; January: 282–93.

Greenhalgh T, Robert G, MacFarlane F, *et al.* Storylines of research in diffusion of innovation: a meta-narrative approach to systematic review. *Soc Sci Med.* 2005; 61: 417–30.

Greenhalgh T, Wood GW, Bratan T, *et al.* Patients' attitudes to the summary care record and Healthspace: qualitative study. *BMJ.* 2008; June: 1–11.

Ham C. *Health Policy in Britain*. Basingstoke: Palgrave MacMillan; 2004.

Hammer M, Champy D. *Reengineering the Corporation*. Cambridge, MA: Harvard Business School Press; 1990.

Hampton R. Groups push physicians and patients to embrace electronic health records. *JAMA.* 2008; 299(5): 507–9.

Harrison MI. *Implementing Change in Health Systems: market reforms in health systems in the UK, Sweden and the Netherlands*. London: Sage Publications; 2004.

Hayrinen K, Saranto K, Nykanen P. Definition, structure, content, use and impacts of electronic health records: a review of the research literature. *Int J Med Inform*. Online version; 2007.

Health Reform Summit Committee. Opportunities to increase efficiency in health care: statement by Peter R Orszag. *HRSC on Finance*. United States Senate. 16 June 2008.

Heathfield H, Pitty D, Hanka R. Evaluating information technology in healthcare: barriers and challenges. *BMJ*. 1998; 316: 1959–61.

Hendy J, Fulop N, Reeves BC, *et al*. Implementing the NHS information technology programme: qualitative study of progress in acute trusts. *BMJ*. 2007; 334: 1360. Online First, doi:10.1136.

Hendy J, Reeves BC, Fulop N, *et al*. Challenges to implementing the national program for information technology: a qualitative study. *BMJ*. 2005; 331: 1–6.

Herzlinger RE. The failed revolution in healthcare: the role of management. *Har Bus Rev*. 1989; 67(2): 95–103.

Hippisley-Cox J, Pringle M, Cater R, *et al*. The electronic patient record in primary care: regression or progression? A cross sectional study. *BMJ*. 2003; 326: 1439–43.

Hunt VD. *Process Mapping*. Chichester: Wiley; 1996.

Information Commissioner's Office. *The Information Commissioner's view of NHS Care Records*. London: ICO; 2007.

Institute of Medicine. *Crossing the Quality Chasm: a new health system for the 21st century*. Washington DC: Committee on Quality Healthcare in America, National Academy Press; 2002.

Janz BD. Information systems and healthcare II: back to the future with RFID: lessons learned, some old, some new. *Commun AIS*. 2005; 15: 132–48.

Jeffcott MA, Johnson CW. The use of a formalised risk model in NHS information system development. *Cognit Tech Work*. 2002; 4: 120–36.

Johns ML. Privacy and security of health information. In: Carter JH, editor. *Electronic Health Records*. Philadelphia: ACP Publishing; 2008. pp. 295–333.

Kaplan RS, Norton DP. The balanced scorecard: measures that drive performance. *Har Bus Rev*. 1992; Jan–Feb: 71–9.

Kim MI, Johnson KB. Personal health records. *J Am Med Inform Assoc*. 2002; 9(2): 171–80.

Klein R. *The New Politics of the NHS*, 4th ed. Harlow: Longman; 2001.

Kohn LT, Corrigan JM, Donaldson MS. *To Err is Human: building a safer health system*. Washington DC: National Academies Press; 1999.

Kyu Kim K, Michelman JE. An examination of factors for the strategic use of information systems in the healthcare industry. *MIS Quarterly*. 1990; 14(2): 201–15.

Lee ML. A conspicuous production theory of hospital behaviour. *South Econ J*. 1971; 38(1): 48–58.

Luftman J. Assessing business IT alignment maturity. *Commun AIS*. 2000; 4(14): 1–51.

McNulty T, Ferlie E. *Re-engineering Healthcare: the complexities of organizational transformation*. Oxford: Oxford University Press; 2002.

McNulty T, Ferlie E. Process transformation: limitations to radical organizational change within public service. *Org Stud*. 2004; 25(8): 1389–412.

Majeed A. Ten ways to improve information technology in the NHS. *BMJ*. 2003; 326: 202–6.

Majeed A, Lester H, Bindman A. Improving the quality of care with performance indicators. *BMJ*. 2007; 335: 916–18.

Makoul G, Curry RH, Tang PC. The use of electronic medical records. *J Am Med Inform Assoc.* 2001; 8(6): 610–15.

Mandl KD, Lee TL. Integrating medical informatics and health services research. *J Am Med Inform Assoc.* 2002; 9(2): 127–32.

Mohan J. *Planning, Markets and Hospitals.* London: Routledge; 2002.

Moore MH. *Creating Public Value.* Cambridge, MA: Harvard Business School Press; 1995.

National Audit Office. *Improving IT Procurement. Report by the Comptroller and Auditor General.* HC 877 Session 2003–4: 5 November. London: HMSO; 2004.

National Audit Office. *The National Programme for IT in the NHS. Report by the Comptroller and Auditor General.* HC 1173 Session 2005–6: 16 June. London: HMSO; 2006.

National Audit Office. *Delivering Successful IT-enabled Business Change. Report by the Comptroller and Auditor General.* HC 33–1 Session 2006–7: 17 November. London: HMSO; 2007.

National Audit Office. *The National Programme for IT in the NHS: progress since 2006.* London: National Audit Office; 16 May 2008.

National Patient Safety Agency. *Right Patient – Right Care.* NHS, NPSA; 2004.

Nerenz DR. What are the essentials of systems integration? *Front Health Serv Manage.* 1992; 9(2): 58–61.

Ondo K, Smith M. Outside IT: the case for full IT outsourcing. *Health Finan Manage.* 2006; 60(2): 92–8.

Payne TH, Rhia GG. Managing the life-cycle of electronic clinical documents. *J Am Med Inform Assoc.* 2006; 13(4): 438–45.

Pfeffer J, Sutton RI. Evidence based management. *Public Manage.* 2005; September: 14–25.

Pollock A. *NHS plc: the privatisation of our healthcare.* London: Verso; 2005.

Porter M, Teisberg EO. *Redefining Healthcare.* Cambridge, MA: Harvard Business School Press; 2006.

Rifkin DE. Electronic medical records: saving trees, saving lives. *JAMA.* 2001; 13: 1764–9.

Rigby M, Budgen D, Turner M, *et al.* A data-gathering broker as a future-orientated approach to supporting EPR users. *Int J Med Inform.* 2007; 76: 137–44.

Rossi PH, Lipsey MW, Freeman HE. Expressing and assessing program theory. In: *Evaluation: A systematic approach,* 7th ed. Thousand Oaks, CA: Sage Publications; 2004.

Scott R, Rundall TG, Vogt TM, *et al. Implementing an Electronic Medical Record System: successes, failures, lessons.* Oxford: Radcliffe Publishing; 2007.

Scott WR, Ruef M, Mendel PJ, *et al. Institutional Change and Healthcare Organizations.* Chicago: University of Chicago Press; 2000.

Summers P. *The Transition to Centralised Information Technology in Health: a case study of the University of Birmingham experience* [MPA dissertation, unpublished]. University of Warwick. October 2007.

Thomas RL. Learning the alphabet of healthcare IT. *Health Finan Manage.* 2006; 60(3): 100–2.

Wanless D. *Securing our Future Health: taking a long-term view. Final report of an independent review of the long-term resource requirement for the NHS.* London: DoH; April 2002. Available at: www.hm-treasury.gov.uk/Consultations_and_Legislation/wanless/consult/wanless_final.cfm.

Willcocks L, Currie WL. Pursuing the re-engineering agenda in public administration. *Public Admin.* 1997; 75(4): 617–50.

Wyatt JF. Four barriers to realising the information revolution in healthcare. In: Lenaghan J, editor. *Rethinking IT & Health*. London: Institute for Public Policy Research; 1998. pp. 100–22.

CHAPTER 2

Information systems (IS) integration approaches in healthcare: a critical review

David Finnegan and Khairil Azhar Abdul Hamid

INTRODUCTION

Current socioeconomic market conditions have pushed organisations to rethink their resource utilisation and act lean. Efforts to minimise the waste within technology, processes and effort are gaining popularity more than ever before. In order to capitalise on these benefits of technical innovation, integration of technical applications and processes has become paramount, yet complex. The delineation and application of an information system integration strategy in healthcare is not straightforward. Nevertheless integration themes are going from strength to strength. Beretta (2002) sees integration as a precondition for building competitive advantages. Braganza (2002) buttresses this by emphasising the positive effects of integration in respect of better responses to market changes and better relationship, with customers and suppliers.

There are numerous definitions of integration. In order to review IS integration in healthcare we need to unearth a suitable definition for the subject. An often-cited view of IS integration sees it as a technical state involving the connectivity of interdependent computer systems that physically and logically link the information resources of different organisational units (Hasselbring 2000; Gulledge 2006). Others argue that IS integration is defined as a function of the structural configurations of the organisation that support optimal decision making (Fiedler, *et al.* 1996).

Some scholars have a macro-level view of the role of integration as a strategic tool through which the integration of information and data add value to uniquely idiosyncratic aspects of an organisation (Wyse and Higgins 1993). Others still lament that these aforementioned perspectives neglect the social aspects of integration and ignore the importance of integrating people and their ideas within information systems (Waring and Wainwright 2000; Finnegan and Willcocks 2007).

Many authors, however, construct their views around various combinations and aspects of integration, be it from elements of a strategic, social, organisational or technical nature. This is often where the lines blur when delineating various meanings and interpretations of systems integration. There is evidently a high level of ambiguity and complexity associated with different ideas of IS integration.

To promote a debate on IS integration, this chapter reviews the literature, with particular focus on healthcare. First, we look at concepts and approaches surrounding the implementation of integrated systems from the generic IS and management literature. We consider how information systems are characterised and identify the key challenges relating to their development and integration. Second, we consider specific contributions from the IS and health informatics literature. There is already significant relevance in addressing this topic as an area of research. For example, the adoption of integrated electronic health record is high on the national agendas of many countries. In the United Kingdom, the development of a nationwide electronic record for the National Health Service is being constructed based on a government pledge to deliver high-quality personalised health services designed around the patient (Department of Health 2002). Similarly, other western European nations such as the Netherlands, Denmark and Finland are actively encouraging the adoption of electronic health records (Rigby, *et al.* 2007). In the United States the former and current administration has called for the provision of universal health records for every US citizen. This has led to the newly created Office of the National Co-ordinator for Health Information Technology (Hillestad, *et al.* 2005; Bernstein, *et al.* 2007; Shortliffe 2005).

DEFINITIONS OF INTEGRATION

Integration has been defined in several ways. For Gulledge (2006), the conceptualisation is expressed as a technical concern understood in terms of the physical and logical interconnections of computer-based information systems that communicate and share data. Finnegan and Willcocks (2007) and Waring and Wainright (2000) advocate a multifaceted deliberation of the term that accounts for organisational issues to be adopted. The concept of integration remains intricate and befuddled with varying definitions ranging from that of a process (Wyse and Higgins 1993; Hasselbring 2000; Waring and Wainright 2000; Gulledge 2006), a system or product (Waring and Wainwright 2000; Gulledge 2006), or a condition (Fiedler, *et al.* 1996; Evgeniou 2002).

The starting point of any examination of the topic is that integration represents the interconnection and linkages between isolated information systems artefacts (Wyse and Higgins 1993; Fiedler, *et al.* 1996; Hasselbring 2000; Waring and Wainwright 2000; Wainwright and Waring 2004; Evgeniou 2002; Gulledge 2006; Mendoza, *et al.* 2006). Even within the parameters of this definition, there are different schools of thought as to which of the varied technical approaches achieve integration. Gulledge (2006) and Mendoza, *et al.* (2006) acknowledge the implementation of point-to-point linkages, known as interfacing, which pass data between systems and applications. This can either qualify as integration methods themselves or features of an integrated system. This approach by the authors can be seen as an infrastructural standpoint towards integration.

Wyse and Higgins (1993), Hasselbring (2000), and Mendoza, *et al.* (2006) consider integration as a much deeper systems-oriented concern that reflects the need for more clearly defined workings of information technologies and data use in line with specific business processes. This personifies an IS integration approach towards the processes of the organisation but still maintains a stronger focus on technical interests. Most authors, however, contend that integration encapsulates much more than a technical panacea. Wainwright and Waring (2004) view integration as an organisational issue dealing with the changes to the way people work. However, as it involves complex and highly subjective aspects of how people, decisions, ideas and activities in organisations are integrated with technology, it is important to clarify the interconnectedness of these terms. For example, Weber and Pliskin (1996) attempt to link organisational performance of recently merged banking institutions with the ability for these previously autonomous organisations to integrate their IS in the face of either newly found cultural synergies or conflicts. Cultural aspects are deemed important as information systems are believed to increase the levels of formal and informal communication and collaboration among organisational members. Their systematically collected evidence has shown that integration may also be considered in terms of a cultural fit. Such arguments illustrate the importance of the organisational and social aspects that define the characteristics of information systems integration within an organisation.

THE DRIVERS FOR IS INTEGRATION

Central to any discussion of integration and its methodological approaches are the objectives such efforts are intended to accomplish. An important observation from the literature is how information systems may improve the coordination of work, the availability and accessibility of information (Evgeniou 2002; Mendoza, *et al.* 2006) and support organisational and inter-organisational processes (Hasselbring 2000). Information systems integration may further improve organisational performance (Fiedler, *et al.* 1996; Evgeniou 2002), and that information is seen as a resource requirement for efficiency and effectiveness, and also deployed as part of a competitive strategy (Wyse and Higgins 1993; Mendoza, *et al.* 2006). This competitive effectiveness is thus hampered if organisations cannot leverage information that is inaccessible by virtue of being isolated and spread across the various data silos. Integration therefore becomes an enabler for strategic advantage.

INFORMATION SYSTEMS INTEGRATION AS A MULTI-DIMENSIONAL CONCEPT

The discussion thus far has clearly demonstrated that integration is often regarded as a loaded concept that cannot be singularly defined. While technical and strategic implications are more readily expressed in concrete terms, other aspects such as cultural and social features of integration are more abstract and subjective but have been shown to be valid elements in the implementation of integrated systems. Furthermore, the layering of shared and intertwined concepts evident from the approaches suggested in the literature reveals the complex packaging of characteristics and features of integration. In developing further a coherent exploration and guiding the discussion into the methodological approaches for achieving integration, it is suggested that a more structured method be applied to develop categorisations of the different integration strategies by using a broader heuristic lens.

Khoumbati and Themistocleous (2006) and Khoumbati, *et al.* (2006) choose to evaluate benefits derived from the use of IT along operational, managerial, strategic, IT infrastructure and organisational dimensions, citing the evaluation model developed by Shang and Seddon (2002). Wainwright and Waring (2004) opt to examine integrated IS implementation along the four domains of technical, systems, organisational and strategic analysis. Hasselbring (2000) also applies his analysis of systems integration along the business (organisational), application (systems) and technology (technical) dimensions. These authors demonstrate how the application of appropriate categorisations can clarify and organise discussions and findings from the literature into more lucid and articulate analyses. Therefore the heuristic method employed in the following sections follows the line of reasoning already adopted in the previous discussion. This necessitates an examination of integration approaches along three recurrent themes apparent in the literature, namely the dimensions consisting of: the technical and systems, the organisational and social, and the strategic channels of investigation. We discuss these below.

TECHNICAL AND SYSTEMS-ORIENTED APPROACHES

The technical and systems-based approaches to integration are commonly characterised by very specific goals that invariably aim to unify organisational IS and databases (Mendoza, *et al.* 2006). These approaches make disparate applications interoperable (Gulledge 2006), by incorporating various technical artefacts into a coherent system that appears to function as a single system in order to integrate organisational and inter-organisational processes (Wainwright and Waring 2004, Hasselbring 2000). However, this portrayal may not be considered accurate in the opinion of all observers. Gulledge (2006) classifies the point-to-point interconnections between autonomous components, to facilitate the communication between different applications, as one valid method within the repertoire of integration. Wainwright and Waring (2004) do not regard this as true integration because it reflects the individual nature of these components without regard as to how the system functions as a whole. For them, integration requires integrated interoperability. Moreover, they contend that interfacing is a mere means of communication and does not allow for systems integrated in this manner to collectively arrive at a decision. However, it is not clear just where the line is drawn when qualifying what is or is not integration. Gulledge (2006) highlights that sophisticated interfacing through the shared use of services across enterprise applications achieves resource integration by sharing business logic that beneficially obviates reduplication, something that may not have been considered by Wainwright and Waring (2004).

ORGANISATIONAL AND SOCIAL-ORIENTED APPROACHES

Although systems integration and enterprise systems approaches have developed detailed technical solutions towards IS as a whole, the application of such methods must account for organisational factors. This has often been a noted concern in the IS-related literature (Finnegan and Willcocks 2007; Finnegan and Currie 2008; Wyse and Higgins 1993; Hasselbring 2000; Waring and Wainwright 2000; Wainwright and Waring 2004; Mendoza, et al. 2006). For example, Wyse and Higgins (1993) argue for the need to extend the concept of systems integration beyond the preoccupations of interfacing and concentrate on interconnecting people in the organisation to the technologies that allow them to be strategically competitive. Their approach advocates a managerial assessment of the organisation's current level of integration defined in terms of relevancy of integrated data to strategic interests. This, although pertinent to the concerns of integration, does not acknowledge social aspects of how integration may be perceived or accepted by these organisational members it is meant to serve.

It is often within this macro-level analysis of the organisation that IS integration approaches invariably emerge in terms of organisational procedural and structural strategies (Wainwright and Waring 2004). This emphasis is recognisable through initiatives that advocate schemes such as business process re-engineering (Hasselbring 2000) or the conformance to structural typologies (Fiedler, et al. 1996; Evgeniou 2002) or structural reorganisation such as divisionalisation, delayering, and downsizing (Wainwright and Waring 2004). These studies tend to regard organisational structures along functional groupings and thus have limitations when applied to more innovative structural forms such as matrix organisations. The main objective, however, is to align the structure of the organisation with IS systems and to achieve organisational integration.

Fiedler, et al. (1996) studied the close links between IS/IT and organisational structure as a whole. Their findings suggest that functional organisations are adapting their organisational structures towards more information intensive and cooperative structures to match structural IT strategies characterised by vertical information systems and horizontally integrated task relationships within the firm. This view very much orientates integration towards the tasks of cooperation, information sharing and communication that is informed by coordination theory and contingency theory.

Yet there is also an acknowledgement that the organisational dimension of integration must account for social factors, the earlier case of cultural synergy from Weber and Pliskin (1996) being such an example. The authors contend that culture is not easily modifiable and can impact the cooperation with and commitment to the success of any IS integration initiative. Indeed, the role of other social factors in terms of effective leadership, user involvement, knowledge and communities in approaching integration help determine the success of these initiatives (Wainwright and Waring 2004; Mendoza, *et al.* 2006) that may be informed by a number of social theories. What all these different viewpoints highlight is the critical impact and importance that organisational change will have on the organisation as systems are integrated into the entity.

STRATEGIC APPROACHES

According to Wainwright and Waring (2004) strategic approaches are about adapting already established and mature strategic management tools and methods to the problems of integration. It is also within this vein that Wyse and Higgins (1993) have argued for the technical and data integration aspect of systems integration to be regarded as a strategic concern. In addition, they argue that managerial focus should emphasise the formalised methodologies to evaluate and plan the integration of information systems in aid of strategic business requirements. These views are aligned to the belief that IS integration strategy now equates to business strategy such as their shared importance to the competitive positioning of firms.

This dimension of IS integration is orientated towards evaluating how the strategic benefits are managed by the organisation. It has been criticised by both Wainwright and Waring (2004) and Wyse and Higgins (1993) for the over-reliance on outdated top-down bureaucratic planning approaches. However, Wyse and Higgins (1993) propose the same types of planning methods towards integration that they vehemently criticise. The main exception is the added emphasis on the notion of temporality or the timeliness in which the internal and external integration of data and interconnections are achieved.

In spite of these distinctions, it remains difficult to unconditionally separate these strategic options from the details of the technical and organisational approaches. For example, business process re-engineering may be regarded as a competitively driven planned strategic action. Yet its application is considered as an organisational approach towards system integration in understanding, architecting and operationalising organisational workflows. External horizontal integration with alliance partners may also be considered as a macro-level strategic approach to integration yet it is realised through the application of technical enterprise application integration and business-to-business methodologies.

In summary, although integration can be deconstructed into its constituent elements and analysed part by part from a technical, organisational or strategic perspective, its meaning can only be appreciated when all the constituent elements are viewed in relation to each other. The analysis and discussion has approached the literature by asking how integration can be defined and understood. Integration is found to be a highly complex subject that is not easy to define, as evidenced by the literature. Yet there are certain characteristics that describe the general features of integration and these were found to be more amenable to interpretation and analysis when deconstructed into categories. As a heuristic device to guide investigation of the concepts and methods surrounding IS integration, categories comprising the technical and systems, organisational and social, and strategic dimensions were applied to structure and organise findings from the IS integration literature.

What is apparent is that IS integration is a multifaceted concept. Technical and systems integration approaches have been well established and defined to reveal a number of methodological options available that in turn afford varying levels of integration between systems, information and organisational processes. Although granting a number of choices, these approaches can appear very confusing. This is a situation that will likely increase as integration technology advances. Systems integration practices offer the tools and methods to navigate these choices and are meant to bridge the heterogeneous nature of organisational IS integration while enterprise systems seek to centralise and control them to a single model. Even so, in many instances such approaches have been the subject of criticism for lacking a strategic focus of integrating IS to the mission of the organisation. Even then resulting planning methodologies meant to address these concerns have been accused of being overly constraining and static in relation to the dynamic realities of organisational needs.

Then there are the organisational and social aspects to consider (Finnegan and Willcocks 2007). Many observers have noted that IS integration cannot be sufficiently defined as the realisation of a technical solution to achieve strategic organisational objectives. Critical success factors related to successful IS integration initiatives have been shown to have a strong organisational and social component.

What can be concluded from this review is to broadly establish what is known on the subject of IS integration. This overview serves to direct a more focused enquiry in the research of healthcare IS integration.

HEALTHCARE INFORMATION SYSTEMS AND APPLICATIONS

After having touched upon some of the key IS integration debates, we move on to establish the background and context of the need for IS integration within the healthcare sector. This is done by showing the chronology of the themes and scope of the issues involved, in addition to trends that have shaped the application of information systems and technology in healthcare. First, it aims to clarify the historical background and development of IS adoption in healthcare by charting the trends related to the information needs and strategies of healthcare organisations over several decades. Second, it reviews common healthcare IS applications to show the breadth and variety of both clinical and administrative systems, and how these systems still largely operate in isolation. Following this, the arguments for integrating these disparate systems are considered in terms of the benefits that can be potentially realised. These arguments are presented against the rationalisations of management and stakeholder concerns that are often made in favour of integration. Finally, a visual timeline of these developments, synthesised from the historical analysis of the literature, is presented to provide an overall picture of prior research in healthcare IS and potential future directions.

HISTORY OF HEALTHCARE INFORMATION SYSTEMS

Healthcare IS has largely seen deployment and application in the financial control and administrative spheres of the healthcare industry. Throughout much of the 1960s, 1970s and 1980s, healthcare IS has been characterised by systems and applications strongly emphasising a departmental focus towards financial and management control (Hughes and Bays 1991; Rivers and Bae 1999; Southard, *et al.* 2000; Stuewe 2002). Although there were early attempts in the 1960s and 1970s to develop integrated clinical systems, standalone rudimentary electronic medical record systems being one example, these projects did not gain widespread acceptance due to a number of technical and institutional barriers (Stead, *et al.* 2000; Shortliffe 2005). The reasons behind this evolutionary trajectory are not unlike those experienced by other sectors; early computer systems in the 1960s and 1970s were leveraged towards data processing needs to meet the efficiency and automation goals that dealt with routine management tasks. Where additional and more novel analytical and numerical computing was required, it was also often targeted towards financial planning priorities (Southard, *et al.* 2000).

In the competitive US healthcare sector, the 1970s and early 1980s saw the emergence of hospital information systems to address the patient admissions and billing processes, again in response to the automation and routinisation of common tasks, but theses tentative steps began the move towards increased integration of administrative applications (Southard, *et al.* 2000; Stuewe 2002). Clinical needs were not regarded then as equally critical or easy to automate through the application of information systems. Rapid developments in networking and microcomputer technologies began supplanting the centralised mainframe systems and individual hospital departments began to acquire their own systems that saw, in addition to a management focus, increased information fragmentation in healthcare organisations (Rivers and Bae 1999).

In the nationalised health service of the United Kingdom, the situation was not too dissimilar. Since the 1960s, the UK National Health Service (NHS) has accumulated large investments in disparate IS solutions at all levels of the service from its initial forays into mainframe acquisitions (Hughes and Bays 1991). Being a public institution, the NHS is accountable for reporting its use of taxpayer-derived resources and the need to manage and integrate information for financial control would culminate in the Resource Management Initiative launched in 1986 (Wainwright and Waring 2000). Two themes therefore emerge to characterise this early healthcare-computing era: first, the focus towards management IS needs, and second, the rapid increase in IS fragmentation; both were to become progressively more problematic. The subsequent challenges for integration would require strategic and technical solutions.

Market-based and legislative factors were also influential in determining the evolution of healthcare IS. The US healthcare services sector has always been strongly competitive and up till the mid-1980s operated on a 'cost plus reimbursement' fee model to charge patients, but government regulations introduced in 1984 changed the cost of treatment to a fixed-rate system (Johns 1997; Southard, *et al.* 2000). Competitive pressures brought about by this change required hospitals and health-care providers to adapt their business strategies, which also influenced the pressing need for more strategic use of IS (Raghupathi and Tan 2002; Shortliffe 2005).

By the mid-1980s and into the 1990s, upheaval in the healthcare business environment switched the emphasis to managed care and quality of care as competitive strategies that required capabilities to effectively coordinate the medical treatment of patients (Southard, *et al.* 2000; Bernstein, *et al.* 2007). Similarly in the UK, patient demands for greater quality and seamlessness of the care process led the government to unveil supporting regulatory and policy decisions, one of which was the Information for Health strategy in 1998 (NHS Executive 1998). These changes would seek technical solutions to bridge the integration gaps brought about by changes in strategic direction.

This change in direction to a clinical focus in healthcare IS saw the introduction of numerous but disparate IS products. In hospitals, these catered to individual clinical and departmental specialisations such as laboratories, blood banks, pharmacies and radiology. These would require greater efforts to be interfaced to legacy systems in order to automate and integrate processes (Stuewe 2002). The 1990s saw further consolidation and convergence of administrative and clinical systems along with a changing strategic focus in the provision of quality care (Bates 2002; Bernstein, *et al.* 2007). This period saw the application of systems integration methodologies such as best-of-breed integration methods through interfacing and interface engines, and enterprise-wide systems that integrated both administrative and clinical functions through a single product and database as exemplified by technologies such as hospital information support systems (Wainwright and Waring 2000; Stuewe 2002; Khoumbati and Themistocleous 2006).

The trend to provide integrated and seamless healthcare has remained unabated. The chronology and evolution of healthcare IS and integration issues have shown us several things:

➤ The early focus of IS was in financial systems where the investment has been stronger. Bates (2002), for example, notes that billing systems on the whole are far superior to clinical systems.
➤ The shape of adoption has been piecemeal and consists of a variety of heterogeneous applications that have contributed to much fragmentation both in administrative and clinical systems and the existence of legacy systems.
➤ There is an increased strategic focus for integrated systems in the patient care process as reflected by efforts to integrate existing legacy systems and also deploy large-scale commercial off-the-shelf (COTS) systems as an integrated IS product in healthcare organisations.
➤ Quality of care and the coordination of care in an ordered clinical pathway

require that administrative systems, clinical information systems and decision support systems must work in tandem and that the link to patient specific information is crucial to achieving this (Bates 2002; Raghupathi and Tan 2002; Bernstein, *et al.* 2007). Electronic health records as the repository of patient information therefore represent a critical link in the entire system of care.

TYPES OF HEALTHCARE IS

Table 2.1 reflects the breadth and diversity in the number of systems and applications that comprise the modern healthcare IS landscape. It is by no means a fully comprehensive account but shows that various legacy systems exist in any single period of time. The transition to newer technologies and applications are also at various stages in the process. It further shows how information on patients (e.g. identification, medical history, demographic data) and information related to their care (e.g. clinical guidelines, medical test results, best practices, admissions) can be distributed across much of the different application and database infrastructure in hospitals and healthcare organisations and how this has expanded in time.

The variety of systems approaches should not, however, be entirely unexpected, considering how healthcare work is known to be very complex in terms of task and process structure (Anyanwu, *et al.* 2003; Avison and Young 2007), in addition to being exceptionally information intensive (Grimson 2001), and requiring large numbers of people who are often divided by managerial, clinical and other institutional structures, to work together to deliver these services (Khatri 2006). Although there is a great need to accommodate a variety of systems' functionality to reflect the diversity in healthcare practices – hence the proliferation of systems – there is also a strong belief for the need to integrate all the information and workflow processes within healthcare organisations with the resulting drive towards integration strategies.

While the overarching strategic objectives of providing higher quality modern levels of seamless care are certainly pressing – as envisioned by healthcare organisations, decision makers and governmental policy makers, and correspondingly demanded by health consumers – the more traditional objectives of integration for efficiency, cost reduction and overall effectiveness (Avison and Young 2007) remain and these reflect generic integration concerns.

TABLE 2.1 Selected examples illustrate breadth and diversity of healthcare IS systems

Application/System	Citation
Hospital information systems (including modules such as admissions-discharge-transfer systems, scheduling and registration, and electronic patient records – integrated clinical and administrative needs).	Rivers and Bae (1999), Southard, *et al.* (2000), Raghupathi (2002)
Laboratory information systems.	Raghupathi (2002)

Application/System	Citation
Pharmacy systems/drug prescription services.	
Clinical decision support systems.	
Document management systems.	
Data warehousing and analytics (clinical and non-clinical).	Southard, *et al.* (2000), Raghupathi (2002)
Universal electronic medical/health records.	Raghupathi (2002), Bernstein, *et al.* (2007)
Strategic decision support systems (non-clinical).	Bernstein, *et al.* (2007)

THE NEED FOR INTEGRATION OF HEALTHCARE IS

The previous discussion has illustrated the piecemeal and fragmented adoption of various systems that comprise the healthcare IS landscape within and between healthcare organisations. Moreover, hospitals or trusts have their own medical specialisations, socio-technical and IT capacities, organisational cultures, structures, budgetary problems and other crucial influences on actual outcomes (Peltu and Clegg 2008). There are strong strategic drivers for integration in healthcare as a business and managerial concern as well as the imperatives driven by regulatory and governmental policy decisions. However, the move towards greater IS integration will always be partially driven by cost and efficiency measures that aim to increase the effectiveness of inter-organisational processes. These concerns are generic to the goals and aims of IS integration as a whole.

One common theme that permeates the health management, health information systems and health informatics literature is the apparent lack of success derived from the application of IS/IT to significantly improve the delivery of healthcare services (Kaplan 1997; Khatri 2006; Avison and Young 2007). Ever since the advent of computerisation in healthcare, observers have lamented the disappointing results of IS/IT adoption and use, especially when contrastingly transformative gains have been reaped in other industry sectors (Kaplan 1997; Khatri 2006; Herzlinger 2006).

This phenomenon has been noted in a number of subject areas including systems evaluation (Kaplan 1997), healthcare innovation (Herzlinger 2006); technology integration (Grimson, *et al.* 2000; Avison and Young 2007) and technology adoption (Caccia-Bava, *et al.* 2006; Hennington and Janz 2007). Healthcare policy, governance and practice-oriented literature has also highlighted this lag and several authors have trumpeted the call for urgent action through the development of various roadmaps, models and best practices that are hoped will assist the sector to better utilise IS/IT (Lutchen and Collins 2005; Herzlinger 2006; Dixon 2007).

These observations reveal the limitations that the technical systemisation of healthcare processes, through the application of hardware, software, and systems integration, have had. While it has been demonstrated that adoption and integration techniques for healthcare IS have followed the traditional systems integration models – interfacing, integration engines, enterprise systems, and the like – and for many of the same strategic reasons, these approaches should not be evaluated in generic terms. Primarily there are concerns about the efficacy of such methods to the specific needs of healthcare.

For example, Winthereik and Vikkelso (2005) acknowledge that, as healthcare tasks are often ambiguous, complex, involve many different technologies and many different people, and are highly distributed, the need for high levels of information processing often results in the standardisation of communications and work processes through technology solutions. At times this is often unavoidable. Some observers such as Landry, *et al.* (2005) go further and would have us believe that many forms of healthcare work and the skills of their associated personnel are so clearly defined that they will be replaced by technology in short measure; they offer the advancements in expert diagnostics systems as one prediction. Such assertions, however, must be regarded as suspect from what is known of healthcare practice.

As Hartswood, *et al.* (2003) cogently observe in their research on psychiatric practice in a toxicology ward, the affordances of such technologies are often limited in addressing the 'fuzziness' of medical tasks, and the design of technical systems often force the conformance of treatment to rigid forms of practice that do not wholly support desired care outcomes. We might also consider the strategic, managerial and clinical implications of integration to the concept of seamless care. Connell and Young (2007) argue that the scale of complexity of clinical decisions and the level of involvement of multiple medical experts in coordinated care drive the need for more person-to-person interaction to enable, among other collaborative medical tasks, diagnosis, treatment, planning and assessment for example. Health information systems, it is argued, instead facilitate such communication and collaboration through the technology infrastructure and thus lose the tacit aspects of social communication greatly required in medical work. Enterprise systems models that have pervaded much of business and manufacturing sectors exemplify the inadequacy of process integration methods in the service of healthcare.

The argument is that the needs of integration should not therefore be perceived in technological terms alone. Yet even these rationalisations are not as straightforward to apply in practice. Sizeable past investments in healthcare IS that have conformed to proprietary architectures and processes often predicate technological systems integration responses to the problems of fragmentation. Technical and systems integration approaches will likely remain as the glue that binds these disparate systems together. Integrated systems, which have seen success in other sectors, will likely be adapted and experimented upon to better meet the needs of healthcare organisations. In tandem with these developments, there is the need for organisational, managerial and social strategies to complement the technical systems approaches. This has been more evident through management strategies that focus on quality management issues and concerns (Rivers and Bae 1999; Bates 2002) and the need for greater user involvement, training, and participation (Bates 2002; Bernstein, *et al.* 2007).

TIMELINE OF HEALTHCARE IS

A chronological representation of major events in the history of healthcare IS derived from the review of the literature. Figure 2.1 conveys our understanding of the origins of healthcare IS; its major developments and gradual alteration brought about by changing strategic needs of the healthcare sector over several decades; the gradual transition to more clinically focused and integrated forms of administrative, financial and medical information; and the vision for an eventual seamless and highly coordinated provision of healthcare. At the centre of this vision is the premise that a highly integrated healthcare information systems infrastructure and services is the way forward.

The diagram depicted by Figure 2.1 distinguishes between clinical and administrative systems to provide greater clarity in the separation of the dual management-clinical structure (Khatri 2006), which is often noted in the delivery of healthcare services and their corresponding information systems. In practice this delineation is not as clear cut. In the progression of the timeline, increased levels of integration between these two structural strands are acknowledged and made more evident in the diagram. It is apparent that healthcare IS has experienced a fragmented model of adoption. Early emphasis on management control systems that were poorly integrated to begin with now complicate the adoption and integration of clinical systems into the overall IS infrastructure landscape as well as organisational work practices. The healthcare sector has strong strategic and management drivers to improve the use of information and these pre-existing conditions present considerable challenges. While existing technical and systems integration solutions have been applied, their success has been mixed. There has been positive progress, yet criticisms are raised for not paying due consideration to the structural, cultural and institutional conditions within healthcare organisations. The heuristic model of categorising the dimensions of integration into technical, organisational and social systems enables better comprehension of the issues and arguments.

HEALTHCARE INFORMATION SYSTEMS INTEGRATION

The review of IS integration literature has shown that an all-encompassing definition of integration is problematic – its complex make-up is difficult to designate to only a limited set of ideas – thus it has been more appropriate and useful to examine integration by assembling and organising its elements along the core features of its implementation and use. The examination of the concept of integration, under the three general categories comprising the strategic, technical and systems, and organisational and social dimensions, has allowed the analysis to progress more coherently.

The chronology of development and evolution of healthcare IS has provided the contextual background on the need for integration in healthcare organisations. Reasons have not only included the traditional mainstays of increased efficiencies and lower costs, but also to facilitate the expanding strategic paradigms associated with greater patient-centricity, the drive towards seamless and continuous managed

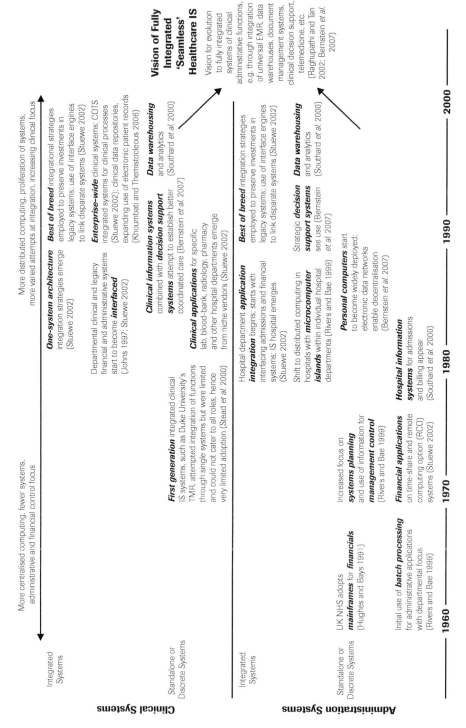

FIGURE 2.1 Healthcare IS timeline of significant developments

care, and the need for increased quality of healthcare services. The achievement of these objectives is seen as contingent upon the highly integrated management and use of information in healthcare delivery. The following review expands and advances the general discussion of integration by examining the approaches and strategies explored within the healthcare IS related literature.

NATURE OF HEALTHCARE ORGANISATIONS

Certain characteristics of healthcare organisations and their work have been observed to impact the decisions taken in approaching the problems of integration. Healthcare work, especially the delivery of medical care, is known to be very complex, often ambiguous and involves many people – health personnel and patients included – interacting within highly distributed organisational networks (Anyanwu, *et al.* 2003; Winthereik and Vikkelso 2005); it intensively uses and generates information (Grimson 2001; Anyanwu, *et al.* 2003) during medical encounters; and it is further complicated by dual management and clinical institutional structures (Khatri 2006; Avison and Young 2007) that are then further fragmented by professional roles and memberships to medical specialisations (Harstwood, *et al.* 2003; Landry, *et al.* 2004; Rigby, *et al.* 2007).

Healthcare work is also very much dependent on close interpersonal interactions between the agents involved in the delivery of care (Connell and Young 2007), and this suggests that a high degree of tacit information and knowledge needs to be exchanged to make organisational coordination, collaboration and inter-working more effective (Berg 2001; Harstwood, *et al.* 2003). The sequence of activities involved in a delivery of healthcare services for a patient involves much more complexity and ambiguity than for example the coordination involved in the value chains of other sectors such as manufacturing or distribution (Avison and Young 2007), especially when clinical pathways cut across many different clinical department or sub-organisations. This demonstrates that the informational needs of healthcare organisations are highly multifaceted and require considerable efforts of integration, and if close coordination is expected, efforts that are appropriate to the unique context of healthcare organisations and their patients.

Yet, as different as healthcare IS needs are, Avison and Young (2007) highlight that the healthcare sector still benefits from the generic models of IS adoption and integration: those approaches that seek to improve process integration in service quality, cost and efficiency; or help to put patients at the centre of focus much like the successful product and customer-centric emphases of other sectors. Even so, the moderating factors of the institutional and social characteristics of healthcare practice indicate that IS integration strategies should place a greater emphasis on human-centred and social aspects during the integration of information systems as the processes and knowledge involved in this type of work are far more dependent upon people to accomplish compared to the automation possible in other areas.

STRATEGIC APPROACHES

There has been no shortage of strategic approaches advocated by strategic management experts on how to achieve the integration of information systems. These have largely involved various planning and assessment programmes that revolve around the need to increase competitiveness, tighten horizontal processes across healthcare organisation sub-units, and improve upon quality outcomes in care. Integration is therefore strategically seen from a service integration perspective. Borne from this has been the emphasis on business process re-engineering (BPR) as a strategic approach to aligning information systems with organisational operations.

Business process re-engineering

Johns (1997), for example, states that competitively reducing hospital costs through the integration of information technology must be done in tandem with the redesign of outdated business and clinical processes. One apparent outcome of the BPR approach is the growing prominence of clinical care pathways that formally delineate and embed within hospital information systems the clinical processes that represent the continuum of care. For Conrad and Shortell (1996) this embodies the healthcare value chain that is implicitly dependent on the effectiveness of information exchange for the coordination of care processes.

These forms of analyses have been shown to be relevant to the strategic consolidation of healthcare systems; one notable example is from the well-documented evidence of the US healthcare integration experience of multi-hospital systems and hospital-physician group mergers in response to the changes to the reimbursement legislation (Conrad and Shortell 1996; Burns and Pauly 2002). Strategic approaches towards IS integration further open up the possibilities for structural integration and business models such as virtual alliances – innovations to horizontal and vertical integration initiatives – that are largely predicated on the efficient and timely sharing of information to coordinate and manage the care processes. Conrad and Shortell (1996) depict this as one way of assembling or rebundling different services in the continuum based upon alliances between care providers, and the acquisition of capabilities required to do this is contingent upon higher investment in clinical and financial information systems.

Competitive analysis

Kim and Michelman (1990) similarly extend the competitive analysis of strategic management approaches to the question of healthcare IS by describing how Porter's (1979, cited in Kim and Michelman 1990) 'five forces framework' can be used to analyse the health organisation's industry position to plan and develop the integration of IS as a competitive weapon. For example, they note the applicability of the framework analysis for raising high switching costs for community physicians referring patients to other hospitals by providing an integrated hospital information system that incorporates all the functionality to support the care of their patients such as checking bed availability and lab schedules.

Quality management and improvement

Total quality management (TQM) and continuous quality improvement (CQI) measures are also strategic approaches to integration. Information systems standardisation through the reduction of unnecessary variation that provides data on cost, quality and care outcomes is seen as an important capability for clinical integration (Conrad and Shortel 1996; Rivers and Bae 1999; Johns 1997). Rigby and Robins (1997) also describe the emerging trends of building healthcare delivery and management systems that are focused on information of human aspects that highlight patient-centric strategies in healthcare IS integration. The reduction of medical errors is also a direct benefit of quality improvements.

Strategic fit and alignment

Strategic fit between IS and organisational objectives has also been the focus of integration approaches that have, from an academic standpoint, been attributed to planning and assessment techniques, incorporating the application of systems maturity models and growth frameworks (Thrasher, *et al.* 2006) to strategic contingency theory and diffusion of innovation theory (Wang, *et al.* 2005).

The review of these approaches is by no means comprehensive, but what they show is that strategic approaches are aimed at aligning, guiding and planning the use of IS resources with the goal of improving organisational performance in support of overall strategic objectives. These macro-level strategic approaches aim to enforce best practices in the adoption and use of integrated information systems. One thing to note is that, although the findings of Thrasher, *et al.* (2007), Wang, *et al.* (2006) and Kim and Michelman (1990) are based on empirical research, the practical bases or contributions of the strategic integration approaches in much of the literature remain unclear.

Technical and systems approaches

The technical and systems approaches adopted for integration purposes have largely been adapted from generic systems integration methodologies. These are to a great extent either in the form of integrated enterprise information systems such as ERP systems – the clinical equivalent of which is the hospital information support system (HISS) (Wainwright and Waring 2000) – or utilise the various interfacing approaches to connect disparate systems. These conventionally fall under either inter-systems communication techniques or subscribe to a common enterprise information architecture. The latter option can also be used to connect islands of enterprise systems through the use of enterprise application integration (EAI) methods. Many instances of these have been adopted in departmentally piecemeal fashion (Grimson, *et al.* 2000).

Technical and systems integration can loosely be classified along these two lines of approach. Integrated systems hold a single database and are intended to be self-contained systems in terms of data and processes that are managed. Hence the issue of fragmentation, it is argued, does not arise as integration occurs *in situ*. The literature is replete with schematised representations of these types of systems, usually in the form of integrated hospital information support systems (HISS) (Kim and Michelman 1990; Wainwright and Waring 2000) that show the various linkages of processes between hospital departments and a single database embedded within a monolithic architected system.

However, the promise of integrated enterprise systems as a solution can only be fulfilled if it is all encompassing and the notion that it is a panacea is not wholly accurate. Fragmentation still results when enterprise systems are implemented much like others types of IS in piecemeal fashion by different departments aiming to pre-serve autonomy. The same integration difficulties still arise when attempting to link these disparate information islands together (Grimson, *et al.* 2000).

More commonly, however, due to the rather chequered adoption patterns common to healthcare, there are a collection of systems integration approaches that are divided along either basic inter-system messaging or more sophisticated sets of methods that allow semantic interoperability. The former is generally not regarded as the ideal choice for integration, as it requires considerable efforts expended in maintaining pairs of interfaces for each connection and raises considerable scalability problems (Grimson, *et al.* 2000). The latter is more sophisticated and is regarded by many as a more complete form of integration (Tsiknakis, *et al.* 2002; Gulledge 2006).

As some observers (Tsiknakis, *et al.* 2002; Khoumbati and Themistocleous 2006) have noted, interfacing methods are the most commonly deployed form of integration. This is particularly apparent when legacy systems need to be integrated into the wider organisational IS landscape or where a best-of-breed strategy is called for. Heterogeneous IS has therefore been the most problematic integration issue in healthcare organisations (Khoumbati, *et al.* 2006). Hence much of the healthcare IS literature has been found to be devoted to studying the methods and impacts of systems integration.

The wide degree of variance of these apparently generic approaches creates some degree of confusion for the adopters. One observation that can be made is that technical integration tends towards enforcing standardisation and uniformity that decreases the amount of variance that is often equated with fragmentation. The number of standards, methods and approaches described in the healthcare integration literature is quite large and can be a source of confusion (Khoumbati and Themistocleous 2006). The following section proposes to demystify and categorise these approaches.

SYSTEMS INTEGRATION

Systems integration is very much the standard means to achieve technical integration of clinical systems in healthcare organisations. Central to the capabilities for system integration is the adherence to technical standards (Khoumbati, *et al.* 2006). Not all systems integration approaches are equal in the levels of integration achieved and each require trade-offs. Not surprisingly, there are debates surrounding which methods should be employed; for examples *see* Khoumbati, *et al.* (2006) and Ciccarese, *et al.* (2005).

Finnegan and Currie (2008) and Stead, *et al.* (2000) echo this argument, criticising that many commercial products are unable to interoperate with each other through common information architectures. While Ciccarese, *et al.* (2005) may regard basic messaging as affording sufficient functionality in clinical workflow applications, Anyanwu, *et al.* (2003) remind us that large-scale integration of workflow is contextualised by the complex and data and people-intensive nature of medical processes. Therefore some methods are not up to the task of wide-scale integration.

The above debates which contribute to the productive dialogue of technical and systems integration strategies are ongoing. However, what is apparent is the importance of protocol standards, architecture standards and process standardisation in healthcare IS integration. Not only do these wide-ranging choices present barriers of consensus on which standards to adopt within and between healthcare organisations (Grimson, *et al.* 2000), but also present added marketplace confusion (Khoumbati and Themistocleous 2006).

SYSTEMS INTEGRATION AND FEDERATED SYSTEMS

Why is systems integration regarded as an important technical approach? The reasons behind this could well be to do more with organisational factors rather than purely technical reasons. It is important to reflect on what is known about the nature of healthcare work and its institutional logics as well as the culture of professional group memberships. Analysis of the literature shows that systems integration simultaneously enables the bridging of heterogeneity while enabling the preservation of autonomy these systems have to whatever organisational subdivision they belong to. The socio-technical advocates often exclaim that the great difficulties in IS integration are frequently of an organisational nature (Berg 2001, Winthereik and Vikkelso 2005; Ellingsen and Monteiro 2006). The less rigid outcomes may well be easier to integrate as they will involve less intrusion between organisational boundaries and reduce the need for organisational change. However, the potential synergies might well be less than in a unified integrated system.

Furthermore, enterprise type systems may also be less attractive to clinical stakeholders as they are often perceived to be tools of management control (Wainwright and Waring 2000; Avison and Young 2007). The apparent failure to effectively deploy HISS in the NHS was related to the added disruption to hospital information (Wainwright and Waring 2000). Difficulties arising from the disruption to existing infrastructure and work patterns are therefore critical concerns. Even the largest integrated healthcare IS modernisation initiative, the in-progress NPfIT of the UK NHS, depends on individual patient administration systems at acute hospital trust level to feed it (Hendy, *et al.* 2005). For such a large-scale integration, a single unified system would be unfeasible to do on account of the diversity and variance in organisational practices.

This leads us to observe that technical approaches can only solve part of the problems of IS integration. Neither is this fact oblivious to some of those that promote systems integration strategies. Ciccarese, *et al.* (2005), for example, argue for greater innovation in integrated clinical decision support systems design. Stuewe (2002) notes that, where systems integration affords best-of-breed approaches, it is less effective when the strategic direction is towards information systems consolidation, citing evidence from the mergers and alliances that occurred within the US healthcare system in the 1990s.

The assumption that technical approaches make is that tighter inter-organisational coupling of processes will yield greater productivity and that workflow can be embedded within computerised systems largely without issue. This aspect is what is most contentious among those advocating a socio-technical perspective of integration; see for example Berg (2001).

ORGANISATIONAL AND SOCIAL APPROACHES

The implications of technology at the organisational and social levels have been the focus of main research streams in the field of IS for the last 30 years and have included, for example, the subjects of user involvement and satisfaction in systems development and use, user acceptance of technology and the diffusion of innovation (Banker and Kauffman 2004). Similarly, strategies relating to the successful integration of IS in the healthcare sector have adopted the recommendations for these concepts and theories to manage the complex processes that influence successful technology integration within the organisation. Some of the main approaches reviewed that have strong organisational and social components are discussed here.

Organisational forms and social structures

The structure of the organisation has been regarded as being strongly influenced by the effects of information systems and technology as improvements in communication and in information and resource sharing enable more fluid functional structures to exist (Fiedler, *et al.* 1996; Landry, *et al.* 2004). While IS has already been known to alter the structural fabric of the organisation, producing decentralised and distributed forms among them (Fiedler, *et al.* 1996), there is also recognition that organisational changes are required to maximise the potential of technological innovations.

Grimson, *et al.* (2001) declares that the strategic process view of healthcare services that is enabled through system integration methodologies can only be achieved with complementary support of appropriate organisational structures. They are, however, vague on the actual operationalisation of such structures. This need to integrate in order to span organisational units is well established from the strategic and technical dimensions but more practicable and lucid solutions are needed (Hasselbring 2000).

Conrad and Shortell (1996) suggest that integrating physicians with the functional infrastructure is in itself a core capability of clinical integration and one way to achieve this is to organise them into groups that facilitate communication and learning. Weiner, *et al.* (2004) rationalises this by way of the increased level of interdependence and coordination precipitated by expanding clinical IS integration, one which inexorably increases the involvement of clinicians with IS concerns as well as their interactions with the staff and managers who provide the IS facilities and strategic leadership.

There is evidence to support the fact that this critical organisational inter-working can be enhanced through structurally based socially oriented interventions. Research by Caccia-Bava, *et al.* (2006) on the absorptive capacity of hospital organisations proposes that the combination of effective communication channels and strong cultural characteristics contribute to the adoption success of new systems. The contention here is that these benefits can be similarly realised by imitating the same structural features of successful hospitals by constructing overlapping shared knowledge structures and establishing boundary-spanning communications channels.

Weaknesses of this study, however, stem from the lack of a richer ethnographic approach towards qualifying culture, relying instead on a competing values framework, and therefore the classification of cultures is somewhat limited. Nonetheless, these types of ideas are not wholly new and find analogies with established theories of knowledge management and its related concept of communities of practice (COPs) (Ward and Peppard 2002).

Organisational culture, knowledge and learning

What further emerges from this line of investigation is the importance of the softer organisational aspects such as culture. As demonstrated by Weber and Pliskin (1996), cultural synergy can itself be regarded as a precursor to successful IS integration. Caccia-Bava, *et al.* (2006) posit that culture can somehow be managed or nurtured towards productive ends, specifically through structural archetypes.

Research of integrated delivery systems by Weiner, *et al.* (2004), however, suggests that the relationship between supportive, integration-friendly culture and management intervention may not be as direct as what Caccia-Bava, *et al.* (2006) propose. Their findings affirm instead that culture – specifically organisational learning culture – requires time to develop within very unique organisational contexts. The main difference between their views is that Caccia-Bava, *et al.* (2006) believe that culture adaptations can be more easily planned for, whereas Weiner, *et al.* (2004) contend that the process is more evolutionary as experience with integration increases.

Weiner, *et al.* (2004) use as their conceptual research framework the integration life cycle model which places the degrees of organisational learning culture alongside a maturity path, starting with the integration stages beginning with emergence, proceeding then to growth, to maturity, and onwards. Those familiar with systems maturity models (Nolan 1979) will immediately recognise the telltale S-shaped curve from such frameworks. Both sets of authors, however, are in agreement that prior learning is the key determinant of effectiveness, underpinning even supportive cultural types. Caccia-Bava, *et al.* (2006) define this as managerial IT knowledge, i.e. that which represents collective shared knowledge and experiences of the organisation.

Weiner, *et al.* (2004) typify this as an organisational emphasis of continuous improvement and shared values that promote thinking and the shaping and redesigning of processes that spans organisational boundaries. This puts a more practical and implementable solution to Grimson, *et al.*'s (2001) call for business process re-engineering that is sometimes perceived as just a buzzword. Ultimately, therefore, debates regarding the degrees to which culture can be planned or nurtured to evolve in beneficial directions may be less relevant compared to managing for its intended outcome, which is a capability for learning that strengthens and grows organisational knowledge to contribute positively towards IS integration success.

Organisational knowledge, learning and capabilities

Much has already been said of the approaches that can facilitate knowledge and learning on the road towards improved organisational and social integration of IS. From a more strategic, albeit organisational outlook, Khatri (2006) encapsulates what has been said of organisational knowledge and learning into the concept of IT capability.

The approach advocated here is that learning should be constructed as an embodied capability within healthcare organisations through enlightened and professionally competent leadership. The aim is to develop inimitable resource endowments premised on the resource-based view of the firm. Whereas the previous approaches have focused on enabling the organisation to move forward in integrating technology innovations into work practice, this prescription aims to create the internal capability that becomes the source of IS/IT innovations themselves.

SOCIO-TECHNICAL AND USER-ORIENTED CONSIDERATIONS

User-led or user-oriented factors have also been the focus in the formulation and recommendations of healthcare IS integration approaches. These strategies take the perspective that integration methods must account for how medical work practices are conducted at the micro level and involve the participation of users during implementation if they are to be successful. Notably, advocates of socio-technically oriented approaches often express exasperation towards the technical and systems view of integration (Ellingsen and Monteiro 2006; Winthereik and Vikkelso 2005).

Ellingsen and Monteiro (2006) are of the opinion that technical standardisation approaches often assume that seamless integration and its automation of horizontal processes can be assured through the dependability of the IS infrastructure for sharing pertinent medical information across intra and inter-organisational boundaries. This, they claim, is a problem borne from the ensconced heterogeneity of healthcare IS that technical and systems integration approaches attempt to bridge through standardisation of technologies and of practice. These types of issues expose some very major divisions and tensions between the idea that IS integration can be conceived and realised from a systems view on one hand, and the idea that IS integration must also be a socially negotiated process on the other.

Winthereik and Vikkelso (2005) attribute this state of affairs partially to the assumption that better inter-organisational communication of information, and hence coordination and collaboration, can be resolved. To an extent it can, if the information exchanged between medical practitioners in support of a patient's care can be satisfied solely by explicitly encoded information.

Their point, however, gains increasing credence if we consider it against the variant and complex nature of healthcare work. In part, integration of IS has to account for the properties of sense making, interpretation and translation of information as much as it has to do with its transmittance. This is apparent in the electronic discharge letter example. The technical implementation of the system by which the hospital informs a patient's personal physician of the outcome of treatment in the hospital actually provides very little by way of affordances that effectively narrate the course of care. This is illustrative of a deeper schism between the social and technical fit of systems that impedes efforts towards tight integration of technology and people.

Socio-technically oriented approaches are therefore predominantly concerned with the involvement of systems users for shaping the development, implementation and use of these systems to fulfil specific work needs. Subjects such as user involvement and satisfaction as well as the factors related to technology acceptance and diffusion of innovations have been acknowledged as important strands of IS research (Banker and Kauffman 2004; Finnegan and Willcocks 2007; Finnegan and Currie 2008). Such approaches may, however, have unintended outcomes that are less desirable.

Berg (2001) argues for deeper systematic approaches towards modelling idiosyncratic work practices and points to successes in deploying ethnographic means for understanding the detailed social processes and working practices of healthcare organisations. Berg (2001) gives an example of a customised systems development initiative and one might argue that similar approaches in relation to COTS-type integration will be quite different as the technology is more constrained to modification and adaptation. Clearly even user-led approaches are not infallible. The trend towards healthcare IS integration further covers distributed sites and institutions. Ellingsen and Monteiro (2006), for example, question the viability of having the type of user-led evolution, as envisioned by Berg (2001). In the light of this movement, they cite that standardisation across multiple settings is inevitable even for a rudimentary level of systems integration to be achieved.

While socio-technical user-led approaches have their importance in the scheme of organisational integration, they cannot be expected to present a complete panacea to the extant problems of IS integration. Furthermore, they require the same management and care in deployment in managing organisational change in the face of integration practices.

CONCLUSION

In conclusion, many of the approaches mentioned in this chapter have not been too dissimilar to generic IS integration strategies. Many of the strategic IS integration models have found their counterparts within the healthcare IS paradigm. For example, performance improvement towards the efficiency and effectiveness of organisational and inter-organisational processes see the BPR analogy mapped to the concepts of seamless and integrated clinical care. Total quality initiatives manifest themselves as the increasingly strategic focus on patient centricity and satisfaction. Competitive advantage and strategic fit similarly occupy the minds of healthcare organisations as they would other sectors.

As for technical and systems integration, healthcare has been considerably constrained by its own institutional characteristics and historical development. While enterprise type systems will continue to be important, there is no denying that the heritage of legacy systems continues to determine major technical integration approaches that are often hindered by a multitude of confusing, competing and non-interoperable standards, protocols and architectures. Even as healthcare institutions strive towards integration, technically they will still require approaches that help maintain autonomy while simultaneously attempting to bridge the various data and application silos entrenched within many organisations.

This has not been helped either by belated investments in clinical systems that are now crucial for shifts demanded by changing market demands, as seen in the United States for example, or regulatory and policy decisions in public health systems, as seen in the UK NHS and some other western European nations. Strategically and technically healthcare has not been very apparent in innovating its own models. Rather it has co-opted and adapted prior generic experiences.

There have, therefore, been accusations by some against the preoccupation with technical integration matters, but this is often unavoidable given the context of complexity and high degrees of variance within the medical field. But it has also been clear that organisational and social measures must be undertaken to successfully integrate the technology with medical practices. Structural reforms, cultural management and user-oriented approaches as well as emphases on learning, knowledge and capabilities comprise several proposed means to assist integration with healthcare organisations. However, evidence of operationalising and realising the benefits from these approaches is mixed.

This chapter has focused on what is known about the possible strategies for achieving healthcare IS integration, while providing useful insights on how these elements can be arranged and organised for definitional clarity and analytical value. It is not, however, entirely clear how to answer the more profound question of how best to evaluate the optimal combination of strategies from this array of approaches for it is apparent that they must synergise and operate in tandem. A multi-strategy approach with several socio-technical contextual elements discussed in this chapter can potentially provide a guideline for the design and implementation of a holistic IS integration in healthcare. The interconnectedness, order and weighting of these strategies can vary depending on the local integration landscape. It is anticipated that further structured analysis of the literature may yield typologies that can be deployed usefully to examine the specific implementation of complex healthcare IS such as electronic healthcare records. It could be useful to conduct empirical investigations using a multi-layered/multi-strategy approach in a multiple case study scenario to draw further conclusions and clarity in the subject area of integration in healthcare.

REFERENCES

Ahgren B, Axelsson R. Determinants of integrated healthcare development: chains of care in Sweden. *Int J Health Plann Manage.* 2007: 22(2): 145–57.

Anyanwu K, Sheth A, Cardoso J, *et al.* Healthcare enterprise process development and integration. *J Res Prac IT.* 2003; 35(2): 83–98.

Aveyard H. *Doing a Literature Review in Health and Social Care.* Maidenhead: Open University Press; 2007.

Avison D, Young T. Time to rethink healthcare and ICT? *Commun ACM.* 2007; 50(6): 69–74.

Banker RD, Kauffman RJ. The evolution of research on information systems: a fiftieth-year survey of the literature in management science. *Manage Sci.* 2004; 50(3): 281–98.

Bates DW. The quality case of information technology in healthcare. *BMC Med Inform Decis Mak.* 2002; 2(7): 1–9.

Beretta S. Unleashing the integration potential of ERP systems: the role of process-based performance measurement systems. *Bus Proc Manage J.* 2002; 8(3): 254–77.

Berg M. Implementing information systems in healthcare organisations: myths and challenges. *Int J Med Inform.* 2001; 64(2–3): 143–56.

Bernstein ML, McCreless T, Cote MJ. Five constants of information technology adoption in healthcare. *Hospital Top.* 2007; 85(1): 17–25.

Bloomfield BP. The role of information systems in the UK National Health Service: action at a distance and the fetish of calculation. *Soc Stud Sci.* 1991; 21(4): 701–34.

Boulton M, Fitzpatrick R, Swinburn C. Qualitative research in healthcare: II. A structured review and evaluation of studies. *J Eval Clin Pract.* 1996; 2(2): 171–9.

Braganza A. Enterprise integration: creating competitive capabilities. *Integrated Manuf Syst.* 2002; 13(8): 562–72.

Brazhnik O, Jones JF. Anatomy of data integration. *J Biomed Inform.* 2007; 40(3): 252–69.

Brown PJB, Warmington V. Data quality probes: exploiting and improving the quality of electronic patient record data and patient care. *Int J Med Inform.* 2002; 68(3): 91–8.

Burns LR, Pauly MV. Integrated delivery networks: a detour on the road to integrated healthcare? *Health Aff.* 2002; 21(4): 128–43.

Caccia-Bava MDC, Guimaraes T, Harrington SJ. Hospital organization culture, capacity to innovate and success in technology adoption. *J Health Organ Manag.* 2006; 20(3): 194–217.

Carnicero J, Blanco O, Mateos M. The application of information and communication technologies to clinical activity: electronic health and clinical records. *Pharm Policy Law.* 2005, 2006; 8: 69–82.

Ciccarese P, Caffi E, Quaglini S, *et al.* Architectures and tools for innovative health information systems: the Guide Project. *Int J Med Inform.* 2005; 74(7–8): 553–62.

Connell NAD, Young TP. Evaluating healthcare information systems through an 'enterprise' perspective. *Inf Manage.* 2007; 44(4): 433–40.

Conrad DA, Shortell SM. Integrated health systems: promise and performance. *Front Health Serv Manage.* 1996; 13(1): 3–40.

Cross M. In sickness or in health? *IEE Review.* 2004; 50(10): 38–41.

Currie G, Brown AD. Implementation of an IT System in a hospital trust. *Public Money Manage.* 1997; 17(4): 69–76.

Currie WL, Guah MW. IT-enabled healthcare delivery: the UK National Health Service. *Inf Syst Manage*. 2006; 23(2): 7–22.

Currie WL, Guah MW. Conflicting institutional logics: a national programme for IT in the organisational field of healthcare. *J Inf Technol*. 2007; 22(3): 235–47.

Davidson E, Chiasson M. Contextual influences on technology use mediation: a comparative analysis of electronic medical record systems. *Eur J Inf Syst*. 2005; 14(2): 6–18.

Davidson E, Heslinga D. Bridging the IT adoption gap for small physician practices: an action research study on electronic health records. *Inf Syst Manage*. 2007; 24(1): 15–28.

Department of Health. *Delivering the NHS Plan*. CM 5503. London: HMSO; 2002.

Devaraj S, Kohli R. Information technology payoff in the health-care industry: a longitudinal study. *J Manage Inf Syst*. 2000; 16(4): 41–67.

Dixon BE. A roadmap for the adoption of e-Health. *e-Service J*. 2007; 5(3): 3–13.

Ellingsen G, Monteiro E. Seamless integration: standardisation across multiple local settings. *Comp Support Coop Work*. 2006; 15(5–6): 443–66.

Evgeniou T. Information integration and information strategies for adaptive enterprises. *Eur Manage J*. 2002; 20(5): 486–94.

Fiedler KD, Grover V, Teng JTC. An empirically derived taxonomy of information technology structure and its relationship to organizational structure. *J Manage Inf Syst*. 1996; 13(1): 9–34.

Finnegan DJ, Currie WL. A centrist approach to introducing ICT in healthcare: policies, practices and pitfalls. *J Cases Inf Technol*, Special Issue on Health Reform Initiatives from around the World; 2008.

Finnegan D, Willcocks L. *Implementing CRM: from technology to knowledge*. Chichester: Wiley; 2007.

Grimson J. Delivering the electronic healthcare record for the 21st century. *Int J Med Inform*. 2001; 64(2): 111–27.

Grimson J, Grimson W, Hasselbring W. The systems integration challenge in healthcare. *Commun ACM*. 2000; 43(6): 49–55.

Gulledge T. What is integration? *Ind Manage Data Syst*. 2006; 106(1): 5–20.

Hart C. *Doing Your Masters Dissertation*. London: Sage Publications; 2005.

Hartswood M, Procter R, Rouncefield M, *et al*. Making a case in medical work: implications for the electronic medical record. *Comp Support Coop Work*. 2003; 12(3): 241–66.

Hasselbring W. Information system integration. *Commun ACM*. 2000; 43(6): 33–8.

Haux R. Health information systems: past, present, future. *Int J Med Inform*. 2006; 75(3–4): 268–81.

Hayrinen K, Saranto K, Nykanen P. Definition, structure, content, use and impacts of electronic health records: a review of the research literature. *Int J Med Inform*. 2008; 77(5): 291–304.

Hendy J, Reeves BC, Fulop N, *et al*. Challenges to implementing the national programme for information technology (NPfIT): a qualitative study. *BMJ*. 2005; 331: 331–6.

Hennington AH, Janz BD. Information systems and healthcare XVI: physician adoption of electronic medical records: applying the UTAUT model in a healthcare context. *Commun AIS*. 2007; 19: 60–80.

Hersh WR. Medical informatics: improving healthcare through information. *JAMA*. 2002; 288(16): 1955–8.

Herzlinger RE. Why innovation in healthcare is so hard. *Har Bus Rev.* 2006; 84(5): 58–66.

Hillestad R, Bigelow J, Bower A, *et al.* Can electronic medical record systems transform healthcare? Potential health benefits, savings and costs. *Health Aff.* 2005; 24(5): 1103–17.

Hsu MH, Chiu CM. Predicting electronic service continuance with a decomposed theory of planned behaviour. *Behav Inf Technol.* 2004; 23(5): 359–73.

Hughes JT, Bayes J. Managing IT: the introduction and adoption of new systems. *Public Money Manage.* 1991; 11(3): 31–6.

Jensen TB, Aanestad M. How healthcare professionals make sense of an electronic patient record adoption. *Inf Syst Manage.* 2007; 24(1): 29–42.

Johns PM. Integrating information systems and healthcare. *Logistics Inf Manage.* 1997; 10(4): 140–5.

Kaplan B. Addressing organisational issues into the evaluation of medical systems. *J Am Med Inform Assoc.* 1997; 4(2): 94–101.

Kaplan B, Duchon D. Combining qualitative and quantitative methods in information systems research: a case study. *MIS Quarterly.* 1988; 12(4): 571–86.

Kaplan B, Farzanfar R, Friedman RH. Personal relationships with an intelligent interactive telephone health behaviour advisor system: a multimethod study using surveys and ethnographic interviews. *Int J Med Inform.* 2003; 71(1): 33–41.

Khatri N. Building IT capability in health-care organisations. *Health Ser Manage Res.* 2006; 19(2): 73–9.

Khoumbati K, Themistocleous M. Evaluating integration approaches adopted by health-care organisations. *J Comput Inf Syst.* 2006; 47(2): 20–7.

Khoumbati K, Themistocleous M, Irani Z. Evaluating the adoption of enterprise application integration in health-care organisations. *J Manage Inf Syst.* 2006; 22(4): 69–108.

Kim KK, Michelman JE. An examination of factors for the strategic use of information systems in the healthcare industry. *MIS Quarterly.* 1990; 14(2): 201–15.

Kuziemsky CE, Jahnke JH. Information systems and healthcare V: a multi-modal approach to healthcare decision support systems. *Commun AIS.* 2005; 16(9): 407–20.

Landry BJL, Mahesh S, Hartman SJ. The impact of the pervasive information age on healthcare organisations. *J Health Hum Serv Adm.* 2004; 27(3–4): 444–64.

Lee AS, Baskerville RL. Generalising generalisability in information systems research. *Inf Syst Res.* 2003; 14(3): 221–43.

Lemmer B, Grellier R, Steven J. Systematic review of nonrandom and qualitative research literature: exploring and uncovering an evidence base for health visiting and decision making. *Qual Health Res.* 1999; 9(3): 315–28.

Lenz R, Beyer M, Kuhn KA. Semantic integration in healthcare networks. *Int J Med Inform.* 2007; 76(2–3): 201–7.

Levy Y, Ellis TJ. A systems approach to conduct an effective literature review in support of information systems research. *Informing Sci J.* 2006; 9: 181–212.

Lutchen M, Collins A. IT governance in a healthcare setting: reinventing the healthcare industry. *J Health Compl.* 2005; 7(6): 27–30.

McDonald CJ. The barriers to electronic medical record systems and how to overcome them. *J Am Med Inform Assoc.* 1997; 4(3): 213–21.

Makoul G, Curry RH, Tang PC. The use of electronic medical records: communication patterns in outpatient encounters. *J Am Med Inform Assoc.* 2001; 8(6): 610–15.

Mark AL. Modernising healthcare – is the NPfIT for purpose? *J Inf Technol*. 2007; 22(3): 248–56.

Mendoza LE, Perez M, Griman A. Critical success factors for managing systems integration. *Inf Syst Manage*. 2006; 23(2): 56–75.

Newell S, Swan JA, Galliers RD. A knowledge-focused perspective on the diffusion and adoption of complex information technologies: the BPR example. *Inf Syst J*. 2000; 10(3): 239–59.

NHS Executive. *Information for Health*. Wetherby: Department of Health Publications, A1103; 1998.

Nolan RL. Managing the crises in data processing. *Har Bus Rev*. 1979; 57(2): 115–26.

National Audit Office. *The National Programme for IT in the NHS: progress since 2006. Vol. 1*. London: HMSO; 2008. Available at: www.nao.org.uk/publications/nao_reports/07-08/0708484i.pdf

National Audit Office. *The National Programme for IT in the NHS: project progress reports. Vol. 2*. London: HMSO; 2008. Available at: www.nao.org.uk/publications/nao_reports/07-08/0708484ii.pdf

Peltu M, Clegg C. Using IT to deliver better NHS patient care: how the socio-technical approach can help NPfIT meet its goals (Paper in preparation). London: British Computer Society; 2008.

Raghupathi W. Information technology in healthcare: a review of key applications. In: Beaver K, editor, *Healthcare Information Systems*. Boca Raton, FL: Auerbach Publishers; 2002.

Raghupathi W, Tan J. Strategic IT applications in healthcare. *Commun ACM*. 2002; 45(12): 56–61.

Rahimi B, Vimarlund V. Methods to evaluate health information systems in healthcare settings: a literature review. *J Med Syst*. 2007; 31(5): 397–432.

Rigby M. Applying emergent ubiquitous technologies in health: the need to respond to new challenges of opportunity, expectation, and responsibility. *Int J Med Inform*. 2007; 76(Suppl.): S349–52.

Rigby M, Budgen D, Turner M, *et al*. A data-gathering broker as a future-orientated approach to supporting EPR users. *Int J Med Inform*. 2007; 76(2–3): 137–44.

Rigby MJ, Robins SC. Building healthcare delivery and management systems centred on information about the human aspects. *Comput Methods Programs Biomed*. 1997; 54(1–2): 93–9.

Rivers PA, Bae S. Aligning information systems for effective total quality management implementation in healthcare organizations. *Total Qual Manage*. 1999; 10(2): 281–9.

Robbins SP. *Organizational Behaviour*. Upper Saddle River, New Jersey: Pearson Custom Publishing; 2001.

Shang S, Seddon BP. Assessing and managing the benefits of enterprise systems: the business manager's perspective. *ISJ*. 2002; 12: 271–99.

Shortliffe EH. Strategic action in health information technology: why the obvious has taken so long. *Health Aff*. 2005; 24(5): 1222–31.

Southard PB, Hong S, Siau K. Information technology in the healthcare industry: a primer. *Proceedings of the 33rd Hawaii International Conference on System Sciences*. Maui, Hawaii, 4–7 January 2000.

Stead WW, Miller RA, Musen MA, *et al*. Integration and beyond: linking information from disparate sources into workflow. *J Am Med Inform Assoc*. 2000; 7(2): 135–45.

Stuewe S. Interface tools for healthcare information technology. In: Beaver K, editor, *Healthcare Information Systems*. Boca Raton, FL: Auerbach Publishers; 2002.

Tange HJ. The paper-based patient record: is it really so bad? *Comput Methods Programs Biomed*. 1995; 48(1–2): 127–31.

Thrasher EH, Byrd TA, Hall D. Information systems and healthcare XV: strategic fit in healthcare integrated delivery systems: an empirical investigation. *Commun AIS*. 2006; 18: 692–709.

Tsiknakis M, Katehakis DG, Orphanoudakis SC. An open, component-based information infrastructure for integrated health information networks. *Int J Med Inform*. 2002; 68(3): 3–26.

Wainwright D, Waring T. The information management and technology strategy of the UK National Health Service. *Int J Public Sector Manage*. 2000; 13(2–3): 241–59.

Wainwright D, Waring T. Three domains for implementing integrated information systems: redressing the balance between technology, strategic and organisational analysis. *Int J Inf Manage*. 2004; 24(4): 329–46.

Wainwright D, Waring TS. The application and adaptation of a diffusion of innovation framework for information systems research in NHS general medical practice. *J Inf Technol*. 2007; 22(1): 44–58.

Wallace M, Wray A. *Critical Reading and Writing for Postgraduates*. London: Sage Publications; 2006.

Walsham G. Learning about being critical. *Inf Syst*. 2005; 15(2): 111–17.

Wang BB, Wan TTH, Burke DE, *et al*. Factors influencing health information system adoption in American hospitals. *Healthcare Manage Rev*. 2005; 30(1): 44–51.

Ward J, Peppard J. *Strategic Planning for Information Systems*, 3rd ed. Chichester: John Wiley and Sons; 2002.

Waring T, Wainwright D. Interpreting integration with respect to information systems in organisations: image, theory and reality. *J Inf Technol*. 2000; 15(2): 131–48.

Weber Y, Pliskin N. The effects of information systems integration and organisational culture on a firm's effectiveness. *Inf Manage*. 1996; 30(2): 81–90.

Webster J, Watson R. Analyzing the past to prepare for the future: writing a literature review. *MIS Quarterly*. 2002; 26(2): xiii–xxiii.

Weiner BJ, Savitz LA, Bernard S, *et al*. How do integrated delivery systems adopt and implement clinical information systems? *Health Care Manage Rev*. 2004; 29(1): 51–66.

Winthereik BR, Vikkelso S. ICT and integrated care: some dilemmas of standardising inter-organisational communication. *Comp Support Coop Work*. 2005; 14(1): 43–67.

Wyse JE, Higgins CA. MIS integration: a framework for management. *J Syst Manage*. 1993; 44(2): 32–7.

Yusof MM, Kuljis J, Papazafeiropoulou A, *et al*. An evaluation framework for health information systems: human, organisation and technology-fit factors (HOT-fit). *Int J Med Inform*. 2008; 77(6): 386–98.

CHAPTER 3

Modernising healthcare: really connecting for health?

Annabelle Mark

INTRODUCTION

Understanding the dynamics of the role of IT in the modernisation of healthcare is enlightened by a focus on the development of the world's largest civil IT programme in the UK NHS. The National Programme for Information Management (NPfIT) developing within the NHS is part of what began in 1999 as a UK strategy to modernise government through innovation and the use of information technology (Cabinet Office 1999). This approach was reaffirmed in the *Transformational Government Enabled by Technology* (IT Strategy Project Team 2005) strategy document that sets this agenda around users, while hoping to increase efficiency. However, problems and delays to the programme, now set out in both government reports and research, suggest that the primary purpose of connecting patients to the healthcare system any time any place, to ensure they are seen safely, securely and successfully, may not be achievable or indeed acceptable. The roll-out of NPfIT and its associated problems are of interest to providers of healthcare in the UK and beyond, so understanding what is happening is of interest on a number of levels, as factual information about what happens, as an exploration of the relevance of theory, as a description of the impact of context, and as analysis and speculation about subsequent developments. Exploring these simultaneously may provide some answers.

GOVERNING AGENDAS

The political language of the UK government has changed since its election in 1997, moving from modernisation to transformation, reflecting perhaps an increasing urgency for achievement by the Labour administration in particular areas. However, ideas that rested on modernisation also reference a past era of modernism (Bauman

2006) that itself disconnected the past from the future and was concerned with, among other things, the fitness for purpose of whatever was being designed, be it buildings or technology. Key questions are: Whose purpose is government serving? Why does this now need transforming through a specific focus on users? Who are these users in both theory and practice? Further: What evidence in relation to NPfIT is there that this project is achievable or desirable in the form it is now taking? Answers to these questions from both research and political rhetoric appear confused, perhaps because of a failure to think through the aims and objectives of modernisation and how it has been enacted in healthcare (Blackler 2006); however, such confusion is not confined to the UK as a recent international review of the electronic health record (EHR) shows (Häyrinen 2008).

In the UK a top-down approach dominated by political and IT industry perspectives was initially justified by the effectiveness of the IT procurement process, which itself has now fallen into some disrepute because of the withdrawal of some suppliers and the disingenuousness of others (The Committee of Public Accounts 2008) in failing to deliver products. The initial aggressive commercial management of the sector by the NHS, through Richard Granger, to secure a shared market between suppliers was contrasted with the weakness of the stakeholder engagement or both professionals and the public, reinforcing an impression that this was about a contest between public sector and private industry, rather than provision for patients.

The transformational government agenda behind the programme requires effective leadership for both projects and their associated change process (Jones and Williams 2006). This has been enacted through what is known as transformational leadership (Bass 1990; Alimo-Metcalfe and Alban-Metcalfe 2005) and is associated with four components, namely idealised influence, inspirational motivation, intellectual stimulation, and individualised consideration, all of which are important to a project such as NPfIT. However, it can lead to the manifestations of charismatic leadership in a destructive manner (Tourish and Pinnington 2002); such behaviour can damage both policy and implementation as well as those individuals involved, as the NPfIT project demonstrates.

Contextually, events in the UK, both politically and organisationally, have changed: politically with the change in leadership of the ruling party, and organisationally with the sudden and collective departure of many of the top team in the NHS in 2006, and at the start of 2008 with the departure of Richard Granger as head of NPfIT or Connecting for Health as it had become. These changes are also highlighted in the two reports on NPfIT from the National Audit Office in June 2006 and May 2008 (Comptroller and Auditor General 2008; Comptroller and Auditor General 2006). Even the credibility of these official value-for-money approaches was cast into doubt because of political delays in publication of the first one (Collins 2006); this also raised questions about whose interests were being served. This concern was evidenced by two open letters to the House of Commons Health Select Committee from a group of 23 UK academics published in *Computer Weekly* on 11 April and 10 October 2006. They suggested that concrete objective information was not available to external observers, confirming that this project may be subject to one of the five paradoxes of IT evaluation that 'the greater the spend on I.T. the worse I.T. evaluation became' (Seddon, Graeser and Willcocks 2001).

Evidence from the Public Accounts Committee hearing on 16 June 2008 (The Committee of Public Accounts 2008) indicates that this remains the case and there is no intention to commission a truly independent evaluation; independence in this sense means that final reports are not subject to any submission, screening or approval by funders before publication of outcomes. Instead, an internal evaluation mechanism was put in place and in April 2006 The NHS Connecting for Health Evaluation Programme (NHS CFHEP) was set up 'To commission, manage and bring to a successful conclusion, a programme of urgent research on behalf of National Programme for Implementing Information Technology (NPfIT) and its stakeholder communities, using its own funding' to provide expert insight on issues of implementation. Nevertheless, the need to establish credibility for their programme and to answer critics is confirmed in the titles of their published research so far, such as the UCL Report 'Summary Care Record Early Adopter Programme – an independent evaluation'(Greenhalgh, *et al.* 2008).

Other more longitudinal work undertaken through the NHS Service Delivery and Organisation programme (Hendy, *et al.* 2007) also claims to provide independent findings, but the scarcity of work not funded by or ultimately reported to the Department of Health, such as the work by Currie and Guah (Currie and Guah 2007), is so far rare, and so provides a degree of independent insight not found elsewhere. Questions that seem immediately pertinent to the snapshot of events described in this research are those articulated by Dawson (Dawson 1999) as 'what do we know?' and 'what can we learn?'. The research was based on a four-year study funded by the Engineering and Physical Sciences Research Council and reflects an ever-changing environment in which this necessarily historical perspective (Torfing and Sorensen 2002) using institutional theory may provide lessons for the future. Some of these lessons, in retrospect, may be that other theoretical perspectives are required because of the changing context and content of what is being studied. Furthermore, it is necessary to learn from previous experiences of implementation, and IT implementation in particular, in both public and private sector domains, but as Huxley suggested, 'That men do not learn very much from the lessons of history is the most important of all the lessons that history has to teach' (Huxley 1960).

CONTENT AND CONTEXT

Whatever has been discovered, or discovered again, by the research, we also now know that, since completion of the study, two significant indicators of key issues have led to policy developments; these are: a focus on the role and purpose of the electronic health record; and the clarity of costings both past, present and future. Following on from the publication of the National Audit Report (Comptroller and Auditor General 2006), the Department of Health in the UK set up a Summary Care Records Taskforce (Department of Health 2006) to aid introduction of the electronic patient record (EPR) by addressing patient and public concerns. This taskforce reported the need for a more sensitive and pragmatic approach to design and implementation. This is indicative of Currie and Guah's (2006) conclusion that the outcome of NPfIT as a project is not clear, primarily because it is a politically and socially contentious innovation which engenders a range of interpretations across different social, political, organisational and professional groups. As if to further confirm this, the taskforce chair Harry Cayton, Director for Patients and the Public, was subsequently appointed as chair to the National Information Governance Board to oversee the quality of information governance in the NHS, to offer advice on confidentiality and security of patient information, to monitor the implementation of the NHS Care Record Guarantee and to advise the Secretary of State. This confirmed the need to demonstrate a move away from the political, professional and commercial interests towards the user/patient agenda that is now at the declared heart of policy.

Furthermore, following the academic and industry concerns, the House of Commons Select Committee on Health undertook its own review (Health Committee House of Commons 2007) into NPfIT and expressed similar concerns over matters of principle: for example, it recommended 'We note that in France patients will own their national summary record. This approach gives patients more control over who can access their record and more opportunity to influence and take control of their own care. We therefore recommend that Connecting for Health consider a similar model for the SCR in England (Paragraph 123). This proposal is now accepted by government for further investigation' (Secretary of State for Health 2007). Concerns over matters of practice in the management and delivery of systems are also now addressed through the Chief Executive of the NHS review of Connecting for Health, including its management of NPfIT (Timmins 2006).

What the government and institutional responses demonstrate are the conflicting institutional logics described by the research (Currie and Guah 2007), and which are still present in the latest study of the Summary Care Record implementation (Greenhalgh, Stramer, Bratan, et al. 2008), which reiterates the lack of a shared understanding and agreement on which institutions and whose logic matters because, as Brennan (Brennan 2005) suggested, this is not simply a plan to computerise our medical records; it is a project to transform the way the NHS works. The focus, however, has been on a set of timetables and cost targets in relation to four distinct developments, of which only one is a product, that is the NHS Care Records, and three are processes critically dependent on the role of the various stakeholders in each process: the electronic appointment booking, electronic transmission of prescriptions and IT infrastructure and networks.

However, it is the location, form, content and ownership of the care record that has proved critical, not least because its role and purpose was ill considered by the institutions involved at the outset, that is government, its agents and the IT industry, and reflect international concerns over matters of security and confidentiality in similar developments elsewhere (Coiera 2007; Detmer and Stein 2006; Terry and Francis 2007). The clarity provided by the four-part UK descriptor of what is important has been seductive to both politicians and patients who have a vested interest in what is happening to this public investment, but who only recently realise how institutional agendas have intervened by subverting the original purpose to provide safer treatment at the point of need. Indeed, if institutional studies and the associated theory that underpins the Currie and Guah research still only provided an account of how institutions govern action (Lawrence and Suddaby 2006) through the role of rational formal structures alone, it would not be sufficient to the task of understanding the progress of the implementation of the NPfIT in the NHS. However, if it is indeed more than this, as Currie and Guah, using the work of the new institutionalists, suggest it is, then institutions are the product (intentional or otherwise) of purposive action (Jepperson 1991) as patterns of sequenced interaction supported by specific mechanisms of control. NPfIT is the latest example of this, representing both part of this purposive action and as a new mechanism of control in itself for a range of stakeholders. Institutions, in this view from Jepperson, are also the product of specific actions taken to reproduce, alter and destroy them. The NHS, when seen from this perspective, while enduring as a value within the UK social context, and a brand within its increasingly commercial context, is constantly reframing its policy purpose and thus simultaneously reproducing, altering and destroying institutions within itself not least because where such 'reproductive activity' increases, the question becomes one about the stability of the institution and its purpose as a whole. NPfIT as part of the Connecting for Health project, as it has now become, is also part of this dynamic as well as being prey to its consequences. One example of these consequences that demonstrates the contentiousness of such government-led initiatives is the process by which the technical capability of the NPfIT project was assessed.

As part of the first report of the National Audit Office investigation, QuinetiQ were commissioned to carry out a process capability study, reporting in 2005. QuinetiQ is a company formed from the greater part of the former government defence agency DERA when it was split up in June 2001. As a privatised company, QinetiQ is now one of the largest defence research organisations in the world and has been the subject of controversy resulting in National Audit Office criticism for the private profits made in the process of its transfer from public ownership (Report by the Comptroller and Auditor-General 2007). In undertaking the NHS review QuinetiQ, not surprisingly, used a model reserved for the government in the UK which was not subjected to the same external evaluation and academic rigour as other models in the public domain, although the report assures us they do meet the two published international standards set out in BS ISO/IEC 15288:2002 and BS ISO/IEC 15504–2:2003. Such reassurances are, however, questionable when literature that is informing their report is inappropriately out of date; for example, in relation to organisational behaviour they cite a 1991 edition of a standard text *Organisational Behaviour* – an introductory text by Hucksynski and Buchanan for which there is currently a 2006 sixth edition. It is important if confidence in the outcome, its process and its costs is to be maintained by both the public and staff (Comptroller and Auditor General 2006) that a more open and academically rigorous process of evaluation takes place. In the absence of this there seems to be a potentially negative correlation developing between the quality of IT evaluation and enhancement in IT performance. Unless this is addressed, it will demonstrate what Seddon, *et al.* suggest is the fourth paradox in IT evaluation (Seddon, Graeser and Willcocks 2001), that is that IT evaluation techniques seem rarely to improve.

DEVELOPING RELEVANT CONTEXTUAL INFORMATION

It is important that research in this area incorporates (Mark 2006a) the exploration of a number of issues pertinent to such developments in healthcare, notably:

➤ behaviour, that is, what people do as well as what they say they do
➤ the emergent (but not expected) outcomes
➤ the conflicting agendas between different interest groups, and
➤ the poverty in pragmatism that arises when research seeks to establish in the short term what does and does not work, notwithstanding the possible reversal of such outcomes when reviewed over time and/or space.

Comparative research across national boundaries is also only just beginning in relation to electronic patient records, for example through the IMaGE project (Hinds, *et al.* 2006) that arose from key issues highlighted in the UK eDiaMoND project to pool and distribute information on breast cancer treatment, screening and diagnosis. Such international initiatives will prove an important influence in the shaping and reshaping of national agendas in both information management and healthcare.

Further concerns around the development of medical records and the way data is transferred and interpreted have arisen because of a completely different set of activities driven by a new set of institutional logics, that is, the outsourcing abroad of the transcription of medical record notes by cash-strapped hospitals and GPs (Mulholland 2006). As Dave Prentis from the trade union UNISON points out, these providers are being targeted aggressively by companies who encourage the use of cheaper labour to undertake this task in places such as India and South Africa; this demonstrates the space/time separation that is a feature of the new modernity (Bauman 2006), providing another dimension to both safety and security issues. This outsourcing trend is not confined to the UK, as it is estimated that currently about 10% of US notes are written in this way, usually by trainee doctors rather than expertly trained medical secretarial staff. Proving responsibility and liability for transposed errors is difficult enough within the UK over time, and when things go wrong such international transfers only confirm further that the fragmentation is extending now over space. Patient information held within medical records is developing in many new ways, which may not improve them. However, the primary questions for consideration are, therefore, who owns the record and what interest do they have in its accuracy. Evidence from France, highlighted in the House of Commons Select Committee Report (Health Committee House of Commons 2007), would seem to suggest that ownership by individuals rather than governments will be the key to real security not just within the UK but also across nation states in Europe and beyond (Detmer and Stein 2006).

PROGRESSING PROBLEMS

The volume of activity involved in NPfIT is very large indeed; during the Currie and Guah research it was serving upwards of 50 million citizens with 325 million consultations in primary care, 13 million outpatient appointments and 5.6 million inpatients in one year. This activity is now being driven by the need to keep pace with the changes and developments required to provide safe and effective healthcare in the 21st century in which IT plays an integral part within the wider government agenda. It is also leading the way internationally in terms of the size and volume and attempted integration of the activity by virtue of the scope of the NHS (Anderson, *et al.* 2006; Detmer and Stein 2006).

However, what is described as the challenge of affordable healthcare, which Currie and Guah suggest this investment must support, is of itself a statement of only one set of institutional logics that have bedevilled the NHS since its inception, highlighting the complexity of the question, which can be summarised as affordable for whom – the public as patient or taxpayer? This issue is playing an increasingly important role in the current implementation, not least because of the changing financial climate for UK healthcare in general and NPfIT in particular. Affordability, however, is itself a loaded term suggesting that the unaffordable is unsustainable and may influence others across the world also struggling with this issue (Hendy, Fulop, Reeves, *et al.*). The language itself arises from a range of commercial and political interests that see themselves disadvantaged by the NHS, and continue, as Pollack (2005) showed, to reinterpret and often misrepresent its economic and social effectiveness. Indeed the NHS is historically no more daunting financially, in relative terms now, than at its formation (Wanless 2002; Webster 2002) yet what is affordable depends on whose institutional logics are at work, and whose interests are being served.

The need to understand the changing nature of demand (Mark, Pencheon and Elliott 2000) and its interpretation by patients, professionals and policy advisors alike, means the issue is further compounded by the different but related context of clinical activity that is an essential part of the process of NHS care. In contrast, within the clinical domain the development and institutionalisation of IT has followed a very different trajectory, particularly within the centres of clinical excellence such as the teaching hospitals, highlighting the conflicting institutional logics at work between and within healthcare organisations. Developments such as MRI scanning (Mayor 2003) are examples of the UK's world-class leading-edge utilisation of technology. Such developments, however, throw a negative comparative light on the failure to grow at the same speed as the information management systems and processes required for the patient as they traverse the organisations over time and now through space. However, the original NPfIT objective of providing access to individual records anywhere in the UK for patients and professionals is now also being confounded by:

➤ the independent status of foundation trusts who do not have to participate
➤ the widening credibility gap in the capacity to both deliver the system and ensure its security
➤ increasing fragmentation of provision across the public voluntary and private

sectors as part of the policy agenda for the separation of provision and delivery of healthcare

➤ increasing separation between the self-governance of the separate parts of the UK, as Scotland and Wales choose different, and in the case of Wales, perhaps more successful strategies in delivering records, e.g. in general practice and diabetic care .

These disparities have enabled both the maintenance of boundaries and hierarchies to the benefit of some and may have facilitated the construction of 'cultural dopes' (Hirsch and Lounsbury 1997) among others, such as patients and some professional groups.

GOVERNANCE AND FINANCE

The critical part played by governance systems at organisational levels in the institutional context of healthcare within recent years is demonstrated in the development of clinical and research governance strategies (Howarth and Kneafsey 2005; Nicholls, et al. 2000) within NHS organisations. Both have their own internal institutional logics and are part of the strategy, as Currie and Guah suggest, to exercise control over the professional groups. However, there is a failure to acknowledge the behavioural impact of such changes in policy as others have also found (Greenhalgh, Stramer, Bratan, et al. 2008; Hendy, Fulop, Reeves, et al. 2007). The consequent recursive nature of structure and the action of agents that results from this, as set out by Giddens' (1984) structuration theory, can provide further insight, as Scott (2005) suggests, showing through this interactive and recursive model a replacement for former more determinist approaches. Giddens' approach, according to Scott (2005), provides a more balanced conception of the relation between freedom and order. Structuration theory thus also provides further perspectives on the process of the interplay between parts in ways that institutional theory has yet to fully resolve. This change is achieved through what Giddens (1984) describes as the instantiation of the new context through the process of agents enacting and thus continually reinforcing or reproducing these new structures that both enable and constrain them and underpins much of their behaviour rather than declared policy of government.

The failure to reflect on the behavioural consequences in relation to NPfIT of this process is critical to understanding. Added to this are the subsequent changes to organisational structures and policy purpose, with a declared move towards a patient-centred approach (Department of Health 2004), which may still be at odds with motivating forces in practice; this has had detrimental effects on both the organisational structure and its agents. It is furthermore expressing the tension between distributed and centralised power that changes over the life cycle of governments, but is often justified with a post-hoc rationality (Weick 1995) that attempts to provide some coherence and rational purpose to actions. For example, the rapid reshaping and renaming of healthcare organisations as part of what Jepperson (Jepperson 1991) analyses as the institutional need to reproduce, alter and destroy themselves means that organisational life cycles are extraordinarily truncated, and often distinguished only by their instability (Mark 2006a). This was demonstrated by the scrapping of the NHS Modernisation Agency in 2005, following the Gershon review of public sector efficiency (Gershon 2004). The agency was initially given responsibility for helping local trusts deliver the change management agenda associated with the NPfIT, so the subsequent changes which attempt to localise this activity may prove problematic in relation to relevant expertise and commitment (Hendy, Fulop, Reeves, *et al.* 2007).

In 2003 the NHS Confederation had estimated that the costs of managing these changes introduced by IT will be least as much as delivering the IT itself, while the British Computer Society's Health Informatics Committee (December 2003) estimates the costs of critical business and other changes as being four to eight times the cost of procuring systems. While this responsibility for local organisational delivery has transferred in name to others, notably strategic health authorities, from 1 April 2007, as part of the NPfIT Local Ownership programme, much of the organisational knowledge and memory associated with it has been dispersed or lost. This is part of a wider problem for the NHS where a number of organisational indicators have demonstrated these dysfunctions (Mark 2006a), such as:

➤ a reduction in organisational citizenship behaviour in part because of the breaking of the psychological contract (Coyle-Shapiro, Kessler and Purcell 2004)
➤ an increase in what Caddy (2001) has described as 'Orphan Knowledge', that is knowledge forgotten, separated or isolated within the organisation because of the dislocation of both individuals and organisations
➤ a known increase in stress and symptoms of burnout in staff working within healthcare leading to dysfunction at all levels (Halbesleben 2008)
➤ the loss of what Goffman (1959) called the 'display rules' and Hochschild (1983) has more recently developed as the 'feeling rules' of the organisation, where shared understandings of behaviour enable the organisation to operate effectively.

Connecting for Health may have a virtual policy purpose for the future, to make such instabilities less problematic through a technology infrastructure that makes organisational boundaries open; however, where such boundaries cross between public and private sector providers from buildings to IT, to delivering services, things may become more rather than less complex because the primary motivational forces differ. An example of this is embedded within the research by Currie and Guah, who quote a Director of ICT thus:

> In the past, the hospital was owned by the state. Now that we are part of the private finance initiative (PFI), the buildings are privately owned. If someone wants a new socket in their wall, I can no longer go and fit one in. I have to ask the leaseholders of the building to do this, and the cost is five times as much.

This changes relationships within the organisation as everyone is either a provider or purchaser in this internal market.

This raises broader issues about the motivational forces at work and how they are changing behaviour. So, for example, on the 4 Ps model (Figure 3.1), while the effect of PFI hospitals is to move motivation from the public probity quarter into the private profit quarter, the reverse may be said of the effects on IT suppliers who have now had to justify their decisions to the Public Accounts Committee (The Committee of Public Accounts 2008), which may in part be why some suppliers have left the project and others are struggling.

Expenditure has also risen significantly. In an interview with the *Financial Times* in 2006 (Timmins 2006), the Minister responsible, Lord Warner, confirmed that declared costs only represented the national contracts for the systems' basic infrastructure and software applications, and when training staff, buying PCs and upgrading and assimilating existing systems over the decade-long programme are included, the figure was now £20 billion; however, such cost inflation is common across similar systems in other parts of the world (Charette 2006). This confirms the political simplification that has been at the heart of the costings and targets that is now being deconstructed as part of what Lawrence and Suddaby (Lawrence and Suddaby 2006) describe as the creation and dismantling of the mythology (around NPfIT) that skilled actors, such as politicians, can manipulate during processes of institutional stasis and change. However, institutional theory still lacks a detailed

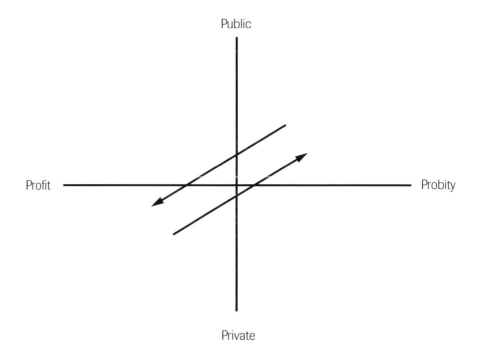

FIGURE 3.1 Motivation in the mixed economy: the 4 Ps Model

understanding of precisely how such mythologies are communicated to and appropriated by such actors and may provide the mask of safety for these inherently risky political adventures (Jones and Williams 2006).

Further evidence from this interview shows the Minister continuing to dismantle the mythology by stating that the extra money did not mean the programme would cost more than expected. Instead it reflected the full expense of switching existing IT spending from outdated systems to the new ones, through companies who have been vested (Roy 1981) with rights to supply what Currie and Guah suggest is 45% of the market share so far for the programme. The vesting of rights in this way is therefore shown, as Lawrence and Suddaby (2006) suggest, to be not only about the breaking up of state monopolies to create new actors and new field dynamics, but also enables blame to be distributed away from government as part of Jepperson's (Jepperson 1991) purposive action to create patterns of sequenced interaction supported by specific mechanisms of control. The most recent manifestation of this is in the development of the Local Implementation agenda following the Chief Executives Review, which may be a little too late to ensure that blame, too, can be distributed away from centralised policy to local and private sector institutions responsible for delivery of the technology. Both groups of actors have been required to appear before the public accounts committee in its pursuit of probity on behalf of the public purse, so now conflating the previously distinctive motivational forces that separate public and private sector institutions as described above in Figure 3.1.

ELECTRONIC PATIENT RECORDS

The introduction of electronic patient records was for a long time bedevilled by policy, professional and ethical issues that often failed to remain faithful to patient interests (Rector, Nolan and Kay 1991). This has been somewhat ameliorated by the separation into the summary care record (SCR) and the detailed care record (DCR). However, the fierce dispute within the medical profession over what should be included on the record, and how patients' data should be added (Watson and Halamka 2006) and transferred securely is far from resolved (Greenhalgh, Stramer, Bratan, *et al.* 2008). This dispute with those representing both patient and citizens' interests in the collection and storage of data will be monitored in health by the governance committee chaired by Harry Cayton, Director for Patients and the Public. However, the transformational government agenda that traverses government and private sector organisations will continue to demonstrate the conflicting institutional logics that can derail such programmes. Originally, it was proposed that the summary record would include major diagnoses, operations and recent tests, as well as current medications and allergies. It was also proposed that patient data would be added on an 'opt-out' model, implying that consent to have the basic data added would be assumed, but with patients retaining the right to opt out. This is now replaced by government acceptance of the Taskforce recommendations (Cayton 2006) that envisages that the process for creating summary care records – that initially contain a small but important amount of patient information: current medications and allergies and adverse reactions – will follow from a robust public information programme in the early adopter sites that will inform patients they have a defined and realistic period of time to review their proposed summary record by viewing it on HealthSpace or by asking to see a printed copy provided by their GP should they wish to. Patients would be invited to correct or amend their record and offer explicit consent for their record to be shared or to opt out of sharing, should they wish to.

After a realistic period, it would be assumed that those patients who have chosen not to view their summary care record are giving implied consent for it to be shared in appropriate settings.

The taskforce also noted that there may be people who do not want their summary care record to be shared or uploaded and how this might be achieved will be considered by an advisory group drawn from patient, clinical and managerial stakeholders to oversee the future development of the summary care record. The taskforce also noted that until it is possible to 'seal off' parts of the record it should only include non-sensitive information, and handling any sensitive information should be agreed with patients. The taskforce agreed that in time, as the system matured, the content of the record should become more complete. However, preliminary research on the SCR roll-out indicates that this is a more complex problem and it is too early to determine any form of measure for success despite a desire by many professionals and patients to support the concept (Greenhalgh, Stramer, Bratan, *et al.* 2008).

The British Medical Association's family doctors' committee rejected the earlier proposals from government, saying patients' consent should be sought, but indications that a compromise may be found (Cross 2008) will show whose institutional logics prevail. However, at the same time many hospital doctors favoured a much richer summary record, thus demonstrating the conflicting logics even within the medical profession. More interestingly, in October 2006 it was announced that NHS Direct, the national health helpline, had consolidated all its five million patient records into one single database and upgraded its call centres across the UK to create a 'virtual contact centre'. The move was designed to make sure that patient enquiries can be easily handled anywhere, regardless of their origin, in much the same way that the EPR will. So which institutions and whose logics are in control here, and what is the relationship between them from the patient's perspective?

The EPR is only one quarter of the activity set out in the national programme for IT (NPfIT) in 2002. The remaining three are about improving process rather than data capture, through investment in electronic booking, prescription transmission, and infrastructure and networks. This division is important in terms of external appearances as a modernised and transforming organisation (Cabinet Office 1999; IT Strategy Project Team 2005). In this sense problems may be more those associated with institutional entrepreneurship (DiMaggio 1988), particularly when considering the role and development of NHS Direct in parallel with NPfIT. Institutional entrepreneurship is important because it focuses attention on how new institutions arise and the manner in which interested actors work to influence their institutional contexts through such strategies as technical and market leadership, lobbying for regulatory change, discursive action, and shifting the focus of institutional research towards the effects of actors and agency (Lawrence and Suddaby 2006).

This compares with the narrower conceptualisations found in statements of institutional theory that have delineated key sets of concepts and relationships that, while relevant theoretically to the institutional structures and logics, organisational forms and conduct in the introduction and implementation of NPfIT, may oversimplify the world of practice. This shift is increasingly important in healthcare organisation in the UK and Europe where the rise of entrepreneurialism as a solution to health provision dilemmas has yet to be fully understood (Saltman, Busse and Mossialos 2002). Of particular concern in these developments is the impact of corruption and the potential lessons that must be learnt from deregulation of public utilities. The role of actors in the transformation of existing institutions and fields is important within institutional research where the ability of actors, particularly those with some key strategic resources or other forms of power, such as IS systems development or professional roles, will have significant impacts on the evolution of institutions and fields in healthcare (Greenwood, Suddaby and Hinings 2002). The most recent third way between the motivations found between the traditional conceptualisation of public probity and private profit is the notion of social entrepreneurship that seeks to combine the public good with innovation (Hartigan and Billimoria 2005), but has yet to demonstrate its role as a credible alternative to the motivation for private profit and public probity.

MORE INTERESTING TIMES?

The basic question that is posed by political economy, critical to an understanding of UK healthcare, remains: whose interests are being served and why? This is as much about the absence of power, because of destabilised environments and the loss of knowledge, as it is about who has power (Currie and Guah 2007). Power is not a stable resource as it moves between actants, be they politicians, the NHS, suppliers and the public, depending on such dynamics as electoral and contractual timetables and obligations as well as personal and organisational motivations. There is also the question of intentionality in terms of the political future of the NHS, tempered by the espoused institutional and policy level aversion to risk and centralising tendencies of the state. Connecting for Health and its forebears, while giving direction, is essentially centrist, but runs contrary to the decentralised nature of UK healthcare provision based, for example, on general practice and its operational independence which had led to the proliferation of disparate systems. Rationalising this into the five types of electronic patient record, which the NHS executive initially said needed to be built first, was a good start in recognising difference. It addressed the separate needs of the professions and organisations in healthcare, in mental health, acute hospital care, GP primary care, community services and primary care, but not necessarily the needs of the patients themselves. In this sense the UK experience is contrary to the current US experience that also informs both the research by Currie and Guah and IT and UK government policy.

In the US laws vary from state to state, so standardisation is not possible and the

US is, anyway, some way behind in the development of electronic health records (Detmer and Stein 2006). However, it may be of future interest in the UK because NPfIT is an English development, and the devolution of Scotland and Wales has meant they are increasingly divergent, ensuring that diversity will grow further than that between public and private sector provision alone, constructing a very different landscape of healthcare. This too is the reason why basing the research, as Currie and Guah did, on the work done in healthcare by Scott, *et al.* (2000) in San Francisco, while seeming to have less comparative relevance to the current UK environment, may have more significance to its future. The cultural and historical imperatives are, however, different, notwithstanding the insightful conclusions drawn from that work that have informed this UK study. Changes to US perspectives may be indicative of the more widespread international thrust towards patient ownership (Detmer and Stein 2006; Terry and Francis 2007) of their records, but a comparison of one state's legislation in relation to the UK shows they are already heading in the right direction. For example, in the state of California the health record is the physical property of the healthcare provider/facility, but patients have a right to:

➤ review and/or have a copy of that record – in the UK this is true with the exception of those parts that involve a third party or if the doctor feels it will cause the patient psychological harm
➤ ask to have the medical record corrected – in the UK the patient can ask to have their opinion as to accuracy inserted, but neither patient nor doctor can alter the notes
➤ not have medical information disclosed to others unless they direct the provider to do so or unless the law authorises or compels it – in the UK this applies, but only a judge or the force of law, for example under the notifiable diseases legislation, can make disclosure a requirement without the patient's permission.

Furthermore, the institutional logics which informed the original developments in the UK paid attention to those institutions constructed for policy purposes only. They did not look to organisations or networks for patients, nor did they look at those provided by, for and to professions. However, the latter groups in particular display a longevity far more important and significant to organisational change than the organisations in which they operate, and for that reason alone gain credibility because of their role and purpose as professional practitioners, which is why the UK project now has problems.

Indeed the stabilising aspects of the policy purpose of the NHS, together with the role of professional organisations, provide evidence of what Scott (2001) describes as the issue of institutional persistence, to which little attention has been paid and for which little evidence is agreed. Destabilising healthcare organisations by constantly changing them is a function of both political action and finding an access point to intervene in the far more significant institutions of professional practice. The purpose in healthcare is to simultaneously create, maintain and disrupt the institution, to redefine the allocation of material resources or the social and political capital needed to create new institutional structures and practices (Lawrence and Suddaby 2006); it is achieved through advocacy and defining and vesting in specific people and roles and constructing identities. Such identities are not only difficult to impose on well-established professional groups such as doctors, but may not be appropriate from a professional or patient perspective, especially if it is the alternative interests of technology alone which people believe are being served.

Many of the other activities are described by Lawrence and Suddaby as both cognitive and affective in their process and intent and represent a closer examination of institutional work. Indeed, unlike rule-based work that underpins so much in the information management field and which depends on some actor to enforce compliance, normative work relies on cultural and moral force which is embedded in communities of practice. It is this failure to recognise the differences that are implied both ontologically and epistemologically, in theory and practice, that may be at the heart of the current impasse in the UK (Mark 2006a).

INNOVATING PRACTICE

Innovation is, as the Minnesota longitudinal studies of technology found (Van de Ven, *et al.* 1999), neither sequential nor orderly, but is best characterised as a non-linear dynamic system. The system consists of a cycle of divergent and convergent activities that may be repeated over time and at different organisational levels. This divergent-convergent cycle is found to be the underlying dynamic that explains the development of corporate cultures for innovation, and while resource investments and organisational structure enable this innovation cycle, external institutional rules and internal focus provide the boundaries, but the critical lesson remains to 'go with the flow', because, as Hinings (Hinings 2006) says in relation to healthcare, the problems arise because of a mismatch between the design of the change and what is actually required to facilitate innovation through a terrain that is highly uncertain, loosely coupled and riddled with unanticipated consequences.

Pragmatism can also inform the scope and structure of developments, as EPR developments in the Lombardy region of Italy demonstrate, building as they do on this notion of institutional persistence, in the context of a national culture more attuned to fragmented localised groups and communities. In Lombardy an innovative integration project using the Ensemble platform and based in Vimercate Hospital near Milan was implemented in just three months. The project, led by Lombardy Informatica, is responsible for the Regional Service card programme with a wider remit than health that utilises existing IT resources. As the CIO Giovanni Delgrossi, a winner of the Intersystems DEVCON Ensemble Innovator Awards 2006, says:

> It avoids the 'rip and replace' solution by pulling and consolidating patient data from existing systems in all of its member hospitals and clinics. It also reads medical information from smart cards that have been issued to each citizen, and from a central data repository for the Lombardy region.

> (www.intersystems.com/devcon2006/innovator.html)

Member hospitals are able to continue using the applications they already have in place; for example, two are based on Oracle, one uses applications that were developed internally with Caché, and one uses Caché-based packaged applications from the InterSystems' partner Trak Health. The difference now is that all these varied applications 'talk'. By 2006, smart cards had been distributed to approximately 9 million citizens, 2500 pharmacies, and 145 000 healthcare organisations. In addition, because the Regional Service Card programme complies with decisions made in 2003 by the European Commission, there is the potential for extending the programme across all of Italy, and even to the pan-European level. The objective is to improve the quality of treatment while also improving the overall efficiency of healthcare delivery which, while distributed between agencies, is also owned by the patient through the service card.

The current lack of work on understanding what can be maintained from existing systems has become critical as the NPfIT timetable has faltered badly and patient safety is compromised because the UK has been mesmerised by the idea of a simple superstructure. However, as Huxley reminded us (Huxley 1960), the search for success is found as much within knowledge of failure as a review of alternative successes. What the Italian example provides is also a reminder that it should not be the technologists, professions and institutions who should be at the heart of the solution but the self-interest of the individual patient within their cultural context. The problem of the motivation and discourse in NPfIT is a centralist approach to an individualist issue. In this sense it is not radical enough, although the contextual change in policy (Department of Health 2004) that puts the patient at the heart of healthcare does provide an opportunity to look again at the issue. Furthermore, a reconsideration of the patient journey in UK healthcare (Mark 2006b) shows that responses to electronic patient records will involve the interplay between rational and emotional processes.

As the cognitive theorists suggest (Frijda 1988), patients act on the bases of physical responses and the use of past experience to understand the present and much depends on their individual attitude to risk, especially if Lupton is right in her assertion that risky behaviour increases in response to the intensification of control and predictability of modern life (Lupton 1999). Sorting these factors is complicated by both the patient and organisational perspectives and the utilisation of emotions that take place within the wider society for instrumental purposes (Mark, Pencheon and Elliott 2000). Furthermore, the legislative changes required to allow patients greater ownership of the medical record, in whatever format it might be converted into, must also enable the transfer of data by patients (or not) between different providers in the UK and eventually anywhere in the world. So, for example, given the extent of ownership of mobile phone technology in the UK (Wright 2006) currently running in excess of 80% and the emotional significance attached to that technology by individual owners (Vincent 2006), it provides an obvious portal through which to access such personal information as healthcare notes however and wherever they might be stored. Because of this, the research methods to understand what happens would also need to be reconsidered and the use of Actor Network Theory (ANT) (Blackler 1999), that is, a combined theory and method that looks at micro interactions of human and non-human actants, including technologies, would become more appropriate. The emphasis changes because what ANT illuminates is that not all actors behave in the same way or, if they do, for the same reasons.

CONCLUSION

In conclusion, institutional logics are changing because of changes to the role of public and private organisations in the provision of health services in the UK (McLaughlin, Osborne and Ferlie 2002). Many of these alternatives for healthcare provision are international in scope, so there is a convergence of policy ideas across national boundaries as indicated in the lessons being learnt about the role and purpose of electronic patient records, especially when these are in the interests of the individual patient. In the UK at present the institutions and professions of healthcare have both the expertise and the information about individual patients, thus the interests are weighted against the patient; this is being reinforced by the construction of NPfIT through what Dale (Dale 2001) describes as the objectified disembodiment rather than the embodied subjectivity (Dale 2001) of patient experience. The instantiation (Giddens 1984) of IT through NPfIT and whatever follows or develops from it must incorporate both of Dale's elements if it is to succeed as a valid, reliable and trusted tool of the patient, the NHS community and the international providers of healthcare.

REFERENCES

Alimo-Metcalfe B, Alban-Metcalfe J. Leadership: time for a new direction? *Leadership.* 2005; 1(1): 51–71.

Anderson GF, Frogner BK, Johns RA, *et al.* Health care spending and use of information technology in OECD countries . *Health Aff.* 2006; 25(3): 819–31.

Bass BM. From transactional to transformational leadership: learning to share the vision. *Organ Dyn.* 1990; 18(3): 19–32.

Bauman Z. *Liquid Modernity.* Cambridge: Polity Press; 2006.

Blackler F. Organising for incompatible priorities. In: Mark AL, Dopson S, editors, *Organisational Behaviour in Health Care: the research agenda.* Basingstoke: Macmillan; 1999. pp. 223–42.

Blackler F. Chief executives and the modernization of the English National Health Service. *Leadership.* 2006; 2(1): 5–30.

Brennan S. *The NHS IT Project: the biggest computer programme in the world . . . ever!* Oxford: Radcliffe Publishing; 2005.

Cabinet Office. *Modernising Government.* Cm4310, London: HMSO; 1999.

Caddy I. Orphan knowledge: the new challenge for knowledge management. *J Intellectual Capital.* 2001; 2(3): 236–45.

Cayton H. *Information Governance in the Department of Health and the NHS.* London: Department of Health; 2006.

Charette R. EHRs: electronic health record or exceptional hidden risks. *Commun ACM.* 2006; 49(6): 120.

Coiera EW. Lessons from the NHS National Programme for IT. *Med J Aust.* 2007; 186(1): 3–4.

Collins T. Report fuels calls for new NHS IT review. *Computer Weekly.* 20 June 2006: 1–4.

Comptroller and Auditor-General. *The National Programme for IT in the NHS.* HC 1173, London: HMSO; 2006.

Comptroller and Auditor-General. *The National Programme for IT in the NHS: progress since 2006.* HC 484, London: HMSO; 2008.

Coyle-Shapiro JA-M, Kessler I, Purcell J. Exploring organizationally directed citizenship behaviour: reciprocity or 'it's my job'? *J Manage Stud.* 2004; 41(1): 85–106.

Cross M. Health department and BMA may reach compromise on records system. *BMJ.* 2008; 336: 1398–9.

Currie W, Guah M. A national programme for IT in the organizational field of healthcare: an example of conflicting institutional logics. *J Inf Technol.* 2007; 22: 235–48.

Dale K. *Anatomising Embodiment and Organisation Theory.* Basingstoke: Palgrave; 2001.

Dawson S. Managing, organising and performing in health care: what do we know and how can we learn? In: Mark AL, Dopson S, editors. *Organisational Behaviour in Health Care: the research agenda.* London: Macmillan; 1999. pp. 7–24.

Department of Health. *Putting People at the Heart of Public Services: the NHS Improvement Plan. 80.* 2004.

Department of Health. *Minister Announces Taskforce for Electronic Records.* Department of Health 2006/0265. London: Department of Health Press Office; 2006.

Detmer D, Stein E. *Learning from Abroad: lessons and questions on personal health records for national policy.* Washington DC: AARP Public Policy Institute; 2006.

DiMaggio PJ. Interest and agency in institutional theory. In: Zucker LG, editor. *Institutional Patterns and Organizations: culture and environment.* Cambridge, MA: Ballinger; 1988. pp. 3–22.

Frijda NH. The laws of emotion. *Am Psychol.* 1988; 43(5): 349–58.

Gershon SP. *Releasing Resources to the Front Line: independent review of public sector efficiency.* London: HM Treasury; 2004.

Giddens A. *The Constitution of Society.* Stanford, CA: Stanford University Press; 1984.

Goffman E. *The Presentation of Self in Everyday Life.* New York: Overlook Press; 1959.

Greenhalgh T, Stramer K, Bratan T, *et al. Summary Care Record Early Adopter programme: an independent evaluation.* London: University College London; 2008.

Greenwood R, Suddaby R, Hinings CR. Theorizing change: the role of professional associations in the transformation of institutionalised fields. *Acad Manage J.* 2002; 45: 58–80.

Halbesleben JRB. *Handbook of Stress and Burnout in Health Care.* New York: Nova Science Publishers; 2008.

Hartigan P, Billimoria J. Social entrepreneurship: an overview. *Alliance.* 2005; 10(1): 18–21.

Häyrinen KSKNP. Definition, structure, content, use and impacts of electronic health records: a review of the research literature. *Int J Med Inform.* 2008; 77(5): 291–304.

Health Committee House of Commons. *The Electronic Patient Record.* Eighth report. London: House of Commons; 2007.

Hendy J, Fulop N, Reeves BC, *et al.* Implementing the NHS information technology programme: qualitative study of progress in acute trusts. *BMJ.* 2007; 334: 1360.

Hinds C, Jirotka M, Mustafizur R, *et al. Ownership of Intellectual Property Rights in Medical Data in Collaborative Computing Environments.* First International Conference on e-Social Science; 2006.

Hinings B. Concluding thoughts. In: Casebeer A, Harrison A, Mark AL, editors. *Innovations in Health Care: a reality check.* Basingstoke: Palgrave Macmillan; 2006. pp. 248–50.

Hirsch P, Lounsbury M. Ending the family quarrel: toward a reconciliation of 'old' and 'new' institutionalisms. *Am Behav Sci.* 1997; 40: 406–18.

Hochschild AR. *The Managed Heart: commercialisation of human feeling.* Berkeley: University of California Press; 1983.

Howarth ML, Kneafsey R. The impact of research governance in healthcare and higher education organizations. *J Adv Nurs.* 2005; 49(6): 675–83.

Huxley A. A case of voluntary ignorance. In: Huxley A. *Collected Essays 1959.* London: Chatto and Windus; 1960.

IT Strategy Project Team. *Transformational Government Enabled by Technology.* London: Cabinet Office, HMSO; 2005.

Jepperson RL. Institutions, institutional effects, and institutionalism. In: Powell WW, DiMaggio PJ, editors. *The New Institutionalism in Organizational Analysis.* Chicago, IL: University of Chicago Press; 1991. pp. 143–63.

Lawrence TS, Suddaby R. Institutions and institutional work. In: Clegg SR, *et al.,* editors. *Handbook of Organization Studies,* 2nd ed. London: Sage Publications; 2006.

Lupton D. *Risk.* New York: Routledge; 1999.

McLaughlin K, Osborne S, Ferlie E. *New Public Management: current trends and future prospects.* London: Routledge; 2002.

Mark A. Notes from a small island: researching organisational behaviour in healthcare from a UK perspective. *J Org Behav.* 2006a; 27: 1–17.

Mark A. Emotional affects: developing understanding of healthcare organisation. In: Zerbe W, Ashkanasy N, Hartel CEJ, editors. *Research on Emotion in Organizations, Volume 2: individual and organizational perspectives on emotion management and display.* Oxford: Elsevier; 2006b.

Mark A, Pencheon D, Elliott R. Demanding healthcare. *Int J Health Plann Manage.* 2000; 15(1): 237–53.

Mayor S. Nobel prize in medicine awarded to MRI pioneers. *BMJ.* 2003; 327: 827.

Mulholland H. Overseas transcription errors 'putting patients' lives at risk'. *Guardian.* 21 June 2006.

Nicholls S, Cullen R, O'Neill S, *et al.* Clinical governance: its origins and its foundations. *Br J Clin Gov.* 2000; 5(3): 1–9.

Pollack A. *NHS Plc: the privatisation of our healthcare.* London: Verso Books; 2005.

Rector AL, Nolan WA, Kay S. Foundations for an electronic medical record. *Methods Inf Med.* 1991; 30: 179–86.

Report by the Comptroller and Auditor General. *The privatisation of QinetiQ.* HC 52 2007–8, National Audit Office; 2007.

Roy WJ. The vesting of interests and the determinants of political power: size, network structure and mobilization of American industries, 1886–1905. *Am J Soc.* 1981; 86: 1287–310.

Saltman R, Busse R, Mossialos E. *Regulating Entrepreneurial Behaviour in European Health Care Systems (European Observatory on Health Care Systems).* Buckingham: Open University Press; 2002.

Scott WR. *Institutions and Organizations*, 2nd ed. Thousand Oaks, CA: Sage Publications; 2001.

Scott WR. Institutional theory: contributing to a theoretical research programme. In: Hitt MA, Smith KG, editors. *Great Minds in Management: the process of theory development.* Oxford: Oxford University Press; 2005.

Scott WR, Ruef M, Mendel P, *et al. Institutional Change and Healthcare Organizations.* Chicago, IL: University of Chicago Press; 2000.

Secretary of State for Health. *The Government Response to the Health Committee Report on the Electronic Patient Record.* CM7264. London: HMSO; 2007.

Seddon P, Graeser V, Willcocks L. *IT Evaluation Revisited: plus ça change . . .* Eighth European Conference on Information Technology, Oriel College, Oxford, UK; 17–18 September 2001.

Terry NP, Francis LP. Ensuring the privacy and confidentiality of electronic health records. *Uni Illinois Law Rev.* 2007; 2: 681–736.

The Committee of Public Accounts. Uncorrected transcript of oral evidence. Minutes of evidence taken before the Committee of Public Accounts, Monday 16 June 2008. *National Programme for IT in the NHS: progress since 2006.* HC 737–I. London: House of Commons; 2008.

Timmins N. Plans for NHS files are late by two years. *Financial Times.* 30 May 2006.

Torfing J, Sorensen E. Nordic studies of power and democracy: towards a constructivist analysis of governance from below. In: Torfing J, Sorensen E, editors. *European Economic and Political Issues.* New York: Nova Science Publishers; 2002. pp. 1–18.

Tourish D, Pinnington A. Transformational leadership, corporate cultism and the spirituality paradigm: an unholy trinity in the workplace? *Hum Relat.* 2002; 55(2): 147–83.

Van de Ven AH, Polley DE, Garud R, *et al. The Innovation Journey.* New York: Oxford University Press; 1999.

Vincent J. Emotional attachment and mobile phones. In: Bertschi S, editor. *Thumb Culture: the meaning of mobile phones for society.* Transcript Verlag, Transaction US; 2006.

Wanless D. Securing our future health: taking a long-term view. *The Wanless Review.* London: HM Treasury; 2002.

Watson N, Halamka J. For and against: patients should have opt out of national electronic care records. *BMJ.* 2006; 333: 39–42.

Webster C. *The NHS: a political history.* Oxford: Oxford University Press; 2002.

Weick K. *Sensemaking in Organisations.* Thousand Oaks, CA: Sage Publications; 1995.

Wright A. Mobile phones could soon rival the PC as world's dominant internet platform. *IPSOS.* 18 April 2006.

CHAPTER 4

Integrating healthcare with ICT

John Powell

WHAT IS E-HEALTH?

Consider the near future. Diana Johnson is a 48-year-old woman with diabetes. She recently experienced some palpitations and logged on to her myNHS website profile to find out what she should do. After reading some background information she filled in some tick box responses and was directed to an online chat session with a health advisor. Unfortunately, it seemed that her palpitations may be more serious than she thought and she needs to be examined by her consultant. She books this via a secure Internet site and is emailed some advice as to how she can look after herself in the meantime. She is also e-mailed a questionnaire about her cardiovascular health which she submits online. On the day of the appointment Diana completes the e-check in at home and is allocated her appointment time. At the automated reception her iris is read and her electronic medical records, test results and X-rays are retrieved. The hospital no longer has hard copies of any of these. An RFID (radiofrequency) tag is dispensed in the form of a plastic bracelet to be worn for the duration of the hospital visit. The movements around the hospital of all patients, equipment and drugs are tracked centrally. Diana remembered her appointment as she received an automated SMS text message reminder the day before.

While Diana awaits her outpatient appointment for her diabetes check-up she can read her electronic health records on the provided screens and can enter new data (for example, on her current pattern of diet and exercise). Tailored health advice is provided automatically to her as she does this and various algorithms can give her risk estimates for (for example) how likely it is she will suffer a heart attack depending on how she modifies her current behaviour. It is the first time the consultant has seen her face to face for three years as, in the interim, she has been a patient of his virtual diabetes clinic. She has attended the virtual clinic using a web-browser on her mobile telephone, and her glucose meter reader has regularly transferred her blood sugar readings to the hospital via a wireless network. At the appointment the consultant is concerned with her recent palpitations so he issues her with a 'Smart Vest' to take home. While she wears the vest it measures her ECG, pulse and blood pressure and transmits the readings to the hospital in real time via a wireless network. Fortunately, the results indicate that Diana's heart is, in fact, in pretty good shape. However, it does seem that she may be suffering from anxiety disorder with panic attacks. She is directed to an online screening tool which confirms the diagnosis and she immediately begins a course of computerised cognitive behavioural therapy on the Internet. She also joins a virtual support group for other people with diabetes who have anxiety disorder.

Such an integrated scenario is the vision of the proponents of e-health, for whom new information and communications technologies hold the key not simply to automating previously manual processes, but for revolutionising the way in which the entire healthcare system works, and shifting the balance of both power and responsibility from healthcare professionals to patients. There are many recorded definitions of e-health, from the succinct, 'use of the internet or other electronic media to disseminate health related information or services' (Gustafson and Wyatt 2004) to the aspirational:

> an emerging field in the intersection of medical informatics, public health and business, referring to health services and information delivered or enhanced through the Internet and related technologies. In a broader sense, the term characterises not only a technical development, but also a state of mind, a way of thinking, an attitude, and a commitment for networked, global thinking, to improve healthcare locally, regionally, and worldwide by using information and communication technology (Eysenbach 2001).

Such has been the uncertainty of the scope of e-health, the NHS Service Delivery & Organisation Programme-funded two-year-long research projects simply to map the field in advance of more focused calls for proposals. There are even two review articles published that have identified the range of e-health definitions used worldwide (Pagliari, *et al.* 2005).

Oh, *et al.* (2005) found that the common features among the 51 definitions that they identified were 'health' and 'technology'. In the Pagliari, *et al.* (2005) study, the authors conclude that e-health is more specifically about health and the 'internet and related technologies'. Thus the main area of debate is whether e-health is specifically concerned with the Internet (and related technologies), or if it encompasses a broader perspective of all information technologies. Certainly the term has only come into use in parallel with the Internet revolution and clearly has associations with Internet-specific terms such as e-business and e-marketing. The broader definition brings the term more into overlap with the field of health informatics, and it is interesting that several researchers in this field have now adopted the term e-health as perhaps having more currency in the early 21st century. Of course these minor distinctions about the degree to which all ICTs are included or not under the banner of e-health become less important as technologies converge. One definition that has merit due to its simplicity is that used by the World Health Organization, 'e-health is the use of information and communication technologies (ICT) for health' (*see* www. who.int/kms/initiatives/E-health/en/).

E-health then encompasses services such as health-related Internet information sites, automated online therapy, e-mail consultations, online pharmacies, telE-health, home monitoring systems and virtual clinics. It also includes information technology-based health system developments such as NHS Connecting for Health and similar initiatives in other countries, which will bring profound changes to the organisation and delivery of healthcare, including shared electronic records, computerised decision support systems, electronic prescribing and electronic booking of appointments.

The importance of information technology to the future of healthcare is now widely accepted. The Wanless reports on long-term trends and recommendations for the future of UK healthcare prepared for HM Treasury describe information technology as holding the key to the better coordination of care, and even bringing such benefits as allowing health professionals more time to spend with their patients (Wanless 2002, Wanless 2004). Medical schools now teach IT skills. E-health has found its way to the top of the health service research agenda with the new Office for Strategic Coordination of Health Research establishing e-health (for them, this constitutes realising the research benefit of the NHS IT system (*see* www.parliament. the-stationeryoffice.co.uk/pa/cm200607/cmselect/cmsctech/978/97804.htm).

The major players in the computer industry are taking a keen interest in e-health. Alongside this there appears to have been a shift in the commercial sector of healthcare information technology from being technology-centred to becoming patient-centred, and embracing the e-health agenda. This can be seen in how the marketing outputs have changed over time. At the 2006 MedNet conference in Toronto, a Microsoft video was played showing their vision of IT-enabled future healthcare – showcasing state-of-the-art hardware such as curved flatscreens and wireless tablet PCs. The presenter proudly declared how 'almost all of these technologies are available now'. In 2008 Microsoft produced a new vision for the future of healthcare (*see* www.microsoft. com/industry/healthcare/media/health07_hires.wvx), which continues to feature a range of technology 'solutions', but where the emphasis has clearly shifted onto the patient, supported by technology, taking control of their health and healthcare to maximise their well-being. A good example of this shift in control is the Microsoft product HealthVault which is a free online patient-controlled health record.

WHY IS E-HEALTH IMPORTANT?

In the 21st century the NHS in the UK, and healthcare providers in other developed countries, face some major challenges. Three key challenges are listed below. E-health is seen as providing answers to each of these key challenges:

1 providing for an ageing population with increasing prevalence of (expensive to treat) chronic illness
2 improving patient safety and reducing errors

3   educating patients to become informed consumers taking an active role in their healthcare.

The demographic transition to an ageing population living longer with chronic disease means not only that healthcare providers have to find the resources to care for these people, but also that there are fewer younger people to provide informal care or to fund the welfare state through taxation. Pharmaceutical companies are investing heavily in developing new drugs for the major chronic conditions such as cancer, heart disease and dementia, and they need to recoup their investment. Information and communication technologies (in various guises of e-health, tele-care, tele-health, etc.) are seen as an answer to these issues. The topic of telecare in particular has been one of technology being the answer to many of the problems healthcare currently faces. E-health solutions are posited as relatively cheap methods of delivering care and support, both remotely and with automation. This includes remote monitoring and remote consultation delivered by healthcare practitioners, as well as self-monitoring tools to support self-management. The goal is the main-tenance of independent living for those with chronic illness and a reduction in the use of secondary care.

E-health has the potential to improve healthcare services in many ways. It is seen as a key element in knowledge management initiatives (for example, lean healthcare) implemented to improve patient safety. Technology could reduce errors, improve patient experience and reduce costs. Much of the discussion about the ability of tech-nology to solve human problems has been positive, with little criticism of e-health, which carries risks as well as benefits. Again the discourse here has predominantly been a positive one of technology solutions for human problems, and it is rare to find rhetoric from publicly funded agencies critical of the e-health agenda. Yet little attention has been paid to the evidence that e-health interventions carry risks as well as benefits. Similarly, e-health applications sometimes fail to work in practice due to problems with implementation and professional resistance (Car, *et al.* 2008).

The third major theme in healthcare in developed countries at the start of the 21st century concerns consumerism and the empowerment of the patient. As discussed above, e-health in general and the Internet in particular are seen as vital in facilitat-ing this. The quantum change in accessibility of information brought about by the Internet revolution has coincided with the move to shift the balance of power from professionals to patients. Health information on the Internet now allows consumers to make informed choices about their health and to access the esoteric knowledge previously only available to health professionals. In a seminal paper in 1999 the sociologist Michael Hardey highlighted the challenge to professionals that this new access represents (Hardey 1999). Web 2.0 developments such as health-related virtual communities allow patients to contact each other, which can facilitate empowerment through universality (knowing one is not alone), installation of hope (knowing that others get better), and the empathy and understanding of others in the same situa-tion (Powell 2007). Health services are beginning to harness the benefits of informed, expert patients who can take control of their own healthcare, facilitated by giving patients access to their online health record. Such informed, empowered patients can then begin to self-manage their conditions at home, perhaps helped by remote monitoring and virtual consultations.

BARRIERS TO AN INTEGRATED E-HEALTH FUTURE

E-health may not be a technological panacea but, nonetheless, information and communications technologies do have the potential to bring profound changes to the ways in which healthcare is delivered and patients manage their own health. In this section we consider some barriers to overcome for e-health to realise the potential of a fully IT-enabled, integrated health service. The e-health applications that can deliver this vision will bring fundamental changes to working practices and organisational culture in the health service. The NHS Connecting for Health programme and similar initiatives in other countries are therefore as much about change management as about IT implementation. New e-health tools do not so much face technological barriers as socio-technical ones, which are concerned with the interaction between people and technologies. These barriers threaten both public and professional confidence in the widespread use of e-health applications. Next, we examine five barriers in more detail.

Some socio-technical barriers to e-health adoption include the following:

1   concerns over security and confidentiality
2   effects on working practices
3   access issues and the digital divide
4   issues of regulation, quality and trust
5   demonstration of effectiveness and efficiency.

SECURITY AND CONFIDENTIALITY

One barrier to the implementation of e-health solutions is the widespread concern about the security and confidentiality of electronic data. As an illustration of this concern, one of the major hurdles that the NHS Connecting for Health programme has had to overcome in England is professional resistance, led in particular by general practitioners, to the transfer of patient data to a national electronic record system. The key role of GPs in raising concerns is based both in their historical role as 'custodians of the record' giving them a sense of ownership of patient records, and also in the fact that UK primary care practices have been at the forefront of IT innovation, often in contrast with the NHS as a whole, and many GPs have developed particular interests in healthcare information technology.

Some have expressed their fears that a national database of records would be vulnerable to malicious use by hackers or rogue healthcare workers, and that the risk of a system failure potentially affecting the whole NHS records system was too great. Supporters of this argument point to multiple failures in large scale public sector IT programmes, and to various high profile security lapses concerning public data. Much of this debate has crystallised on the issue of 'opt in' or 'opt out' consent for patients to allow their records to become part of a national electronic record, with those in favour of the 'opt in' model arguing that the public needs to be fully informed before agreeing to the potential risks of such a system, rather than have their records uploaded by default. Those on the other side of the argument point to the lack of security in current paper-based systems, where confidentiality is protected more by the difficulty in finding particular sets of notes, rather than by a proper information governance structure with appropriate access controls. Nevertheless, concerns about the security and confidentiality of electronic data have been a significant factor hindering the adoption of e-health tools.

EFFECTS ON WORKING PRACTICES

Car, *et al.* (2008) undertook a major systematic review of the impact of e-health on the quality and safety of healthcare. They examined 67 systematic reviews and 284 randomised controlled and controlled clinical trials. While they found clear evidence that some e-health systems can improve the quality of care and reduce errors, other initiatives can in themselves lead to errors. For example, a study in the *Journal of the American Medical Association* found that computerised physician order entry (CPOE) systems could cause patient medication errors (Koppel, *et al.* 2005). The authors concluded that such systems needed to improve their design to incorporate how they would actually be used in practice, not in an idealised setting.

One UK example can illustrate how human factors can derail the best intentioned and robust technological solutions. In response to concerns of security and potential confidentiality breaches, the NHS Connecting for Health programme has designed a secure sign-in process requiring both a smart card to be physically placed in a card reader, and the entry of a password. Once access is gained, an individual health worker will only be able to view records with which they have a 'legitimate relationship', as determined by their job role and location. The system also keeps an audit trail of who accesses what, to allow retrospective identification of inappropriate access. Yet such a secure sign-in system has subsequently been accused by frontline workers of leading to delays in the delivery of healthcare. As a consequence there are many reports of healthcare workers bypassing the secure sign-in process, and undermining the audit safeguards, by leaving terminals signed in throughout a working day, allowing any member of staff to use them. In this case a process designed to maximise security has perversely led to a failure of access controls due to the human dimension and the impact that the e-health system had on working practices.

ACCESS AND THE DIGITAL DIVIDE

Even in 'Broadband Britain' there is a significant digital divide in Internet access between the 'have-nets' and the 'have-nots'. Access is not simply about having a computer with the right software and connection – it's also about having the ability to use the Internet in a productive way. This includes both computer literacy (ability to use the PC) and also e-health literacy (ability to access, interpret and use the health information found online). The most prominent digital divide is by age group. Despite media hype about 'silver surfers', the prevalence of Internet use decreases with age. There are also divides by educational level, income group and literacy, with better educated, higher earning individuals with higher levels of literacy more likely to use the Internet for all reasons including their healthcare (obviously these variables are interrelated). If the Internet is to be the mechanism for empowering individuals to take control of their own health, and for delivering new services such as accessing test results and treatments such as online therapy, then healthcare providers need to be aware of which groups will be excluded and whether these are the same groups who suffer exclusion from traditional health services. The most widespread information technology platform with good penetration in hard-to-reach groups is the mobile telephone, and increasingly health services are using mobile telephone technology, such as SMS messaging alerts, as appointment reminders or to support behavioural interventions such as smoking cessation.

The digital divide is not only about Internet access. Within healthcare settings some professional groups (such as doctors) have better technology access to IT facilities than others, and there are also differences between settings. In general primary care practitioners have good access, whereas some non-acute secondary care settings, such as mental health trusts, have poor access to computer systems. These differences reflect historical differences in IT investment as well as cultural differences in working practices.

REGULATION, QUALITY AND TRUST

One specific area of e-health that has caused concern to health professionals in particular is the unregulated nature of the healthcare Internet. The biomedical literature has been dominated by worries about the threat of poor quality information on the Internet leading to harm for patients. Numerous studies have been devoted to this topic. With colleagues I undertook a review of these in 2002 when we identified 79 studies (Eysenbach, *et al.* 2002). I am now aware of at least a further 100 studies which would fit our inclusion criteria. Much of this research has been of low rigour and frankly tells us little other than 'the quality of information on the web is variable'. Information quality has always varied, and poor quality health information has always been accessed – whether in out-of-date textbooks or in conversation with peers. The difference the Internet makes is twofold – a quantum increase in accessibility, and the possibility for sources to appear more authoritative than they are. Despite a moral panic about the risks of online information, there is a notable absence of any consistent evidence showing patients coming to harm from health-related Internet use. Research suggests that, although in practice patients do not pay as much attention to the authority of the source as they say they would do (Eysenbach and Köhler 2002), they do trust sources that they would trust in 'the real world', such as official health service websites and charity sites. Furthermore, studies of lay health behaviour suggest that patients are generally sensible in finding information from a variety of sources and doing their own triangulation.

A further issue concerning regulation is the lack of a regulatory system for e-health applications (such as computerised decision support systems) in contrast to the systems in place to regulate pharmaceutical products and medical devices. On the one hand this can facilitate adoption at a local level by removing some of the regulatory hurdles that these other interventions have to overcome; on the other hand it means that e-health applications can come into practice without rigorous evaluation of harms and benefits, and this links to the final socio-technical barrier.

DEMONSTRATION OF EFFECTIVENESS AND EFFICIENCY

A key challenge for the proponents of e-health interventions is to demonstrate their effectiveness and efficiency compared with the status quo. For interventions this requires evidence from randomised controlled trials, and for system-wide changes there is a need to use both qualitative and quantitative health services research methods to demonstrate the value of e-health. The evidence-based healthcare movement of the 1990s and beyond has created a legacy whereby new developments in healthcare will be greeted with scepticism until they have shown benefits in terms of the quality of patient care and/or in health service costs. The systematic review by Car, *et al.* (2008: 18) again demonstrates that some of the major e-health applications have limited evidence behind them. They say:

> The empirically demonstrated benefits relating to introduction of EHRs are currently limited to improved legibility, time savings for some professionals (nurses), and the facilitation of higher order functions such as audit, secondary analysis of routine data and performance management. Time taken for doctors to enter and retrieve data has in contrast been found to increase; studies have furthermore found that the time disadvantage for clinicians to record and retrieve information did not attenuate with increased familiarity and experience with using EHRs.

A robust evidence base for the benefits of e-health applications is central to achieving widespread adoption.

CONCLUSION

If e-health overcomes the barriers described above, the landscape of healthcare provision could radically change. This chapter began with a case history vignette of a future health scenario. This vignette was described as representing the near future, and much of what was described is being implemented in the more advanced health settings. Many health systems in industrialised countries are implementing information technology programmes that will see the digitalisation of the majority of routine tasks, from patient administration systems to electronic booking of appointments, electronic prescribing, electronic health records, systems for archiving and retrieving images and pathology test results. Practitioners are being helped with decision support systems. Providers are beginning to deliver services online to patients in their own homes. Such services include online consultations and Internet therapy. Internet-enabled devices are being developed to allow remote monitoring of both physiological and social functioning. Personalised, wearable healthcare is arriving with the development of smart clothing with embedded sensors. Mobile health (Mhealth) is using platforms such as mobile telephones and PDAs to deliver tailored health information and advice to patients, and to receive direct feedback. Ultimately, pervasive technology may achieve the goal of creating expert cyberpatients, fully informed about their health, remotely monitored by a health provider, who only becomes aware of them when an intelligent system detects a need. First, though, healthcare providers need to fully understand the true harms and benefits of e-health applications and engage with healthcare workers to understand the impact of new technologies on working practices and patient care, to ensure that the potential of e-health is fully realised.

REFERENCES

Car J, Black A, Anandan C, *et al. The Impact of E-health on the Quality and Safety of Healthcare. A Systemic Overview and Synthesis of the Literature. Report for the NHS Connecting for Health Evaluation Programme.* March 2008.

Cooksey D. *A Review of UK Health Research Funding.* London: HM Treasury; 2006.

Crocco AG, Villasis-Keever M, Jadad AR. Analysis of cases of harm associated with use of health information on the internet. *JAMA.* 2002; 287: 2869–71.

Eysenbach G. What is e-health? *J Med Internet Res.* 2001; 3(2): e20. Available at: www.jmir.org/2001/2/e20/

Eysenbach G, Köhler C. How do consumers search for and appraise health information on the World-Wide-Web? Qualitative study using focus groups, usability tests and in-depth interviews. *BMJ.* 2002; 324: 573–7.

Eysenbach G, Powell J, Kuss O, *et al.*. Empirical studies assessing the quality of health information for consumers on the World Wide Web: a systematic review. *JAMA.* 2002; 287: 2691–700.

Gustafson DH, Wyatt JC. Evaluation of E-health systems and services. *BMJ.* 2004; 328: 1150.

Hardey M. Doctor in the house: the internet as a source of lay health knowledge and the challenge to expertise. *Soc Health Illness.* 1999; 21: 820–35.

Koppel R, Metlay JP, Cohen A, *et al.* Role of computerized physician order entry systems in facilitating medication errors. *JAMA.* 2005; 293: 1197–203.

Leong KC, Chen WS, Leong KW, *et al.* The use of text messaging to improve attendance in primary care: a randomized controlled trial. *Fam Pract.* 2006; 23: 699–705.

Oh H, Rizo C, Enkin M, *et al.* What is e-health (3): a systematic review of published definitions. *J Med Internet Res.* 2005; 7(1): e1. Available at: www.jmir.org/2005/1/e1/

Pagliari C, Sloan D, Gregor P, *et al.* What is e-health (4): a scoping exercise to map the field. *J Med Internet Res.* 2005; 7(1): e9. Available at: www.jmir.org/2005/1/e9/

Powell J, Clarke A. Investigating internet use by mental health service users: interview study. *Stud Health Technol Inform.* 2007; 129: 1112–16.

Rodgers A, Corbett T, Bramley D, *et al.* Do u smoke after txt? Results of a randomised trial of smoking cessation using mobile phone text messaging. *Tobacco Contr.* 2005; 14: 255–61.

Wanless D. *Securing our Future Health: taking a long-term view.* London: HM Treasury; 2002.

Wanless D. *Securing Good Health for the Whole Population.* London: HM Treasury; 2004.

World Health Organization Global Observatory for E-health webpage. Available at: www. who.int/kms/initiatives/E-health/en/

CHAPTER 5

The National Programme for IT (NPfIT): is there a better way?

Sean Brennan

INTRODUCTION

Early in 2004, the British Government announced the award of eight enormous IT contracts with a combined value of more than £6 billion. The companies selected would introduce new IT systems and processes to Europe's largest public sector organisation, the National Health Service (NHS) in England. The contracts, which were originally due to run for seven years, until December 2010, are now more than half-way through, but at this stage, as 2008 is ticked off the calendar, all is not well with the National Programme for IT (NPfIT). Both the programme and the agency NHS Connecting for Health (NHS CfH) set up to deliver the programme have received considerable and sustained criticism from many sources since its inception. This chapter builds on the author's book, *The NHS IT Project: the biggest computer programme in the world . . . ever!* (Brennan 2005) and a published article in the *Journal of Information Technology* entitled 'The biggest computer programme in the world ever! How's it going?' (Brennan 2007). It seeks to identify why this programme has attracted such high levels of criticism and whether there might have been 'another way'.

THE NATIONAL PROGRAMME FOR IT
NPfIT: NISPs, NASPs and LSPs

One thing that the programme has delivered in abundance is a long list of new acronyms. NISPs, NASPs and LSPs are just three: three groups of providers who will work closely together to deliver integrated services across the NHS in England. National infrastructure services providers (NISPs) will deliver infrastructure components nationally. These include BT and the New NHS Network (N3). The national application service providers (NASPs) will deliver national applications such as the Choose and Book service and the National Care Records Service (NCRS): the National Data Spine and the Electronic Transfer of Prescriptions (ETP) – now called 'The Electronic Prescription Service' (EPS). Local service providers (LSPs) will be responsible for delivering the local aspects of the National Care Record Service (NCRS).

These new creatures, local service providers, were created for contracting purposes – the Department of Health divided the country into five 'clusters' of strategic health authorities and ran competitions in each to select a dedicated LSP who would deliver the integrated NCRS solutions/service across that patch.

The five clusters initially established were:

1 London
2 North East, Yorkshire and Humberside
3 South East and South West
4 East of England and East Midlands
5 West Midlands and North West.

WHAT DO THEY PLAN TO DELIVER?

National Care Record Service (NCRS): the Data Spine

The Care Records Services is the core service in the programme. This is the part of the programme involved with managing the process of patient care in hospitals and the community, and with the collection of information about each patient's care. It is expected to bring a number of benefits to the NHS, including access to integrated patient data, prescription ordering, proactive decision support and best practice reference data.

Phase One of the NCRS specification (which was expected to have been delivered by December 2004), stated that all clinicians should be able to browse the Internet and view basic clinical information about their patients online. At this time one third of hospitals should have been supporting electronic X-rays. Phase Two was expected to give clinicians access to a more comprehensive patient record including specialist results, GP prescribing history, hospital discharge summaries and clinical documentation. It is sad to reflect that it was initially intended by 2008 to have delivered comprehensive, community-wide patient records with support for care pathways and appointment scheduling across different NHS organisations as well as inpatient and outpatient prescribing in hospitals. There has been slippage.

The national part of the National Care Record Service, the Data Spine, was not going to simply be a repository for clinical information but also an active component of any transactions undertaken locally. Yes, not only will the Spine control who has access to which patients' clinical information, but it will also be the gatekeeper to any local clinical functionality delivered through the LSP's NCRS service. This means that nothing can be done in any local LSP without the user going through an authentication process within the Spine. The Spine also maintains each patient's 'demographic' data – and keeps the personal information about every member of the population up to date: address; registered GP, change of names etc. as previously described in the NHS Strategic Tracing Service. It is not just a national record – the Spine really is the supporting infrastructure for the rest of this ambitious programme.

Electronic Transfer of Prescriptions (ETP)

In September 2003 the Electronic Transfer of Prescriptions (ETP) was added to the specification for NCRS and renamed the Electronic Prescription Service (EPS). This service, despite its name, is *not* about prescribing but about the movement of electronic prescriptions between GPs, community pharmacists and the National Prescribing Pricing Authority (PPA). While it will reduce some of the administrative burden in managing repeat prescribing, more importantly it will collect feedback from the pharmacies, which will enable clinicians to know if their patients are collecting their medications. In certain cases, GPs will be able to devolve the routine management of repeat prescriptions to community pharmacists.

Finally, it will drastically reduce the bureaucracy associated with the data flows associated with prescriptions. At present, the paper prescription, completed and signed by the GP, is cashed and dispensed by the community pharmacist, and ultimately ends up with the Prescribing Pricing Authority in Newcastle where the handwritten data is manually input into the PPA database. This provides useful medication information, which is then available to local GPs and primary care trusts. By computerising this manual process the evidence suggests that there are considerable opportunities to reduce fraud by up to £3 billion per annum.

Choose and Book

The e-booking system will operate across the NHS and it is intended to give patients more choice and control over their hospital appointments. GPs and other clinicians are able to book patient appointments and consultations immediately rather than waiting for an appointment letter. In the early days of this development, this task was often delegated to GP reception staff. It was during these early days that Choose and Book raised considerable amounts of antibodies among practice staff, although now that the technical 'clunkiness' has been reduced, its true potential has become more apparent.

The New NHS Network (N3)

A rapid, secure, robust and reliable network is an essential component of the national programme, without which the national implementation of clinical IT will not happen. This network must be robust and have enough capacity (bandwidth) to enable rapid and efficient communication within and between NHS participants.

NCRS: local solutions

It will be the active components of what is collectively known as the NCRS that will deliver the greatest clinical benefit. Yes, a sharable national electronic record will also give benefit, but the real clinical benefit is the implementation of electronic prescribing, electronic order communications, integrated care pathways and ultimately telemedicine, and remote home care support. All these components, when coupled to clinical decision support tools, have the capacity to radically improve the effectiveness of clinical care and reduce clinical risk.

WHAT IS THE PROGRESS OF NPfIT?

It soon became increasingly obvious to the NHS and to other observers that the scale of the NHS NPfIT was far greater than anything the UK public sector has ever seen. Was the programme too ambitious? Plans published by NHS Connecting for Health (CfH) in January 2005 indicated than by April 2007, 151 acute hospital trusts were expected to have implemented patient administration systems of varying degrees of sophistication. By mid-2008 less that two dozen had been deployed.

While there were concerns over what would eventually be delivered (would it be ready in time, and what would the total cost be to the NHS?), we should not lose sight of how great an achievement the establishment of this programme was. For the first time, health IT had risen right to the top of the political agenda, with significant commitment from the very top of the office – Number 10.

This 'success' should be seen in the context of the previous 20 years of health informatics when there had been successive attempts to raise the profile of NHS IT. Although these successive initiatives regularly extolled the value of effective IT to good healthcare management, the adoption of clinical IT in the NHS had been patchy at best. On reflection, might it have been enough to raise the profile of NHS IT, assign the funding, and let the various NHS organisations get on with it? Or did it need a huge top-down programme to push the solutions into an unwieldy NHS?

We have seen what was originally planned and even the less sensitive ones among us will have detected a fair degree of hostility to date with the programme from various sectors. This chapter will identify a number of key issues and ask if there was a better way. (For the sake of brevity, a number of elements of the programme are not included in this commentary although their delivery is key to the overall strategy (e.g. GP to GP record transfer and Quality Management and Analysis Service (QMAS) and Secondary Users Service (SUS)).

A NATIONAL CARE RECORD

So great has been the focus in the National Programme on the need for a single patient record, accessible by any clinician anywhere, that it is easy to forget that the original objectives of previous NHS IT strategies did not include a *single* national electronic record. This may be a very desirable outcome, but it was originally a secondary objective, and not until NPfIT was it seen as the main driver. As Frank Burns, author of *Information for Health* and one of the original architects of the NHS IT programme, explained in 2002, 'There was never a business case made for a national EHR. The real benefits of clinical IT is in the use of computerised decision support and local shared records' (Brennan 2002a).

Despite that, the National Programme had wanted a very aggressive timetable and greatly underestimated the complexity of what was proposed. There are some who believe that, despite the initial pain, the NHS NPfIT had taken the right route in nationally mandating tough standards and adopting a service orientated architecture (SOA), the potential benefits of which are now being seen.

This approach requires the definition and national adoption of a service orientated architecture (SOA) for healthcare, comprising centrally provided national services – including the Spine 'business services'. These include patient ID, security, and authentication, which can then be utilised by interoperable administrative and clinical applications. This is a very ambitious approach but one which will eventually eradicate the haphazard and random way that the NHS has implemented clinical systems. Coupled to the relaxation of the monolithic LSP contracts, this standardisation could in the future support a pragmatic Best of Breed model.

In August 2006, the first implementation of the Summary Care Record within the NHS CRS was activated. In line with the policy of the Clinical Leads for a phased introduction to gain professional and public confidence, this release contained only one key clinical record deliverable – the GP part of the Summary Care Record. The GP Summary Record is derived from practices that have a National Programme-compliant clinical computer system and with data that meets defined quality criteria. The data quality had to be assessed and approved before a practice can upload its patient data. When a practice meets these two criteria, a local public information campaign precedes the upload explaining precisely which practices are about to have patient data uploaded to the Spine.

Predictably, the programme got embroiled in issues around the confidentiality of these 'national' records, controversy that eventually saw a bit of a U-turn by the programme. Previously the consent to create the summary record was sought before the record was created. Now a more sensible and pragmatic model has emerged which requires consent to share the record but not its creation. The dilemma for us all is: what can we put in place to safeguard our own personal interests while at the same time ensuring appropriate clinical and social care information is shared?

We all were rightly disgusted with the events that resulted in Victoria Climbie's death in 2000. We all were rightly ashamed that 'the system' had again let down a vulnerable child and probably all of us hoped that it would not happen again. The lack of shared information between healthcare professionals and between health and social services had a direct influence on this tragic outcome, and yet, whenever people try to overcome this deficiency they are hit with the confidentiality counter-argument. We must work though this and soon. The development of a huge national record database, however, is not necessarily the answer. Even though the aims of the Data Spine are now considerably less than they once were, this national repository is still a fundamentally different approach to that advocated by people like Frank Burns who said that the real and genuine benefits (and therefore savings) should be at a local clinical community level – building from the bottom up. Sharing health and social information locally could have saved Victoria. The view that a national record is something that should not be considered until these local systems are in place and working have become directly opposed to the direction of travel selected by the NPfIT which originally envisaged everything being stored on a national electronic database. Perhaps this was the price that had to be paid to get political, and thereby significant financial, support. This concept of a national record sat quite nicely with a government wishing to be re-elected wearing the 'Modernising the NHS' and 'Patient Choice' badges.

THE DELIVERY MODEL

This issue raises key questions: Was this centralised, top-down model the best approach? Would a catalogue of accredited interoperable systems have been a better model?

In 2002, the author interviewed Sir John Pattison, the man who first accepted responsibility for designing the National Programme (Brennan 2002b). One of the issues discussed was the delivery model planned for the programme. Sir John envisaged the appointment of local service providers who would have responsibility for identifying the right IT solutions and delivering them to NHS organisations within a geographical area (later to become the five 'clusters' and subsequently reduced to three). But, was this the most effective model for delivery?

Sir John was asked: 'Could not the existing process be improved simply by developing national business cases, providing ring-fenced monies, and accrediting solutions?' He was forthright in his response:

> There is an issue of capability. What we are proposing is extraordinary in scale and it is precisely the scale of the programme that requires this additional layer. It is needed to ensure not only that the technology solutions are available and accredited, but to underpin those implementations with comprehensive change management. We know that some enthusiasts will forge ahead whatever model is adopted, but it is the generality that require more support and facilitation. The traditional procurement model is not designed to do this and the scale of what we are proposing needs this extra change management facilitation layer (Brennan 2002b).

The view, then, of those running the programme was that the NHS and the solution suppliers did not have enough IT expertise or staff resources to implement the complex clinical IT required of the programme. In addition, the acknowledgement that this was not just an IT project also highlighted the need for organisational change skills that were not readily available in the NHS. The introduction of the LSP layer was expected to deliver this support. The jury is still out on the LSP model, although it is generally acknowledged that this comprehensive programme could not have been delivered with the existing IT support structure in the NHS. Some of the frustrating delays have been the lack of a proven product and in those areas where such a thing actually existed (e.g. some of the PACS products), good numbers of successful implementations have indeed been achieved.

Why did we need to change? What were the problems with the old (procurement) system?

Even the greatest critics of the NPfIT would not advocate going back to the old ways of buying computer systems for the NHS. The old procurement system was time-consuming and costly – for both the NHS and their suppliers. Considerable effort went into identifying the local user requirement, and into getting local clinical and management buy-in. This requirement would then be advertised in the *European Journal* and a lengthy and costly beauty parade started. Even these local community-focused projects required considerable effort to manage the procurements and could probably never have delivered what all the parties wanted anyway. Compromise is always necessary in these processes, and it is difficult to reach total agreement on a single system or suite of systems. It is interesting to note, therefore, that even in the old procurement model it was rare for all the users to come to a consensus, and equally rare for many clinicians to become involved in the decision-making process. An NHS trust employing hundreds of doctors might typically find that two or three doctors, one nurse, and if they were really lucky someone representing the views of the allied healthcare professions (e.g. the physiotherapists) would have the time or the interest to get embroiled in a computer procurement.

In the event, none of the big collaborative procurements ever made it through to completion. The National Programme intervened. So now the pressure of commercial competition had virtually disappeared from the NHS in England. The rigid landscape of solutions and cluster contracts offered by CfH effectively prohibited local NHS trusts from selecting their own systems, although the recent introduction of the additional services contracts has relaxed that rigidity a little. Called the Additional Supply Capability and Capacity Services (ASCC), under the ASCC procurement there is a series of IT framework contracts to provide access to a broader-based supply community necessary to continue to deliver the National Programme for IT as it develops. Connecting for Health suggested that:

> The existing contractual arrangements have worked well. However, the increasing size, complexity and duration of the NPfIT are such that these existing arrangements are likely to require enhanced additional capability and capacity. The Authority has reviewed the current range of services and the likely future requirements with a view to acquiring such additional supply capacity and capability to complement and support these existing contractual arrangements.

In addition, to support the ongoing business of the Authority, there may be requirements for:
1   new local or national systems in support of policy decisions
2   substitution for failed performance
3   specialist knowledge and services necessary for the NHS and wider healthcare service.

By adopting a service orientated architecture (SOA) (E-health Insider 2007a), the programme had hoped it was building a plug-and-play environment, and this would have been fine, but the exclusivity of the initial LSP contracts meant that the choice of applications to plug and play with was restricted to products in the LSP portfolio.

With the SOA architecture it could be argued that once an LSP-preferred supplier fails to deliver to contract, alternative products could now be considered. However, this is an option that requires failure, and hardly qualifies as a positive 'user choice' experience.

DID WE NEED THESE CENTRALLY NEGOTIATED CONTRACTS?

Whenever the National Programme is accused of wasting public money, one defence usually emerges: the contractors, we are told, will only be paid when they deliver the goods. Suppliers to the National Programme are paid when they deliver completed products and services that are fully accepted by the NHS to be safe, reliable and fully functional. All completion risk lies with the contractors. They are liable for any costs that arise. Deliver the programme efficiently and on time and they will (possibly) earn big profits. Deliver wastefully, or late (or not at all) and they stand to make thumping losses. Witness Accenture, originally LSP for two clusters, who exited the programme in 2006 after setting aside $450 million to cover losses on the programme. They were followed in 2008 by Fujitsu's shock departure. Prime contractors are also responsible for managing their own subcontractors' performances, particularly the software suppliers, and so the responsibilities and risks flow down. The NHS, it was argued, could not lose.

But there is also another way that the NHS is set to benefit financially from the programme. A major tactic in the aim of the NHS Connecting for Health to secure best value has been the enterprise wide arrangements (EWA) negotiated with suppliers involved in multiple prime contracts across the NHS. Estimated savings of more than £70 million have already been made through the EWA process. In total, central purchasing of core systems and services by NHS CfH will save the NHS in England an estimated at least £3.8 billion over 10 years. In fact, independent analysts Ovum have estimated that £4.4 billion is being saved through central procurement of IT systems by NHS CfH compared with what could have been achieved by individual NHS organisations purchasing the same systems separately.

This is the first time the NHS has been able to exercise its full weight to drive down prices and benefit from economies of scale for IT products in this way. This approach has the knock-on effect of putting more money for patient care into the pockets of NHS organisations across the country. Unless the NHS starts to pick up the bills of the LSPs, it is doubtful that the complaint that the National Programme is wasting public money can really be justified. Money is being wasted, that is for certain, but it is the share capital of the big consultancy companies that won the right to deliver the programme that is being hit. Yes, there have been considerable costs to the NHS too, with its own armies of management consultants and lawyers, but so far the cold equations of the contract have applied. Where solutions have not been delivered, contractors have not been paid.

The real cost to the NHS if the programme fails, however, is time. The NHS, as has previously been stated, has been demanding clinical IT for decades. Were the Programme to fail, the NHS would be put back a decade.

LOCAL VS. NATIONAL

Could local communities have simply bought their EPR provider products from a catalogue? This approach had been successful in primary care computing, with GP systems being subjected to a rigorous accreditation process. Allowing local choice of the major clinical systems within secondary care may well have ensured greater commitment from local clinicians to avoid them thinking the system was being imposed on them. A model based on local communities could well have been more successful with their implementations if more local choice had been possible, although the NHS would not have benefited from the bulk-buying discounts. A national approach has several problems, not least that a myriad of small suppliers have been pushed out of the picture. Perversely, it was often these smaller suppliers who generally had a good record of delivering clinical IT to the NHS.

ONE SIZE FITS ALL

One size fits all may not deliver what is needed. As Frank Burns said in the BJHC interview in 2002:

> 'I do get nervous that there are people far away from the reality of implementing the strategy and very far away from the culture in the NHS who have this notion that they can simply contract at a national level, for a national solution. I am sure there are still people who think that. I personally think it would be a disaster if ever such an approach were attempted. Integrating healthcare records over the lifetime of an individual, through a whole series of ill-health events, involving a combination of agencies and dozens of different professionals, is complex and requires excellent technical solutions and vast degrees of cultural and organisational change. To suggest you can build that and roll it out in the same way that you would roll out a supermarket check-out system displays, to me, incredible naivety that would make you seriously concerned about their understanding of the complexity of healthcare' (Brennan 2002a).

That is the dilemma. One size will not necessarily fit all. Every healthcare organisation is different. Maybe they should not be as different as they are, but changing the nature of our healthcare institutions may be a bigger challenge than making the IT systems flexible enough to support the different ways they choose to work. Forcing a single solution (with no local tailoring) onto these busy clinicians will not work and this aspect itself is a potential risk to the programme.

RIP AND REPLACE

Many would argue that the policy of replacing existing PAS systems with new PAS systems was a waste of perfectly good working applications. Sitting a clinical module on top of these legacy systems and integrating to specialist clinical modules may have been a workable alternative model. This approach, often referred to as 'Best of Breed', uses existing 'legacy' applications like the PAS or specialist modules, and simply adds an integrated generic clinical application on top. NCRS consists of the National Data Spine (and all its functional components) and those NCRS elements that will be delivered locally. The local elements are those sometimes referred to as the 'doing' systems, including local GP systems with their array of clinical functionality, and those in hospitals and other community settings which include functionality such as electronic requesting of radiology examinations/ordering of laboratory investigations with electronic laboratory reporting and electronic prescribing and medicines administration. Could we not have used these legacy systems (such as the existing workhorse patient administration systems) or existing radiology or laboratory information systems and layered on a generic clinical 'doing' workstation system?

The 2008 Health Informatics Review now seems to think we can. It is a shame this was not seriously considered at the start of the programme but, hey-ho, we are where we are! Would it have been possible to have some local choice of clinical systems (which had to be compliant to some agreed national accreditation/standardisation scheme), while developing an integrated clinical workstation application which would have been a national NHS product?

The answer may well have been 'no', but the lack of a transparent discussion of these options contributed to the festering criticism we continue to see today. Perhaps it was considered. Perhaps it was concluded that, contractually, it would have been too difficult to agree contracts where every site runs different combination of systems, and perhaps this would have meant that the 'bulk-buying' discounts would not have been so generous and therefore the NHS would have lost the £4 billion discounts. We will never know.

WILL THE PROGRAMME DELIVER WHAT THE NHS NEEDS?

Information for Health (1998) identified a sensible and pragmatic strategy for health IT. The same people who criticise NPfIT would probably have applauded sites such as Wirral NHS Trust and Queen's Hospital, Burton. Both sites had invested their own resources in integrated trust-wide IT systems and both are still working examples of the benefits that effective systems can deliver to a busy NHS trust. Is this not what NPfIT is trying to do? Is not the Wirral and Burton functionality exactly what has been bought through the LSP contracts? The fact that it has not yet been delivered (or even built) does not mean the requirement is wrong. NPfIT has simply taken that vision and contracted it out to suppliers through a new delivery model – the LSPs.

LIGHT AT THE END OF THE TUNNEL?

Exactly a decade on from the release of the Information for Health strategy, there have been two eagerly awaited publications: The Darzi Report and the Health Informatics Review. The Darzi Report (Department of Health 2008a) made it very clear that the central push to increase the quantity of clinical care given through our NHS now gives way to a bigger push to ensure that care is of the highest quality. Patient

Recorded Outcome Measurements and pathways of care are central to the success of this approach and therefore the NPfIT's information technology infrastructure is a fundamental requirement for delivering this Darzi quality agenda. Anyone who was expecting the Darzi report to require a fundamental shift in direction of travel for the programme will be disappointed. His vision of the future requires exactly the IT infrastructure that NPfIT is attempting to deliver. No change in direction required. Equally, anyone expecting the Health Informatics Review of July 2008 to require a radical shift in IT strategy will also be disappointed. It removes the dust of a decade, reinforces the need for good informatics people at all levels and suggests that interim solutions are OK. However, there is a need for interim initiatives so that patient information can be made available across different IT systems, different care providers and different care settings ahead of strategic systems' delivery. The recommendations respond to the need for speedy achievement of benefits, taking account of differing local priorities and variations across SHAs (Department of Health 2008b).

The review also includes the usual stakeholder wish-list, which reinforced those of the 1998 strategy with the request that solutions be responsive; solutions should be responsive to local needs and priorities. There may be real and legitimate differences in terms of requirements and priorities because of the specific healthcare needs of a local population, or because of the systems currently in place.

The review seems to have seen some light with regard to how this complex IT can be delivered, adopting the principle of 'don't let perfection be the enemy of the good', with the acknowledgement that there are 'effective local systems currently in use delivering benefits to patients today and that we need the opportunity to use these as interim solutions elsewhere if there is a sound business case and a roadmap to the strategic systems'. This will bring a collective sigh of relief. Someone has at last seen common sense. The reason for this other way is because the delivery of systems is late and there is an issue of timing: 'In some cases, benefits need to be achieved for patients and clinicians sooner than waiting for the strategic systems. Timescales must be realistic. Solutions are needed for the interim pending delivery of the strategic systems' (Department of Health 2008b).

The report goes on to suggest that local organisations have to take greater responsibility for implementation and subsequent transformational change through strong local leadership from management and clinicians. This local leadership must be complemented by strong national leadership where it is needed.

In a commentary of this new review for *E-Health Insider* (17 July 2008), Lyn Whitfield suggested that it is not just family silver that can be found in the loft!

Some of the older NHS IT hands may be planning a trip into the loft this weekend to dig out any local implementation strategies (LISs) that have survived from the days of the 1998 information strategy, Information for Health. Because five years after the national programme tried to take control of NHS IT in general and care records services in particular, the focus of the latest Health Informatics Review is – possibly – nearly – back on local action. The review, led initially by former Department of Health interim chief information officer Matthew Swindells, is careful to say that the 'overall direction' of travel is towards the development and deployment of 'strategic' information systems by local service providers. But it also says there is a need for 'interim' solutions 'to make patient information available across different IT systems, care providers and care systems' while the wait for the strategic solutions grows ever longer.

Enter the Clinical Five

In particular, the review says there is a need to get a 'Clinical Five' set of elements in place in secondary care. These are a patient administration system with 'integration with other systems and sophisticated reporting', order communications and diagnostics reporting, letters with coding, scheduling for beds, tests and theatres, and e-prescribing. Those older NHS IT hands might find the list eerily similar to some of the EPR 'levels' that IfH hoped to achieve. Meanwhile, the Health Informatics Review launches a new implementation acronym. Local Informatics Plans (LIPs) will lay down the route to the 'Clinical Five'.

What goes around comes around. Why didn't anyone pick up that IfH baton? This review is welcome and while its conclusions come five years late, it is hoped that they are not *too* late.

CONCLUSION

The iconic 'Six Level EPR' model was a reasoned pragmatic solution that was well received by both the NHS and suppliers alike and its time may well come again. This comprehensive and complex IT and change programme cannot be delivered overnight and will not be delivered through a big bang approach. The acknowledgement of the need for an incremental plan will result in the old EPR model being dusted off and tweaked – a makeover called . . . Clinical Five!

The model had articulated a clear and concise incremental approach to what was then called the EPR, which would be built at a local clinical community level. It would consist of integrated clinical and administrative systems building on legacy applications if appropriate to do so. These 'active' systems would produce a passive historical record, held locally. A national summary record could, in time, be fed from these local systems. That simple approach was turned on its head: NPfIT (or the government – or both) decided that the main objective of their programme was a single national electronic record. As previously proposed, this may have been required in order to gain the critical political buy-in (and therefore resources) to the programme. Many of the problems with the programme can be traced to that fundamental reinterpretation of what the NHS needed. It might have been workable if this national record was allowed to evolve over time, so long as the programme's primary objective was left untouched – to put in place effective, workable local systems that support the way that healthcare professionals work in local organisations. This view was also reflected by the BCS Primary Care Group who submitted to the National Audit Office in January 2005 that:

We support the view that systems in health and social care should allow appropriate sharing of information and workflows across organisational boundaries. We do not believe that it is necessary or practical to try and achieve this by implementing a single monolithic solution, for the following reasons:

1   No system can be all-encompassing, and we can already see problems at both the geographical and functional borders of NPfIT which will force us to find ways of sharing information and workflows across these borders outside the scope of the planned monoliths.

2   In virtually any other sector (or indeed in healthcare in most other countries) the level of organisational fragmentation is such that there is no choice but to find ways of sharing information and workflows across heterogeneous systems. This means that there is massive effort going into the development of standards and tools to address these problems, and we will soon be able to tap into this work to develop alternative ways to achieve the desired level of integration.

3   Even if the new systems are very good, it is difficult to believe that they will ever serve all of the specialist niches as well as the current best-of-breed systems in those niches do. (E-Health Insider 2007b)

Since the programme's launch in 2002, the LSPs have yet to convince the NHS that they really can deliver solutions and the organisational change required. Is the scale of the challenge just too big for them? There was a stage, in 2003, before the NHS in England was divided into the five arbitrary clusters, when we all expected the delivery model to be much more local. We had 28 SHAs back then, and we expected a process where 28 service providers would be appointed – one for each SHA. To ensure local users are now engaged more appropriately, the programme has introduced another new acronym, NLOP: NPfIT Local Ownership Programme – although some cynics suggest it really stands for No Longer Our Problem! Will the NLOP really mean a shift in decision making downwards to the redefined SHAs or will the major decisions continue to be made behind closed doors and then the NHS expected to act on them?

SO WE COME TO THE FINAL QUESTION: WILL IT WORK?

If NPfIT is about getting the best deal for IT infrastructure for the NHS then, yes, it will be a success. The NHS was a huge spender on IT before the national programme started. Now it gets more, it gets it delivered as a service, and it gets it all at a very keen price. It will get several hundred PAS systems, clinical systems, and all sorts of associated applications delivered down a pipe to the bedside.

Let us try tougher questions:

➤ Will all the software and applications work in the way that they are meant to work?

➤ Will the Spine integrate seamlessly with systems in the five clusters?

➤ Will the security and confidentiality work to everyone's satisfaction?

The answer to these questions is probably 'eventually' – as long as the momentum is maintained and the funding is sustained, one day it will all come together. There is, after all, very little in the programme that is totally conceptually new. But it may all take a lot longer than the NHS expects. New software always seems to take longer to design, build and test than anyone expects. This is an ambitious programme, and there are many obstacles in the path. The main software developers have a lot of code to write. There will be further slippages, renegotiations of deadlines, a general downplaying of expectations, and a long hard slog by the service providers, the software developers, and the NHS alike before it all starts to come together.

There will certainly be scare stories along the way – the press will gather around every hint of failure and will predict catastrophe. But, in the end, this isn't rocket science. It will work because it has to work. The day will come when the systems are in and the project will be signed off. Of course, by then there will be new challenges, new technologies, new obstacles.

Perhaps even this wasn't the question that you wanted answering. If NPfIT is about changing the way healthcare is delivered, there is a third answer to the question 'will NPfIT succeed?' It will struggle. 'That's not what NPfIT is about,' I can hear from some readers, and true, the programme's remit isn't to change the world, just to deliver a service to the NHS, an IT infrastructure for the NHS to use as it chooses. The programme is branded and perceived as a technology initiative. It is a technology initiative. Yet this perception could be its undoing. People might assume it to be non-clinical. It could be perceived as another big PAS project or a HISS, and that would be a shame. The IT offers new opportunities for the delivery of clinical care. But will clinicians see these opportunities to change the way the NHS is delivered? Indeed, will it be seen as an opportunity to them or a threat?

The key purpose of the NHS is to deliver effective clinical care – an objective clearly reiterated in the Darzi Review. Technology will offer alternative ways of delivering that care, so NPfIT is, whether it likes it or not, central to the modernisation of the delivery of clinical care. This is not just about having an electronic record. It is far deeper and grander than that. It is about supporting clinical care with IT, and when you support clinical care with IT, you can then use that technology to influence how that care is delivered. That in turn ensures that the quality of care delivered is maximised and that risk is reduced: the Darzi outcome.

The final major concern is therefore not a technology one, but a clinical one – stimulated by the implementation of technology. During any pre-implementation analysis phase of a large computer project, workflow processes are identified and compared. Imagine the workflow involved in an integrated care pathway. Imagine all the healthcare workers who input into a single pathway. Imagine four different surgeons who have four completely different ways of treating the same condition. Easy, you say, just look at the evidence for which is the correct way to treat that condition and get them all to do it that way. And therein lies the challenge. Changing existing work practices that have evolved over many years will not be easy. Implementing the technology is relatively easy compared to getting agreement on changing clinical practice and implementing integrated care pathways. Simply imposing pathways on these guys (and gals) will not work.

So, back to our final question once again. Will the NPfIT work? Yes, it will deliver the technology to the NHS, but for the NHS to grasp this opportunity, the clinicians need considerable encouragement, a clearer idea of what will be delivered, and evidence of benefit for them or their patients. It still begs the question, 'could there have been a better way to do it?' We will probably never know. Like it or not, NPfIT is now the only game in town. As stated in the opening pages of this chapter, this is a huge and complex undertaking and it is essential for the NHS that this technology is implemented successfully. It must not fail. And to ensure it doesn't, common sense is at last being applied to this ambitious, but sorely needed, programme of work. The mantra 'we are where we are' was used earlier in this chapter. Perhaps it is now more appropriate to say: 'We are now where we need to be'.

REFERENCES

Brennan S. Interview with Frank Burns. *Br J Health Comput Inf Manage*. 2002a; 19(2): 2, 4, 8.

Brennan S. Sir John Pattison speaks to Sean Brennan. *Br J Health Comput Inf Manage*. 2002b; 19(3): 2, 4.

Brennan S. *The NHS IT Project: the biggest computer programme in the world . . . ever!* Oxford: Radcliffe Publishing; 2005.

Brennan S. The biggest computer programme in the world . . . ever! How's it going? *J Inf Technol*. 2007; 22: 202–11.

Department of Health. *Health Informatics Review*. London: DoH; 2008.

Department of Health. *High Quality Care for All: NHS Next Stage Review final report*. Professor the Lord Darzi of Denham KBE. London: DoH; 2008.

E-Health Insider. iSoft director says NPfIT systems 'interchangeable'. E-Health Media Ltd; 3 May 2007a. Available at: www.e-health-insider.com/news/item.cfm?ID_2662

E-Health Insider. *LISs to LIPs with the Health Informatics Review. BCS Primary Care Group Submission to NAO on NHS NPfIT (January 2005)*. E-Health Media Ltd; 2007b. Available at: www.e-health-media.com/comment_and_analysis/333/liss_to_lips_with_the_health_informatics_review

PART TWO

Electronic Health Records

Electronic health records for patient-centred healthcare

Nick Gaunt

INTRODUCTION

That the patient is central to the planning and delivery of healthcare would at first sight seem self-evident. However, health services have traditionally been organised more for the convenience of the provider institution and its staff than for the patient, who is left to make the best of what appears to be a fragmented and poorly coordinated service. This is particularly evident in public-funded health systems such as the UK National Health Service, but even in consumer-led systems such as the United States providers do not present a coherent and consumer-responsive service to all patients. Service users deserve a better healthcare system, one that is responsive to their needs, sufficiently flexible to accommodate their preferences, and that can offer 'seamless' care, in the hope of empowerment and improved quality of care. Patients are becoming more informed about health and disease, largely through greater coverage of such issues in the general media. They are also more familiar with information and communications technologies, especially the Internet and mobile phones, and have come to expect services to be delivered electronically where they can be.

Computerised record systems have been in development in healthcare for several decades and are at last reaching the point where mass adoption of electronic healthcare records and services by healthcare providers is feasible. However, these will not of themselves provide the vision of integrated patient-centred healthcare: systems and services that span multiple providers are necessary and are being developed in a number of countries (Detmer and Steen 2006). In this chapter we explore the nature of patient-centred care and consider how this can be supported by electronic health record systems.

PATIENT-CENTRED HEALTHCARE

Patient-centred healthcare has been defined as:

> An approach to care that consciously adopts a patient's perspective. This perspective can be characterised around dimensions such as respect for patients' values, preferences, and expressed needs in regard to coordination and integration of care, information, communication and education, physical comfort, emotional support and alleviation of fear and anxiety, involvement of family and friends, transition and continuity (USAID 1999).

Patient-centred healthcare requires a significant change in attitude, culture and ways of working and there are many barriers to change (IAPO 2007; Gillespie, *et al.* 2004). Cultural and behavioural factors, including good clinical communication skills, providing appropriate contexts for consultation and respecting the values and preferences of the individual, are dominant factors in the move to patient-centred care (WHO 2004). However, there are also organisational issues: the way that clinics and consultations are provided plays a significant role in enabling and inhibiting patient involvement; the increasing standardisation of care through professional guidelines can conflict with the exercise of choice at the heart of the patient involvement process; and time remains a scarce resource for patient involvement and the efficient management of time and coordination of services is critical (UK Department of Health 2004). Electronic health records and systems can be expected to have an important role in addressing many of these issues.

TABLE 6.1 Some key elements of patient-centred care (adapted from Gerteis *et al.* 1993)

Respect for patients' values, preferences and expressed needs.
Coordination and integration of care.
Information, communication and education.
Shared decision making and support for self-care.
Physical comfort.
Emotional support and alleviation of fear and anxiety.
Involvement of family and friends.
Continuity of care and smooth transition across service boundaries.

ELECTRONIC HEALTH RECORDS AND RECORD SYSTEMS

There are two basic paradigms for health records: those created and maintained by providers of healthcare to assist in their delivery of care, quality improvement, accountability, etc. (variously known as patient, medical or health records); and personal health records that are controlled and maintained by individuals who wish to have their own record of their health and healthcare, to take a greater part in managing their own health (or those of dependants), and to have the ability to choose with whom they share that information.

Both kinds of record have been held on paper since well before the advent of computerisation, and indeed continue to be recorded manually to this day. The paper records kept by medical, nursing and other health professionals have been a mainstay of clinical practice, important documentary evidence of the care process and a means of sharing among care teams. Individuals have often kept paper records of aspects of their own health and care, their immunisations, allergies and medication history, both for their own record and to show to healthcare staff in emergencies, when travelling, or even to ensure better coordination of their care when seeing different providers (Abbott, *et al.* 2001). Brennan (1999) observes the lack of cross-institutional records and communication systems which results in the patient having to convey the treatment plan of one healthcare provider to another. Paper records have of course also been used to share information more formally between patients and their healthcare providers: patient-held maternity records are perhaps the most widely used of these.

Both kinds of record have also seen an evolution of increasingly capable computerised versions: early developments took distinct paths in systems designed respectively for provider institutions (as electronic medical or patient record systems – EMR/EPR) and for the general public (as Internet-based electronic patient-held records – ePHR); more recently there has been a gradual convergence towards electronic health record (EHR) systems that combine provider and patient-contributed content (*see* Table 6.2).

TABLE 6.2 Three major categories of electronic health record systems

	Electronic patient record (EPR)	Electronic personal health Record (ePHR)	Electronic health record (EHR)
Record scope	Detailed records of episodes of care in one institution.	An individual's records of their own health and healthcare.	Longitudinal records of health and healthcare, often only in summary.
Record origin	Generally entered by and maintained within a single institution.	Personally entered and maintained, possibly copied or imported from EPR.	Composite records abstracted from either EHR or EPR, or directly entered by providers and individual.
Main users	Professionals in the institution.	Individual and/or their family or carers.	Professionals and individual.
Focus of system	Supporting care provided within the institution.	Supporting the individual to maintain a healthy lifestyle and take a greater role in managing their own care.	Supporting care that is shared between providers and coordinated around the patient.

ELECTRONIC PATIENT RECORD SYSTEMS

Electronic patient record (EPR) systems contain the detailed records of encounters between patients and their healthcare providers. They are typically held within computer systems serving one institution or a small group of institutions and are designed primarily around that institution's workflow and the needs of its healthcare staff. EPR rarely contain data entered by patients but their right to review the information in their electronic records is usually fulfilled only within the confines of the healthcare institution, although online access through the Internet is beginning to be offered (Winkelman and Leonard 2004; Fisher, *et al.* 2007). Such personal health record 'portals', which are based upon an institution's EPR, have been called electronic integrated personal health records (eiPHR). They are most valued by patients when accompanied by services such as medication refills, receipt of post-attendance summaries, a secure means to contact their doctor and other care providers, and access to relevant educational resources and advice (Pyper, *et al.* 2004; Tang and Lansky 2005; Ralston, *et al.* 2007). While the functionality of eiPHR is similar to those offered in ePHR (see below), they are institutionally based and do not generally include records from other providers. Furthermore, they offer little or no opportunity for patients to contribute to the records themselves. Where this is allowed, it is primarily to add comments on existing entries, to maintain a patient journal, or for self-recording of weight, blood pressure and the like (Cimono, *et al.* 2002; Wald, *et al.* 2004).

PERSONAL HEALTH RECORD SYSTEMS

Electronic personal health record (ePHR) systems are self-maintained records of an individual's health and healthcare. The information may come from healthcare providers, carers or the individual, but it is usually the responsibility of the individual to maintain their records. PHR may also offer the ability for one individual, often the mother, to maintain records for a whole family (Tang, *et al.* 2006; Pagliari, *et al.* 2007). Standalone ePHR emerged as the Internet became popular in the 1990s. Initially, these were merely web-based equivalents of the paper record typically kept by individuals; they still had to enter all their data by hand. Typically, ePHR systems permitted the recording of a variety of data items and offered various services such as lifestyle advice, reminders, secure e-mail and medication refills (*see* Table 6.3). However, data sets were inconsistent and incomplete, the additional functions offered varied between systems and records were not portable between systems (Kim and Johnson 2002).

Users of standalone ePHR found maintaining such a large amount of data to be too laborious and the benefits to be too few. Furthermore, healthcare professionals were often unwilling to trust PHR in their clinical decisions (Tang, *et al.* 2006). It is not surprising that only a very few of these early standalone ePHR remain (Schneider 2001; Kim and Johnson 2002). Currently, ePHR are offered almost exclusively by health maintenance organisations in the US, and by a few national or regional health organisations worldwide (Detmer and Steen 2006). To ease the burden on the individual and encourage sustained use of the system, some ePHR providers offer to manage the transfer of data from EPR systems. However, few of these systems enable easy transfer of records from one ePHR system to another.

TABLE 6.3 Data items and functions offered by ePHR

Personal data and contacts	Health data	Functions
Personal details	Measurements	Linkage of data to advice
Emergency contacts	Allergies	Channels of advice
Carers, proxies	Immunisations	User alerts
Doctors	Medications	Patient communities
Clinics	Surgeries	Lifestyle advice
Pharmacists	Therapies	Health questionnaires
Insurers	Illnesses	Reports
Organ donation preference	Injuries	Pre-visit preparation
Advance directives	Results	Prescription refills
Family/social history	Procedures	Secure e-mail
Appointments	Encounters	
	Plans of care	

HYBRID OR INTEGRATED EHR SYSTEMS

There has also been a gradual integration of record systems from those serving one or a small number of clinicians, through those based on clinical teams or departments, to whole provider institutions and latterly to ones that span primary, community, secondary and tertiary settings or that even span different institutions (e.g. Halamka, *et al.* 2005; Cheung, *et al.* 2007). Systems that integrate records from other EPR or EHR systems to create longitudinal records of care may be referred to as integrated electronic health record (iEHR) systems. Their content is potentially derived from many sources: data may be transferred from the EPR systems of healthcare providers; be entered directly by providers, often from those working in community settings without their own EPR system; and may come from the individuals they are caring for. iEHR implementations are generally developed to support the shared provision of healthcare by a number of institutions (such as members of one hospital group, managed care organisation, regional health organisation or national health system). While one goal of such iEHR may be for patients to experience more integrated care (Ralston, *et al.* 2007), the principal beneficiaries of most iEHR systems remain healthcare providers seeking to improve the efficiency of shared care or to obtain data for public health or research purposes.

iEHR vary in the amount of detail that is transferred from other systems. Some longitudinal records are comprehensive (e.g. Cheung, *et al.* 2007) but many share a minimum set of healthcare data such as diagnoses, allergies, certain test results, medications and treatments. Although standards that define such a 'minimum' data-set are being developed (e.g. the Continuity of Care Record standard – ASTM 2006) there remains considerable diversity in content. Four different summary records are in use in the UK, each with their own datasets (Greenhalgh, *et al.* 2008).

There will be data in each EPR that are only relevant within the context of the originating institution (such as some administrative and scheduling details) and would not be of value if transferred to an iEHR. The practicality and benefit of com-bining the remaining data that comprise the majority of existing EPR is less clear. For example, what is the relevance to EHR users of the potentially large number of sequential blood tests taken while a patient is receiving critical care? Is it necessary to transfer records of each instance of fluid replacement or blood transfusions? Should all digital images and multimedia records be replicated into the EHR? Quite apart from the practical challenges – ensuring standardised terminology and record struc-tures that are necessary for robust data interchange, meeting storage and networking capacity and performance, maintaining data integrity – the value to patient-centred care of collating such a large amount of data has yet to be established. The trend has been to start with a minimum dataset and to increase that as the need becomes evident. However, the value to emergency care of even a summary record is question-able when staff fail to refer to it (Schneider 2001). Lessons have been drawn from the widespread failure of first-generation ePHR (Pagliari, *et al.* 2007; Halamka, *et al.* 2008). The Markle Foundation suggested the following characteristics of an ideal PHR (Connecting for Health 2004):

1 access is controlled by the patient
2 lifelong records
3 contains information from all care providers
4 accessible from any place at any time
5 private and secure
6 transparent (i.e. it is clear who has entered, viewed or transferred each data item)
7 permits easy exchange of information among health providers/organisations.

The same report proposes three models for community-wide integration of health-care records. In the first, the patient acts as the integrator, being responsible for collecting together the necessary data, as was offered in the early PHR systems. The second model uses an intermediary to act as integrator on the patient's behalf, either through an independent vendor who establishes a central database and imports the data from other sources, or through a virtual federation and dynamic retrieval of records. In the third model the personal health record is a by-product of a 'closed' healthcare delivery system, the eiPHR described above.

Recent developments herald a significant convergence in health record systems and may address many of the shortcomings of standalone ePHR identified above.

'Dossia' (www.dossia.org), a non-profit consortium of major employers in the US, is offering its employees, family members and dependants a lifelong personally controlled health record. It is based on Indivo (www.indivohealth.org), an open-source ePHR that supports standards-based communication interfaces to connect to current and future health information systems, can import data from networked medical devices and supports a robust patient access and control model (Mandl, *et al.* 2007). Microsoft Corporation have created HealthVault, a repository for personal health data: it is intended to function as a repository fed from health record systems (such as the New York Presbyterian Hospital EPR) but has a 'connection centre' permitting direct upload of data from other sources, including compatible medical devices such as home monitors. Google Health is a more conventional ePHR platform to which anyone (currently only available to US residents) can subscribe without charge. It too offers interfaces to other health record systems such as the iHealthRecord ePHR developed by the iHealth Alliance (www.ihealthrecord.org) and the Epic EPR system in use in Cleveland Clinic.

These new developments are beginning to blur the distinction between EPR that offer access and services to patients of their own institutions, EHR that offer integration across multiple institutions, and ePHR that individuals control and may share with their providers. They also have the potential to support the concept of health banks acting as universal repositories of healthcare records (Shabo 2006; Ball and Gold 2007). Moreover, they introduce a truly person-centred healthcare record service that might prove to be a key factor in bringing about the transformation of service provision envisioned by patient-centred care.

HOW EHR SYSTEMS MIGHT SUPPORT PATIENT-CENTRED CARE

Healthcare centred around the individual requires EHR systems that:
1   provide holistic records of individuals' health and healthcare that incorporate their own contributions and that can be shared between providers, patient and carers
2   operate effectively across service boundaries, to ensure that individuals experience healthcare that is well integrated with smooth transitions between services
3   ensure accessibility and flexibility of healthcare services, including the choice of provider and options for where care is received (e.g. through scheduling and booking services)
4   support good communication between provider institutions and with the individual
5   provide relevant, trustworthy and personalised information to individuals
6   empower individuals to take greater control over their well-being and healthcare and integrate with individuals' other life activities.

1 Holistic records of well-being and healthcare

As modern healthcare becomes more complex and the number of providers participating in the care of individuals increases, so the problem of disjointed records of care becomes more severe. Typically, the details of care provided by one institution are not available to others who may be managing the same patient. This is detrimental to patient care, particularly in those with long-term conditions who will over time receive care from many different providers. Not having access to the records of prior care can result in inappropriate clinical decisions, needless repetition of diagnostic tests, delays in treatment and poor coordination of care. The patient may have to give the same information many times over, may be given conflicting advice and treatment, has the impression of a disjointed service and can be inconvenienced by poorly timed appointments: at best an unnecessarily poor experience, at worst sub-standard clinical care.

It is not surprising that both patients and their care providers share the ideal of every individual having a holistic record of their health and healthcare: a life-long record that is available whenever and wherever it might be needed to support patient-centred healthcare; that integrates information from diverse sources; that provides sufficient detail to be useful for clinical care; and that is intelligible to the patient. Achieving that ideal is far from easy – there is still little agreement on what the record should contain, who should have access and whether the patient should contribute to it. Healthcare professionals expect to have access to prior records about the patients under their care. Many clinicians believe that, in order to deliver the best possible care, they should be entitled routinely to see all such records, including those made in other institutions. Patients are generally happy for the clinicians with whom they are consulting to see their records, but some will wish to withhold specific aspects of their past care. However, healthcare is seldom delivered by an individual clinician – a team approach has become commonplace, but the patient may not meet or even be aware of the extent of that team. In a single institution the care team can be identified with reasonable confidence; this is not so easy in the context of management of patients with long-term conditions where several independent institutions are contributing care. Who has the right to access a patient's records in this kind of setting is a key constraint on effective implementation of EHR systems.

Sharing the content of healthcare records with patients increases their confidence and involvement in care, improves the quality of the clinical consultation, increases their participation in information and responsibility sharing, health promotion and disease management and can lead to better clinical outcomes (Kirby 1991; Ross and Lin 2003). The greatest benefits have been observed where this shared record is the definitive one in which healthcare professionals make their records rather than keeping duplicate notes elsewhere. While this can be achieved with paper records in some instances, such as maternity records, the lack of access to the record in the patient's absence is a serious constraint. This can be overcome by use of a shared EHR: the creation of Internet-based shared views of EHR (or of multiple EPRs) to which all parties have access can empower individuals with long-term conditions and improve the quality of that care (de Clercq, *et al.* 2001).

Patients benefit even further if they are able to interact with their health record system: to notify or correct errors, contribute their own observations and self-taken measurements to the record, communicate with their clinicians and book appointments (Winkelman, *et al.* 2005). Interaction will surely increase now that there is more general availability of devices suitable for operation by patients in their own home and that are capable of transmitting diagnostic or monitoring data (using Bluetooth or other wireless technologies). The incorporation in devices of standardised interfaces raises the real prospect that data can be sent directly from them into the EHR: for example, both Microsoft HealthVault and Google Health claim to have the capacity to accept data directly in this way. It will soon be possible for patients to procure an assortment of devices, connect them to their own EHR and share the information with providers of their choice. This truly patient-centred innovation of EHR-based telE-health could have the potential to transform the provision of healthcare, particularly to those with long-term conditions or who could then receive intermediate care in their own homes during recovery after discharge from hospital.

2 Coordination and integration of care

While the availability of comprehensive lifelong records is an essential component of patient-centred care, so too is the provision of services to support coordination of healthcare, particularly where care is provided across team or organisational boundaries. Perhaps the most important contribution that EHR systems can make in this regard is to support electronic communication between patients and their care providers, and among their care providers. At a person-to-person level this includes computer-initiated telephone calls, electronic mail, secure messaging sent from within ePHR and, more recently, instant messaging and SMS (these are discussed separately under communication). At a system-to-system level, structured messaging has become well established as a mechanism to share parts or even entire healthcare records. Various standards exist, although the most widely applied is HL7, for which definitions exist for clinical referrals, correspondence, laboratory requests and results and many other messages. XML messages have also been developed, for example to transmit the whole of a patient's EPR from one general practice system to another. One area in which considerable work remains to be done is in the support for inter-institutional workflow management.

In a survey of how healthcare services were understood and experienced by those using them, it was found that the majority were left dissatisfied and unclear about how their needs had been assessed and how services had been arranged. Some were dissatisfied to the point that they were compelled to become proactive in order to ensure that the care provided was adequate (Abbott, *et al.* 2001). Improving the integration of healthcare is evidently a key challenge for patient-centred care: efficient communication and workflow management throughout the patient pathway would be expected to improve the quality and outcome of shared care.

Workflow management systems are widely used to coordinate operational processes in many industries, both within and between businesses, but despite their potential to improve efficiency, quality and user-experience, there are few examples of their application in healthcare. Some institutional EPR systems use workflow management systems to support care pathways for hospitalised patients, but these are generally of a simple nature that allow little or no variation in the sequence of activities. Workflow support for care pathways has been extended into aftercare following discharge (Panzarasa, *et al.* 2002), but usually only where a single EPR has been deployed across primary, intermediate and secondary care. While it is reasonable to expect that workflow management across separate EPR systems would improve patient-centred care, particularly for those with long-term health conditions, such systems are yet to become established practice. Business to business (B2B) and business to customer (B2C) workflow management principles might be applicable to this domain, but there are as yet no standards for how this will be achieved in healthcare. An alternative approach might be to incorporate workflow into EHR systems so that care can be more effectively coordinated across multiple providers. Others have demonstrated the management of clinical workflow based on clinical computerised guidelines systems (Dazzi, *et al.* 1997).

Tailoring care pathways to the needs of individual patients and then coordinating their delivery across different providers is a complex task that is not well supported by the current generation of workflow management systems which are unable to anticipate exceptions and to accommodate dynamic reconfiguration (Klein, *et al.* 2000). Automated workflow is currently confined to supporting processes in the pathway that are stable, well defined and subject to little variation. An area of active development is in the support for ad hoc and adaptive workflows and how these can be assembled to achieve the overall workflow goals within human interaction management systems (Harrison-Broninski 2005). Too little attention has been given to socio-technical issues about the context in which individuals might interact with such systems, particularly with regard to fitting in with their other social activities and networks and how they manage information at home (Winkelman and Leonard 2004; Moen and Brennan 2005). One function that patients do find useful when offered in an EHR is the process for ordering of prescription refills. In the UK, general practitioners are now able to transmit an electronic prescription to a local community pharmacy. This can enhance patient-centred care where the patient is allowed to choose the most convenient pharmacy. In other countries, where the availability of medicines is less strictly controlled, patients can have their requests for prescriptions validated against their EHR and dispensed and delivered direct to their door by pharmaceutical suppliers. There is a potential benefit from allowing dispensing pharmacists to have access to at least a part of the patient's EHR: this would enable details of the product dispensed to be recorded in the EHR, accompanied by any relevant advice that the pharmacist might offer. It also allows the pharmacist to become a more active participant in the healthcare team.

The use of patient-held management plans that identify health problems, explain their causes, recommend actions to overcome them and outline long-term treatment plans and their goals improves compliance and the quality of shared care (Giglio and Papazian 1987; Mellins, *et al.* 2000). Such management plans should be made available to the patient to view through their access to the EHR. Provision of pre-consultation self-assessment questionnaires has also been found beneficial to shared care, improving relationship between patient and health professional and resulting in greater confidence and satisfaction among patients. Patients may prefer to divulge information and seek advice about sensitive or potentially embarrassing medical subjects through such a computerised interaction than by face-to-face discussion with a health professional. However, routine use of such questionnaires during consultations is likely to require significant changes in the physician's working and communication with the patient (Wald, *et al.* 1995). When combined with tailored advice that directed elderly patients to relevant sections of the National Institute on Aging's Age Pages, Wasson and colleagues found that patients felt that their care had improved (Wasson, *et al.* 1999).

Shared assessment is the overall process for identifying and recording the health and social care needs of an individual and for evaluating their impact on daily living and quality of life so that appropriate action can be agreed and planned with the individual. Assessments may be self-administered but are more often undertaken jointly by health and social care professionals in conjunction with the individual. The assessments are then shared between organisations to improve communication and to avoid duplication. Electronic single assessment process (eSAP) systems have been developed in the UK that offer a person-centred approach to health and social care assessment, care planning and review, that are integrated with electronic care records, offer seamless access to assessments and care plans wherever they have been carried out and support secure communication across organisational boundaries. eSAP was developed to support joint health and social care assessment of elderly clients; systems that support assessment for children, and for all adults services, have since been developed, that are based on a Common Assessment Framework (UK Department of Health 2006). These typically integrate multiple databases using service-oriented architectures and might be incorporated within an EHR system.

Despite their potential to improve communication between professionals, to provide seamless integration of health and social care services and to empower the individual, significant socio-technical challenges have been identified that threaten the vision of a standardised approach to shared assessments. More formalised and extended data collection takes more time to gather, detracts from the client relationship and compromises partnership working (Peckover, *et al.* 2008; White, *et al.* 2008). The systems have been designed more for the convenience of professionals than the individual, who can be disempowered as a result.

3 Accessibility and flexibility

In a seminal article on the Semantic Web, Tim Berners-Lee and colleagues described how intelligent software agents and the semantic web might improve the way that individuals negotiate and plan their life to accommodate important healthcare events (Berners-Lee, *et al.* 2001). The essence of the vision is that the individual has access to the necessary information and services; has a choice of time, location and even provider of care; and that healthcare provision is sufficiently flexible to enable negotiation of services to the individual's convenience. With the advent of technologies including the Internet and mobile telephony, service-oriented architectures and patient-accessible records, this vision is coming closer to realisation. However, it also requires healthcare providers to change their culture, organisation and processes to become more responsive to the needs of patients.

An important service to support patient-centred care is the provision of various types of scheduling to coordinate care, especially between multiple providers. Booking systems are now available that allow patients to select time and location of their appointments, not only within one institution, but across multiple providers. The UK NHS Choose and Book service is one such system that offers the patient a choice of service provider and time of appointment for referrals made by their general practitioner. This has been integrated with the NHS 'HealthSpace' ePHR being developed for all residents in England (www.HealthSpace.nhs.uk). Some general practices are offering their registered patients online facilities to book appointments through the practice EPR. Some ePHR, including HealthSpace, offer users a calendar facility in which they can record healthcare appointments and be reminded as the date approaches. These might be of even greater utility and convenience to the patient were they to be fully integrated with their personal calendars that hold all their other appointments. There might even be an advantage in patients choosing to share not only their PHR but also parts of their personal calendar with attending clinicians, so that future care can be planned around their existing life commitments.

Short telephoned reminders to patients to recommend a particular preventative care or an appointment have been found effective in improving compliance with treatments, higher patient satisfaction ratings, fewer missed appointments, reduction in inappropriate follow-up care, and improved attendance for screening (Balas, *et al.* 1997). Written reminders have been found to be more effective than telephone calls for cancer screening compliance, missed appointments, blood pressure screening and immunisation compliance, and automatically generated reminders to patients to attend outpatient clinics are increasingly being sent from EPR systems by e-mail or SMS messages (Balas, *et al.* 1996). Automated alerts have also been used to improve patient compliance with medication (Friedman, *et al.* 1996; Haynes, *et al.* 2000). There are potential disadvantages of automated advice and reminders: patients do not necessarily like being reminded of their risk of illness or advised about appropriate lifestyle changes (Meland, *et al.* 1996); and there is no automatic confirmation that the individual has received such messages.

4 Communication

Providing the patient with a printed summary of a consultation improves their understanding of their care, enhances their relationships with providers, improves satisfaction with care and motivation to comply with treatment plans (Tang and Newcomb 1998). This can be provided at the end of the consultation or soon afterwards, in the form of written notes, computer-generated reports or even audio tapes of consultations. In the UK NHS it is policy to provide to patients copies of all correspondence about them that have been sent from hospital doctors to their general practitioner. Better still, the patient can be given access to the computer-based notes if the consultation is recorded in the EPR since this would be expected to further improve communication and patient involvement.

Patients are increasingly expecting to communicate with their care providers through e-mail. Conventional Internet e-mail is vulnerable to interception and modification, and offers no robust means of authenticating the sender, nor for confirming the safe receipt and opening of messages. These shortcomings can, to a great extent, be circumvented by providing secure communication between patient and their clinicians as a function of the EHR. Patients see integrated messaging to be one of the most important benefits arising from their use of ePHR. It also avoids the potential ethical problems facing clinicians having to respond to unsolicited e-mail from a patient unknown to them and who therefore have no information upon which to base a response other than that provided by the correspondent (Spielberg 1998; Kuszler 2000). It remains to be seen whether it also dispels the concerns that doctors have about issues of liability, disruption of the delicate balance between patient and professional, and the potential flood of additional work that it might bring (Mandl, *et al.* 1998). However, there is growing professional recognition of its potential benefit to improve access to healthcare, let clinicians reach out to patients and increase patient involvement in their own care (Balas, *et al.* 1997; Borowitz and Wyatt 1998; Mandl, *et al.* 1998; Pal 1999).

5 Information and education

Provision of disease and health information to patients is an essential component of delivery of healthcare and preventative medicine, when it can be used to relay information, foster informed decision making, promote healthy behaviour, promote peer information exchange and emotional support, promote self-care and influence demand for health services (Robinson, *et al.* 1998). Increasingly, patients are searching for information about their health concerns on the Internet and may even be better informed than the healthcare professional with whom they are seeking a consultation. The provenance of such information obtained by trawling the Internet is frequently unknown and patients may be unable to distinguish high-quality evidence-based advice from opinion and quackery. For most patients, the limitations of personal knowledge about health problems or healthcare options compromise their ability to judge any decisions made about their health. They may also have a limited understanding of the differences between their own values and preferences and those of the health professionals they consult (UK Department of Health 2004). It is therefore beneficial to patients and providers that health information comes from a trusted source and is available in conjunction with access to their healthcare records.

Online resources such as the NHS National Library for Health and NHS Choices aim to provide accredited patient information, but this is not tailored to the needs of individuals. The Comprehensive Health Enhancement Support System (CHESS) developed by the University of Wisconsin-Madison (http://chess.wisc.edu/chess/home/home.aspx) provides users with up-to-date health information, software to help weigh treatment options, and 24-hour access to medical experts and other patients, all via an Internet connection from home (Gustafson, *et al.* 1992). Several specialist modules have been developed, including breast cancer, asthma, heart disease and HIV/AIDS. 'Information Prescriptions' tailored to the patient's needs either determined from the content of the person's record, or filtered by their preferences, are a useful feature within the ePHR.

While behavioural change can be induced through interactive healthcare systems, not all have been found successful, or have only short-term benefit (Balas, *et al.* 1997). However, applications that have combined health information with interactive role-playing and online support groups have been successful in promoting behaviour change (Alemi 1998). There might be benefit in incorporating such facilities within EHR systems.

6 Autonomy and empowerment

A supportive relationship between healthcare professionals and patients is fundamental to patient-centred care (WHO 2004). At the heart of this relationship is the joint consultation in which patient and clinician work in partnership to develop a common understanding of the patient's values, preferences and needs, and work towards the common goals of optimum healing and recovery. Co-authorship between patient and practitioner is an effective way of conveying more complete, accurate and mutually understandable information and leads to both becoming 'co-producers of quality' in health (Kaplan and Brennan 2001). Many of the features of EHR systems discussed above, and of Internet-based services in general, encourage this joint working and thereby increase autonomy and empower the patient. They also allow consumers to take on a more active role in their healthcare (van Woerkum 2003).

Adapting clinical decision support systems for use by patients may bring major benefits. However, systems providing advice on treatment or lifestyle will need to take into account not only scientific evidence, patient history and local constraints in availability and delivery of care, but also be sensitive to patients' preferences regarding lifestyle and outcomes (Barry 1999; Brennan and Strombom 1998; Leydon, *et al.* 2000). An additional facility provided by ePHR and other Internet services is the ability for patients to create self-help groups and to contact others with the same medical concerns. These may be as informal as simple 'chat rooms', take the form of moderated or unregulated e-mail discussion groups, or groups on social networking sites. Consumer websites have developed support communities whereby patients with the same clinical problem (such as depression or pregnancy) can contact each other and provide mutual support (e.g. www.netdoctor.co.uk and www.surgerydoor.co.uk). Individuals find it helpful for access to such social networks to be provided through the ePHR.

CONCLUSION

Patient-centred care supported by effective ICT systems is still far from widespread: there are many challenges still to be overcome before the vision of the patient at the centre of the healthcare system can be realised (*see* Figure 6.1).

A compelling business case for implementation of EPR, EHR and ePHR still needs

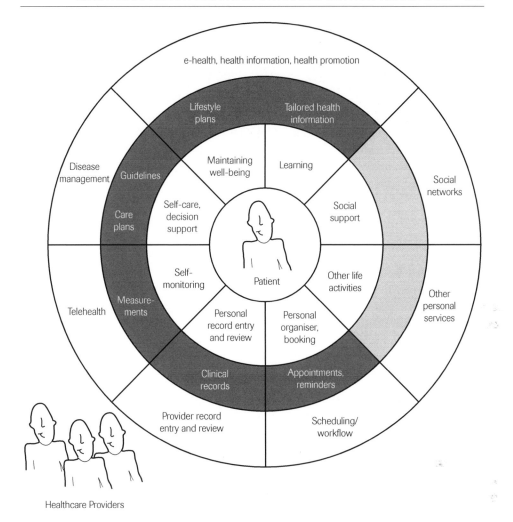

FIGURE 6.1 The patient at the centre of a healthcare system

to be made: more evidence is required from properly designed trials before their real costs and benefits can be established (Walker 2005; Clamp and Keen 2007). Healthcare providers will need to record their clinical notes in EPR systems, a practice that is still uncommon, and then will need to agree to share them with the patients' ePHR system. Vendors of EPR systems will need to agree standards for record interchange and provide suitable interfaces to enable on-demand transfer of records to the ePHR. A means to securely authenticate the identity of individuals making subscription requests will be necessary. While surveys have indicated that the majority of the public would like access to their records, evidence from studies where patients have been offered access suggests that only those with long-term conditions or who have frequent calls upon the existing health services become regular users of ePHR. It remains to be seen whether many individuals are sufficiently motivated or capable of maintaining their own records in these new platforms – experience with early PHRs would suggest that they are not without some assistance from an intermediary to help with the subscription process. There are also concerns that several patient groups, including the poor, elderly or disabled, will be disenfranchised if care shifts to being based on ePHR, thereby deepening the 'digital divide'.

The prospect of greater involvement of patients in their healthcare through the use of ePHR will be realised only if accompanied by changes to the way that health-care is provided. There will need to be greater flexibility; willingness to accommodate patients' needs and preferences, including time and location of care delivery; and openness of clinicians to embrace this focus. There is a wide range of opinions among health professionals about the degree to which patients may be involved in their consultation and care, from protective paternalism, through enlightened self-interest towards a more egalitarian relationship (Elwyn, *et al.* 1999). Willingness to share records with patients, accept the entries they make in them, and to cede con-trol over access to them has been slow to develop and experience from early PHR systems suggests that several key questions remain (Halamka, *et al.* 2008). The very term 'patient-centred care' implies a healthcare provider perspective on the health and care of individuals. Individuals have a far broader interest about their health, well-being and care than merely that offered by healthcare providers. They spend the majority of their life engaged in activities other than healthcare, so naturally are more interested in how care can fit in with their other life needs. This has a pro-found impact on how systems to support patient-centred care are designed: much greater emphasis should in future be given to designing systems around the needs and activities of the patient rather than modelling them on systems intended for care providers.

Concerns over security of Internet-based records abound among the public, patients and healthcare professions. Many countries now have legislation (e.g. Data Protection Acts in Europe and HIPAA in the US) that requires a high standard of protection of health records. ePHR systems should now all be provided with security controls at least as effective as those protecting Internet banking services (security of which the public value more highly than that of their health records). While threats of security breach remain, these are more likely to come from bona fide users of the system than from those attempting to gain unlawful access. There is of course a bal-ance to be struck between the risk of security breach and the benefit that an accessible and shared record can have. Patients with long-term conditions, who have more to gain from using ePHR, are less concerned about security of their record than are the general public.

These challenges are being gradually overcome. Over the past few decades there have been many technological innovations that have each made incremental steps towards patient-centred care: patient-held records of care and management plans; information prescriptions and wellness advice; devices for home monitoring; broad-band network access to homes; Internet services, search engines, social networking and consumer health information sites; Web 2.0, Health 2.0 and Service Oriented Architectures; EPR, ePHR and EHR systems; standards for data interchange; and smart mobile telephony. None of these advances alone has brought about a transformation in the delivery of healthcare but, by building upon them all, the latest generation of ePHR (such as Indivo, Microsoft HealthVault, Google Health) have the disruptive potential to bring about a truly patient-centred healthcare system (Mandl and Kohane 2008). They enable individuals to compile their own lifelong records, stored on the Internet, which are separate but importing data from healthcare provider EPRs and under their own control. The records provide a platform upon which a variety of services can be offered, such as wellness advice, clinical decision aids, disease management tools, and interfaces to consumer healthcare devices.

This personally controlled, platform-based ePHR uses a subscription model whereby individuals assert a claim and request data to be transferred from each of the EPR holding records about them. This removes any reliance on centrally managed data-sharing agreements and networks that are necessary in the otherwise similar 'health records bank' (Ball and Gold 2007). High cost, uncertain business case and complexity of implementation (especially in ensuring security and interoperability) are significant barriers to the formation of health records banks based on such centrally managed networks, even when sponsored by regional or national regulators (Adler-Milstein, *et al.* 2008).

The critical advantage of the personally controlled ePHR model, the one most likely to make this a disruptive innovation, is that the individual, not the health provider, can now make the choice of ePHR system that best suits his or her needs and preferences. Patients with long-term conditions, who are currently dependent on a variety of healthcare providers to monitor and advise on their care, will be early beneficiaries. They will be in a position to adopt a system that, for the first time, puts them in control of their own healthcare, supports home-based monitoring, provides tailored information and advice, allows them to integrate the records from their various care providers, and to share them with whom they choose to plan and coordinate their own care. By creating an open platform upon which services may be offered by many different vendors, one can envisage individuals at last being given an unprecedented choice of applications through which to take greater control over, and feel at the centre of, their healthcare.

REFERENCES

Abbott S, Johnson L, Lewis H. Participation in arranging continuing health care packages: experiences and aspirations of service users. *J Nurs Manage.* 2001; 9: 79–85.

Adler-Milstein J, McAfee AP, Bates DW, *et al.* The state of regional health information organizations: current activities and financing. *Health Aff.* 2008; 27: w60–69.

Alemi F. Virtual managed care organizations: the implications of technology based patient management. *Am J Manag Care.* 1998; 4: 415–18.

ASTM. *Specification for Continuity of Care Record, E2369–05.* West Conshohocken, PA: ASTM International; 2006.

Balas EA, Austin SM, Mitchell JA, *et al.* The clinical value of computerized information services. A review of 98 randomized clinical trials. *Arch Fam Med.* 1996; 5: 271–8.

Balas EA, Jaffrey F, Kuperman GJ, *et al.* Electronic communication with patients: evaluation of distance medicine technology. *JAMA.* 1997; 278: 152–9.

Ball MJ, Gold J. Banking on health: personal records and information exchange. *J Health Inf Manage.* 2007; 20: 71–83.

Barry MJ. Involving patients in medical decisions: how can physicians do better? *JAMA.* 1999; 282: 2356–7.

Berners-Lee T, Hendler J, Lassila O. The semantic web: a new form of web content that is meaningful to computers will unleash a revolution of new possibilities. *Sci Am.* 2001; 284(5).

Borowitz SM, Wyatt JC. The origin, content, and workload of e-mail consultations. *JAMA.* 1998; 280: 1321–4.

Brennan PF. Health informatics and community health: support for patients as collaborators in care. *Methods Inform Med.* 1999; 38: 274–8.

Brennan PF, Strombom I. Improving health care by understanding patient preferences: the role of computer technology. *J Am Med Inform Assoc.* 1998; 5: 257–62.

Cheung N-T, Fung V, Wong WN, *et al.* Principles-based medical informatics for success: how Hong Kong built one of the world's largest integrated longitudinal electronic patient records. *Medinfo.* 2007; 12: 307–10.

Cimino JJ, Patel VL, Kushniruk AW. The patient clinical information system (PatCIS): technical solutions for and experiences with giving patients access to their electronic medical records. *Int J Med Inform.* 2002; 68: 113–27.

Clamp S, Keen J. Electronic health records: is the evidence base any use? *Med Inform Internet Med.* 2007; 32: 5–10.

Connecting for Health. *Connecting Americans to their Healthcare. Final Report of the Working Group on Policies for Electronic Information Sharing Between Doctors and Patients.* Markle Foundation; 2004. Available at: www.connectingforhealth.org/resources/final_phwg_report1.pdf

Dazzi L, Fassino C, Saracco R, Quaglini S, Stefanelli M. A patient workflow management system built on guidelines. *Proceedings of AMIA Annual Fall Symposium.* 1997; 146–50.

de Clercq PA, Hasman A, Wolffenbuttel BH. Design of a consumer health record for supporting the patient-centered management of chronic diseases. *Medinfo.* 2001; 10: 1445–9.

Detmer MD, Steen MA. *Learning from Abroad: lessons and questions on personal health records for national policy.* Washington DC: American Association for Retired Persons (AARP) Public Policy Institute; 2006.

Elwyn G, Edwards A, Gwyn R, *et al.* Towards a feasible model for shared decision making: focus group study with general practice registrars. *BMJ.* 1999; 319: 753–6.

Fisher B, Fitton R, Poirier C, Stables D. Patient record access – the time has come! *Br J Gen Pract.* 2007; 57: 507–11.

Friedman RH, Kazis LE, Jette A, *et al.* A telecommunications system for monitoring and counseling patients with hypertension: impact on medication adherence and blood pressure control. *Am J Hypertens.* 1996; 9: 285–92.

Gerteis M, Edgman-Levitan S, Daley J, *et al.*, editors. *Through the Patient's Eyes: understanding and promoting patient-centred care.* San Francisco, CA: Jossey-Bass; 1993.

Giglio RJ, Papazian B. Acceptance and use of patient-carried health records. *J Am Med Rec Assoc.* 1987; 58: 32–6.

Gillespie R, Florin D, Gillam S. How is patient-centred care understood by the clinical, managerial and lay stakeholders responsible for promoting this agenda? *Health Expect.* 2004; 7: 142–8.

Greenhalgh T, Stramer K, Bratan T, *et al. Summary Care Record Early Adopter programme: an independent evaluation by University College London.* London: University College; 2008. Available at: www.ucl.ac.uk/openlearning/research

Gustafson DH, Bosworth K, Hawkins RP, *et al.* CHESS: a computer-based system for providing information, referrals, decision support and social support to people providing medical and other health-related crises. *Proceedings of the Annual Symposium on Computer Applications in Medical Care.* 1992; 161–5.

Halamka JD, Aranow M, Ascenzo C, *et al.* Health care IT collaboration in Massachusetts: the experience of creating regional connectivity. *J Am Med Inform Assoc.* 2005; 12: 596–601.

Halamka JD, Mandl KD, Tang PC. Early experiences with personal health records. *J Am Med Inform Assoc.* 2008; 15: 1–7.

Harrison-Broninski K. *Human interactions: the heart and soul of business process management.* Tampa, FL: Meghan-Kiffer Press; 2005.

Haynes RB, Montague P, Oliver T, *et al.* Interventions for helping patients to follow prescriptions for medications (Cochrane Review). *The Cochrane Library.* Issue 3. Oxford: Update Software; 2000.

International Alliance of Patients' Organizations. *What is Patient-centred Healthcare? A review of definitions and principles,* 2nd ed. London: IAPO; 2007. Available at: www.patientsorganizations.org

Kaplan B, Brennan PF. Consumer informatics supporting patients as co-producers of quality. *J Am Med Inform Assoc.* 2001; 8: 309–16.

Kim MI, Johnson KB. Personal health records: evaluation of functionality and utility. *J Am Med Inform Assoc.* 2002; 9: 171–80.

Kirby BJ. Patient access to medical records. *J R Coll Physicians Lond.* 1991; 25: 240–2.

Klein M, Dellarocas C, Bernstein A. Introduction to the special issue on adaptive workflow systems. *Comp Support Coop Work.* 2000; 9(3/4): 265–7.

Kuszler PC. A question of duty: common law legal issues resulting from physician response to unsolicited patient email inquiries. *J Med Internet Res.* 2000; 2: e17.

Leydon GM, Boulton M, Moynihan C, *et al.* Cancer patients' information needs and information seeking behaviour: in-depth interview study. *BMJ.* 2000; 320: 909–13.

Mandl KD, Kohane IS. Tectonic shifts in the health information economy. *N Engl J Med.* 2008; 358: 1732–7.

Mandl KD, Kohane IS, Brandt AM. Electronic patient-physician communication: problems and promise. *Ann Intern Med.* 1998; 129: 495–500.

Mandl KD, Simons WW, Crawford WCR, *et al.* Indivo: a personally controlled health record for health information exchange and communication. *BMC Med Inform Decis Mak.* 2007; 7: 25.

Meland E, Laerum E, Maeland JG. Lifestyle intervention in general practice: effects on psychological well-being and patient satisfaction. *Qual Life Res.* 1996; 5: 348–54.

Mellins RB, Evans D, Clark N, *et al.* Developing and communicating a long-term treatment plan for asthma. *Am Fam Physician.* 2000; 61: 2419–28, 2433–4.

Moen A, Brennan PF. Health@Home: the work of health information management in the household (HIMH): implications for consumer health informatics (CHI) innovations. *J Am Med Inform Assoc.* 2005; 12: 648–56.

Pagliari C, Detmer D, Singleton P. Potential of electronic personal health records. *BMJ.* 2007; 335: 330–3.

Pal B. Email contact between doctor and patient. *BMJ.* 1999; 318: 1428.

Panzarasa S, Madde S, Quaglini S, *et al.* Evidence-based careflow management systems: the case of post-rehabilitation. *J Biomed Inform.* 2002; 35: 123–39.

Peckover S, Hall C, White S. From policy to practice: the implementation and negotiation of technologies in everyday child welfare. *Child Soc.* 2008. 23(2): 136–48.

Pyper C, Amery J, Watson M, *et al.* Patients' experiences when accessing their online electronic patient records in primary care. *Br J Gen Pract.* 2004; 54: 38–43.

Ralston JD, Carrell D, Reid R, *et al.* Patient web services integrated with a shared medical record: patient use and satisfaction. *J Am Med Inform Assoc.* 2007; 14: 798–806.

Robinson TN, Patrick K, Eng TR, *et al.* An evidence-based approach to interactive health communication. *JAMA.* 1998; 280: 1264–9.

Ross SE, Lin CT. The effects of promoting patient access to medical records: a review. *J Am Med Inform Assoc.* 2003; 10: 129–38.

Schneider JH. Online personal medical records: are they reliable for acute/critical care? *Critical Care Med.* 2001; 29: N196–201.

Shabo A. A global socio-economic-medico-legal model for the sustainability of longitudinal electronic health records – part 2. *Methods Inf Med.* 2006; 45: 498–505.

Spielberg AR. On call and online: sociohistorical, legal and ethical implications of e-mail for the patient-physician relationship. *JAMA.* 1998; 280: 1353–9.

Tang PC, Ash JS, Bates DW, *et al.* Personal health records: definitions, benefits, and strategies for overcoming barriers to adoption. *J Am Med Inform Assoc.* 2006; 13: 121–6.

Tang PC, Lansky D. The missing link: bridging the patient–provider health information gap. Electronic personal health records could transform the patient–provider relationship in the twenty-first century. *Health Aff.* 2005; 24: 1290–5.

Tang PC, Newcomb C. Informing patients: a guide for providing patient health information. *J Am Med Inform Assoc.* 1998; 5: 563–70.

UK Department of Health. *Patient and Public Involvement in Health: the evidence for policy implementation.* London: UK Department of Health; 2004.

UK Department of Health. *Our Health, Our Care, Our Say: a new direction for community services.* London: UK Department of Health; 2006. Available at: www.official-documents.gov.uk/document/cm67/6737/6737.pdf

USAID, cited in WHO European Observatory Glossary, 1999. Available at: www.euro.who.int/observatory/Glossary/TopPage?phrase=P

van Woerkum CM. The Internet and primary care physicians: coping with different expectations. *Am J Clin Nutr.* 2003; 77(Suppl.): S1016–18.

Wald JS, Middleton B, Bloom A, *et al.* A patient-controlled journal for an electronic medical record: issues and challenges. *Medinfo.* 2004; 11: 1166–70.

Wald JS, Rind D, Safran C, *et al.* Patient entries in the electronic medical record: an interactive interview used in primary care. *Proceedings of the Annual Symposium on Computer Applications in Medical Care.* 1995; 147–51.

Walker JM. Electronic medical records and health care transformation. *Health Aff.* 2005; 24: 1118–20.

Wasson JH, Stukel TA, Weiss JE, *et al.* A randomized trial of the use of patient self-assessment data to improve community practices. *Effective Clin Pract.* 1999; 2: 1–10.

White S, Hall C, Peckover S. The descriptive tyranny of the common assessment framework: technologies of categorization and professional practice in child welfare. *Br J Soc Work*. Advance Access, 16 April 2008.

Winkelman WJ, Leonard KJ. Overcoming structural constraints to patient utilization of electronic medical records: a critical review and proposal for an evaluation framework. *J Am Med Inform Assoc*. 2004; 11: 151–61.

Winkelman WJ, Leonard KJ, Rossos PG. Patient-perceived usefulness of online electronic medical records: employing grounded theory in the development of information and communication technologies for use by patients living with chronic illness. *J Am Med Inform Assoc*. 2005; 12: 306–14.

World Health Organization. *General Principles of Good Chronic Care*. Geneva: WHO; 2004. Available at: www.who.int/3by5/publications/documents/en/generalprinciples 082004.pdf

CHAPTER 7

Integrating electronic health records

Wendy Currie, David Finnegan and Khairil Azhar Abdul Hamid

INTRODUCTION

The purpose of this chapter is to review and summarise the known approaches reported in the literature specifically concerning the integration of electronic health-care records (EHRs). This is motivated by a desire to integrate complex healthcare information systems with a view to improving process and service optimisation. EHRs are viewed as the emerging linchpin in the chain of integrated and seamless healthcare services that aim to place the patient at the centre of the system of care. This section begins with a scene-setting primer regarding the position and role of the medical record and its relation to the developments in electronic health records in the system of clinical care. This is followed by an exposition and analysis of the contributions towards strategies and approaches aimed at achieving integrated care through the adoption of the EHR from the literature base. To aid comparison and clarity, the same heuristic lens is used to categorise these approaches and draw out similarity and themes extracted from the previous review of the healthcare IS integration literature. The aim is to develop a typology that will aid the organisation of knowledge of the subject and further advance discussion of the topic.

FROM PAPER MEDICAL RECORDS TO ELECTRONIC HEALTH RECORDS

The precursor to the EHR is the paper-based patient-centred medical record that was pioneered in the early 20th century (Grimson 2001) and is still widely used today. Although the medical record may serve as a history of a patient's medical condition prior to contact with a healthcare provider, and as a log of changing health conditions as diagnosis and treatment progress, there is no universally standard definition. Carcinero, *et al.* (2005) define the ideal clinical record as the sum total of an individual's clinical history available to any healthcare professional responsible for that person's care. This, however, is a somewhat narrow definition. Grimson (2001) takes a more pragmatic and realistic view that the medical record can be structured in a myriad of ways and has further evolved to incorporate functions that have exceeded its original purpose.

The medical record is also recognised as a means of communicating information about patients between healthcare personnel, as a source of clinical research data for epidemiological study, to provide medico-legal substantiation, and to support administrative and financial operations (Grimson 2001). The medical record is thus a critical component for recording and retrieving information about patients within the healthcare system and also plays an external role. Grimson (2001) argues that the need to manage complex data, while maintaining flexibility for a range of potential uses, presents an impediment to the computerisation of the medical record both on a technical and organisational level. Other studies seem to support this view. Jensen and Aanestad (2007) in a study of Danish hospital surgical wards noted that doctors and nurses forego the use of certain EHR functionality when doing so becomes awkward to incorporate within work routines or when the technology cannot fit the task. This was also highlighted elsewhere by Finnegan and Currie (2008) in a primary care case study where the users (pharmacies) of the technologies relinquished the use of technology and went back to using their personal know-how. Davidson and Heslinga (2007) in a study of US-based primary care practices found doctors reluctant to adopt EHRs, not least because a highly fragmented EHR software market made it difficult for them to acquire a solution able to interface with other electronic information systems required for their practices. Here market-based, technical and organisational factors present barriers to adoption.

These examples show that the complexity of activities in healthcare coupled with the perceived inflexibilities of EHRs make adoption challenging. While not all barriers are the same, given the diversity in global healthcare systems, the complications in integrating the use of EHRs within and between healthcare providers will continue to be challenging. The challenges of EHR adoption, integration and assimilation are therefore numerous. Technical challenges include, for example: difficulty in aggregating existing patient information from fragmented and heterogeneous information systems that often only have data of little clinical value (Grimson, et al. 2000); compatibility issues between existing legacy systems and newly adopted EHR systems (Cross 2004); and lack of standardised data exchange protocols due to fragmented product offerings (Davidson and Heslinga 2007).

No less daunting are the non-technical hurdles. Ensuring that organisational processes are capable of coordinating information between healthcare personnel will continue to be a significant challenge (Grimson 2001). Concerns regarding patient confidentiality (Hendy, et al. 2007) and information governance will also persist. It is widely noted that adoption of electronic healthcare records remains low (Cross 2004; Davidson and Heslinga 2007; Hennington and Janz 2007).

ROLE OF ELECTRONIC HEALTHCARE RECORD IN INTEGRATED CARE

In the light of the issues surrounding EHRs, what then makes their adoption compelling and necessary for healthcare service improvement? In the face of rising demand for more choice and quality in healthcare, the paper-based medical record has severe limitations. It is not easily shared, it is centred upon the institutional boundaries of individual healthcare organisations, it may lack comprehensive medical information concerning the history of treatment given by separate healthcare providers, its information may not be presented in the views and contexts appropriate for different or overlapping clinical needs, it may be vulnerable to errors, it may lack interoperability with other information systems, be restricted in its ability to scale with growing complexity of medical multimedia data (e.g. MRI scans, CT scans, etc.) and it is amenable only to slow manual processing (Grimson, *et al.* 2000; Grimson 2001; Carnicero, *et al.* 2005).

EHRs endeavour to address these limitations through the capabilities of modern ICTs by: enabling clinical information sharing and flows between healthcare bodies, providing a single lifelong record centred on the patient that allows easy aggregation of information from separate episodes of care from different institutions, allowing information to be presented in ways relevant to immediate clinical needs, facilitating technical measures that reduce errors by eliminating manual processes and allowing connections to other clinical information systems and media repositories such as electronic prescriptions and clinical guideline systems (Grimson, *et al.* 2000; Grimson 2001; Carnicero, *et al.* 2005). An example is the health information management needs of the UK NHS. In 2004 there were 650 million drug prescriptions dispensed, nearly 5.5 million individuals admitted to hospital for planned treatment and 4.3 million admissions for emergency treatment. In addition, the NHS in England serves a patient population of approximately 50 million people (NHS Connecting for Health 2005). EHRs can potentially streamline the processes behind those transactions and enable capabilities that were not available before.

APPROACHES IN EHR ADOPTION AND INTEGRATION

Strategic approaches to the EHR are by and large aligned with the general strategies of healthcare IS. As EHRs are considered the central platform by which integrated care is achieved, EHRs are seen as the enablers towards strategic integration of healthcare IS. One recurrent strategic prescription for the integration of EHRs has been that EHRs should be considered as evolutionary changes (McDonald 1997; Wainwright and Waring 2000; Tsiknakis, *et al.* 2002) to allow healthcare organisations to adapt to the pace of change and avoid disruptive change. For example, Tsiknakis, *et al.* (2002) see this from a technical perspective and believe that the integrated federation of the EHR on a national or regional scale of integration can only happen evolutionarily in the light of the great diversity of systems and standards already in place – a loosely coupled systems integration approach.

A review of the technically oriented EHR literature shows a fairly broad agreement that the integration of EHRs should adopt systems integration approaches based on federated linkages between cooperating information systems. Whereas other clinical systems and financial administrative systems may benefit from a centralised control of resources and processes – for example, within a monolithic enterprise systems approach (Wainwright and Waring 2000) – this does not immediately appear viable for the purposes of electronic medical record systems. It is the predominant belief that EHRs should be approached from a systems integration viewpoint because of the widespread heterogeneous, autonomous and distributed nature – exemplified by differing structures, levels of granularity, and coding systems (McDonald 1997) – of healthcare IS systems and databases that are the critical source for much of the data and functionality afforded to EHR systems (e.g. Grimson 2000; Grimson, *et al.* 2001; Tsiknakis, *et al.* 2002; Carcinero, *et al.* 2005; Khoumbati, *et al.* 2006).

This is a logically acceptable assertion when considered against what a huge undertaking it would be to attempt to consolidate numerous disparate systems into a monolithic enterprise system especially in the context of multi-institutional, multi-regional or national efforts in achieving integrated EHRs employing an enterprise resource planning (ERP) approach. The barriers and impediments of starting from a fresh base would be prohibitively expensive and disruptive for many healthcare organisations and governments as differences in legacy systems may be too great to integrate within a single enterprise system.

It is also worth mentioning hybridised alternatives that combine features of the federated and centralised integrated systems ERP approach. For example, enterprise data warehousing (EDW) as a common architecture approach may at first appear to offer a strong advantage as it precisely fulfils the requirements of complex aggregation, combination and structuring of disparate patient data elements from a number of heterogeneous, distributed and autonomous systems into data that conforms to a pre-defined singular format within a single repository while allowing continued autonomy of those systems and their continued independent use of existing proprietary data formats (Grimson, *et al.* 2000; Carcinero, *et al.* 2005; Turban, *et al.* 2008). The strengths of its design are, however, hampered by arduous technical and organisational requirements: complicated and time-consuming data extraction, transformation and loading procedures as well as a necessity for highly expert personnel make it difficult to frequently update data and keep it consistent (Turban, *et al.* 2008). It is ultimately these constraints that limit the ability of EDWs to be deployed as a real-time operational system that is required of patient record systems (Grimson, *et al.* 2000).

EDWs, however, as noted by Raghupathi (2002), Raghupathi and Tan (2002) and Southard, *et al.* (2000), remain strategically important IS for other clinical and administrative needs, for example as decision support systems that analyse historical data for population-centred epidemiological purposes and therefore do not require real-time operational functionality. EHR integration from a technical standpoint is therefore far more constrained in terms of standard choices in systems-based methods, and while enterprise systems or data warehouses do not in most cases present viable choices, the options left do not necessarily guarantee success or ease of deployment.

FEDERATION OF ELECTRONIC HEALTHCARE RECORDS: INTER-SYSTEMS COMMUNICATIONS VS. COMMON ARCHITECTURE FEDERATION

If we accept the premise that the federated approach is the preferred path for the systems integration of integrated health records, for which there is strong evidence to support it, what is the best option for integration? Federation means, at its most basic, the sharing of data and, at an extended level, sharing of integrated processes or services (Tsiknakis, *et al.* 2002). This raises the issue of the need to tightly couple federated systems. McDonald (1997), for example, favours the inter-systems communication approach achieved through systems interfaces, constructed from such standardised healthcare messaging protocols as HL7 or DICOM, but his reasoning has more to do with achieving greater penetration of EHR technology within healthcare organisations than with any technical superiority. In fact, we know that this approach provides only basic communication of data and hence lower functionality and affordances than competing approaches. At best it is able to combine information from disparate systems and provide unified views of patient record data collated from different clinical IS and administrative systems and achieves only functional data integration (Carcinero, *et al.* 2005).

The premise of McDonald's (1997) argument is that the emphasis on EHR architectures and self-contained integrated systems has failed to develop and be deployed quickly enough; hence, as a bridging measure, message-based communication methods should be considered as a first stage of an evolutionary approach. Rigby, *et al.* (2007) have more recently expressed similar sentiments under almost identical reasoning and propose the viability of current generation Internet brokering engines as a solution to support EHR user demands. While the prospect is feasible, there are, however, potentially severe limitations to this approach. McDonald (1997) claims that this approach is useful for a healthcare organisation aiming for multi-site integration, but he neglects to address its applicability in inter-organisational integration, that which represents the true strategic value of EHR integration initiatives, and for which agreement of acceptable standards are notoriously difficult to procure. This apparent advantage for ease of implementation can be disputed. Furthermore, the realities that basic messaging approaches are not scalable throw their long-term viability in doubt. Rigby, *et al.* (2007) admit that semantic interoperability concerns are a critical issue, and while efforts are being made, the maturity of their approach is still at the early stages. This suggests that the strategic and organisational formulas for full-fledged integrated EHRs are underdeveloped.

COMMON ARCHITECTURE: DATA, APPLICATION AND PROCESS INTEGRATION

Would simpler measures proposed by McDonald (1997) or Rigby (2007) further perpetuate the continued and recurrent problem of healthcare IS fragmentation? Such short-term strategies can be argued to lead to further piecemeal, uncoordinated and non-unified solutions in healthcare IS which will perpetuate the cycle of fragmented adoption. It can also be argued that smaller evolutionary steps will better prepare healthcare organisations for future tightly integrated EHR systems by providing much needed learning experiences. For example, even Grimson (2001) appears to revise her earlier views on federation (*see* Grimson, *et al.* 2000) by suggesting that technological debates are pointless, bearing in mind that cross-institutional EHR integration has been lacklustre overall, inferring that immediate goals should build critical mass and broad adoption, much like McDonald (1997). However, Grimson (2001: 118) eventually concedes, 'simply exchanging standard EDI (electronic data interchange) messages is not a long-term solution'. Carcinero, *et al.* (2005) and Tsiknakis, *et al.* (2002) state that the architecture of the EHR must be standardised and therefore proponents of the inter-systems communications position hold the minority view in this debate.

For the universally shareable EHR, the common architecture or model approach is the one favoured by most observers. The strengths of these approaches are in part derived not only from a formally structured and managed systems architecture approach based on agreed technical standards, but as Tsiknakis, *et al.* (2002) note, it is because these approaches also mandate complementary organisational measures in the form of integrated standardised processes, common principles, partnerships and best practices. It does not, however, furnish or provide those measures and so there is also a risk that common architecture approaches will fail without them in place. Common architecture approaches, importantly, afford a sophistication that is more able to be inclusive to the needs of organisational changes and social factors that are critical to the successful adoption and use of EHR and EHR-linked systems.

Ciccarese, *et al.* (2005) report on work developing clinical integration between EHRs and clinical decision support systems that merges patient-specific data with medical protocol knowledge that support clinician diagnosis and treatment. A federated approach was unavoidable, as the authors needed to integrate with heterogeneous systems components and, in particular, legacy systems. An architectural approach was necessary to enable not only the ability to scale, but to enable the construction of a more sophisticated system that intelligently mediates clinical knowledge requirements based on user types. The architectural approach, based on the software engineering precept the Separation of Concerns, formalises both the technical and human interaction aspects of skills and experience within the system. Purely communications-based integration would not so easily be able to model complex organisational and social processes.

Common architecture approaches can be served by commercial application integration engines (also known as EAI tools) as mentioned earlier, although bespoke architectures may be developed to address specialised application integration requirements when needed (e.g. Tsiknakis, *et al.* 2002; Ciccarese, *et al.* 2005). Application integration or EAI has emerged to overcome integration problems at data and process level in healthcare (Khoumbati, *et al.* 2006) by abstracting implementation of shared functions and services, and allowing greater scalability and ease of modification through the use of components (Carnicero, *et al.* 2005).

However, according to an empirical study conducted by Khoumbati, *et al.* (2006) on an EHR integration project at an NHS hospital, the main obstacles to application integration or EAI approaches reported by hospital staff were not technical in nature. Great efforts were needed to garner acceptance from clinical stakeholders and employees that required educating users. Efforts were hampered because of the low levels of organisational learning and experience with the technology as well as the lack of any formal appraisal or evaluation methods to demystify the great number of commercial products adhering to many separate non-interoperable standards. Grimson (2001) similarly observes that organisational and cultural issues present significant impediments to EHR integration. While federated systems integration techniques and common architectural approaches resolve many of the physical and logical data, process and application integration problems related to EHRs mean that organisational change requirements must be confronted as well.

ORGANISATIONAL AND SOCIAL APPROACHES TO THE EHR

In contrast to the technical and systems approaches, the literature concerning organisational and social methodologies towards the integration of EHRs have had less focused attention from the researcher and practitioner communities. Generalist prescriptions of organisational-technology alignment and best practices that accompany the technical-systems literature (e.g. BPR in Grimson 2001; principles, best practices, partnerships, legislation in Tsiknakis, *et al.* 2002) do not necessarily address the vagaries of EHR-based integration or distinguish finely enough its differences with other forms of healthcare IS. Even so, more substantive organisational and social-oriented integration research on EHRs has only recently emerged, and the limited number of studies in the area further underscores that our acceptance of the applicability of some of these findings can only be tentative.

We observe methodological gaps in applying effective organisational strategies for EHR integration purposes. Theoretical approaches and frameworks to understanding the complex social processes and changes that occur during EHR implementation, which may be used as tools for intervention, raise questions about the practicalities for application in a highly complex organisational and social environment. Clearly, any potential solution needs to be operationalised in a resource-constrained organisation, so an appreciation of the relationship between social and technical factors in the integration of EHRs is critical.

Whereas healthcare IS integration approaches exhibit certain categorical features which can be classified under various headings – organisational and social structure, organisational learning and culture, organisational capabilities, and user-oriented strategies – the literature on EHR adoption and integration can also be classified in the same way. This is not to rigidly compartmentalise the literature into narrow classifications, but to recognise the complexity and diversity of themes, topics and approaches. Our intention is to set out a better way of recognising and organising the common elements of these approaches as well as providing a means to compare EHR integration strategies with the general healthcare IS literature. As it is not possible to review all the approaches in depth, we have selected some examples to illustrate the key elements of such strategies.

EHR INTEGRATION AND ORGANISATIONAL STRATEGIES: MANAGING KNOWLEDGE, CAPABILITIES AND PEOPLE

The literature suggests that organisational strategies towards EHR integration are most concerned with the humanistic aspects of technological integration. Those with an organisational and user-based perspective dispute the assumptions of the strategic and technical systems camps that EHRs are largely unproblematic in their capability to afford seamless, automated and high quality healthcare process efficiencies and capabilities. They caution that the sought after benefits of integration must be tempered by the knowledge of organisational inter-workings that operate according to a very different set of dynamics and which are far more unpredictable than what technical systemisation and standardisation attempts to bracket, direct and control.

Hersh (2002), for example, notes that the success of EHR integration is highly dependent upon the usability of the systems themselves, defined as how well it is integrated with clinical workflow and activities, that must demonstrate value if continued patronage of users is to be expected. Berg (2001) describes this as matching system functionalities with organisational working patterns and that the failure to link the two often contributes to failure of such initiatives.

Makoul, *et al.* (2001), for example, compared two groups of physicians: one using desk-based EHR systems in their consultations with patients and one that did not. The EHR-using physicians tended to lessen the amount of interpersonal interaction with patients, as they were mostly concerned with keying information into the system and actually accomplished far fewer clinical tasks than the physicians who were EHR-less. They were given no specific training or guidance on how to simultaneously communicate with patients and use the system as a tool. This resulted in their lower levels of patient-centred activities as well as increased consultation times and without the corresponding improvements in productivity or quality of service. This demonstrates how poor organisational integration can undo the aims of the patient-centric and service quality philosophies that EHRs are meant to enable.

These observations also highlight two pressing needs. First, any approach towards integration must understand the details and requirements of the work processes of healthcare professionals. Second, these approaches should help enact changes that provide the necessary organisational transformations to make the technology work as seamlessly as it is intended. Hartswood, *et al.* (2003) suggest that, in order to achieve inter-service integration, it is important to understand how and why EHRs can work organisationally and how to design interventions to achieve this outcome. The amount of research in this area is sparse, especially for evidence of methods that have seen effective formalised and operationalised application within healthcare organisations. The concept of service oriented integration (SOI) needs further attention and clinical heuristic exploration.

EXAMPLES OF ORGANISATIONAL AND SOCIAL STRUCTURAL APPROACHES

Davidson and Chiasson (2005) explore the assimilation of EHRs during systems development and use through processes that are concerned with adjusting both the social practices that are part of organisational work routines and the technical features of the technology itself. Individualised adaptations of technology and social practices to match idiosyncratic work activities, known as metastructuring of technology (Orlikowski, *et al.* 1995, cited in Davidson and Chiasson 2005), have been shown to be key processes in the contextualisation and assimilation of systems into organisational practice (Davidson and Chiasson 2005).

Davidson and Chiasson (2005) propose that EHR systems can be better integrated into organisational work practices through organisationally sanctioned and managed approaches towards metastructuring, known as technology use mediation (TUM). This is conducted by groups of knowledgeable organisational members. Organising these groups in communities of practice (COPs) where knowledge of the technology and best practices will help other stakeholders to integrate EHRs into their normal routines and practices is important. The implication is that knowledge transferred through appropriate organisational structures may provide an effective means of improving successful EHR integration. Although they have shown advantages in forming and structuring these organisational groups, the resource requirements for deploying this approach are significant as they require several individuals who are actively involved in their own work to participate in shaping and mediating the technology for the benefit of the organisation. While it was noted that larger health organisations such as hospitals were better resourced to deploy such strategies, Davidson and Heslinga (2007) in another study of small physician practices found that TUM was less effective and even ineffective. We can observe from this that organisational and social structural strategies such as TUM often require greater amounts of knowledge worker manpower that small organisations are unable to leverage on. Furthermore, knowledge sharing can be highly convoluted. Previous studies highlight the call for a knowledge sharing culture related to shared benefits (Finnegan and Willcocks 2007). Knowledge can also mean different things for different audiences and therefore delineating knowledge in an integration environment becomes complicated.

EXAMPLES OF USER-ORIENTED AND SOCIO-TECHNICAL APPROACHES

User-oriented approaches are based on a central premise. This is borne from the proposition that understanding the micro-practice patterns of medical work and social behaviours enable users to influence the development and use of EHR systems to better suit their needs or gain their acceptance and lower organisational resistance, and can thus be leveraged to devise technological and practice-based modifications and interventions (Berg 2001; Hartswood 2003; Ellingsen and Monteiro 2006; Hennington and Janz 2007; Jensen and Aanestad 2007). While most authors present research evidence to support claims that socio-technical factors are important in any consideration of EHR integration, there are no clearly defined guidelines on how these principles can be applied, as much of the discussion is theoretically based. Berg (2001) supports the practical measure of utilising ethnographic methods to study work practices before implementing EHRs, yet more work needs to be done in relating theory to practice.

Another example is Jensen and Aanestad's (2007) argument for the managerial implications of understanding how healthcare professionals make sense of the adoption of EHRs. For this, they draw on the sense-making perspective as a counter to the dominant Technology Acceptance Model (TAM) as they claim that EHR adoption is more critically driven by the subtler social and organisational influences that shape collective decisions rather than voluntary individual decisions. As the authors demonstrate from observational and interview data of the study, doctors and nurses undergo certain sense-making social thought processes to conceive or sense the affordances of EHRs in relation to their own work roles and responsibilities and enact different practices surrounding this technology. While we may envision practical value from these insights, the authors continually reiterate that management must guide the EHR adoption process to take into account sense making and conception of healthcare staff about the technology to ensure a smooth implementation.

It is challenging to derive practicable insights in the organisational and social approaches for EHR integration from the current literature. Few authors have substantively shown how their findings and insights might be operationalised as part of an EHR integration strategy. Most of the studies do not relate human agency with the wider organisational and environmental factors that relate to EHR adoption. This area remains largely unexplored and, although similar strategies applied to integration in other industry sectors or to healthcare IS may be relevant, more research is needed about the adoption of EHRs.

What can be concluded from this discussion of EHR integration? First, that the strategic aims and approaches of EHR integration align to what has already been envisioned by the healthcare sector in terms of healthcare IS. Strategic integration approaches the issue of EHRs by promoting the strategic pillars of seamless care, quality care, and patient-centricity. One additional difference, however, is the concept of an evolutionary strategy which is particularly important in drawing out the need for organisational preparedness in the face of potentially transformative technology. This is important as the technical and organisational complexities make integration in healthcare extremely challenging.

From a technical systems standpoint, it can be observed that there is almost unanimous consensus that viable approaches of integrating the EHR are limited. Although the repertoire of systems integration methods provide a number of options, the combination of heterogeneity, autonomous organisations and distributed nature of medical work have resulted in a spread of patient data and medical information that only make federation a practicable option. Although alternatives do exist, such as enterprise type HISS or EDW, the attainment of large-scale cross-institutional records is feasible only through federated systems. Even within this remit, only common architecture approaches conceivably provide the levels of tight coupling that afford the integration of services, processes and other clinical systems. This has serious implications regarding the design and conformance to standards that this approach mandates. Tighter coupling of information systems invariably lead to organisational issues that must be resolved to ensure success of integration.

Research on organisational and social approaches towards EHR integration is less conclusive of how the record can be achieved. However, much of the debate surrounds the importance of organisational competencies and user-orientation. As this area of study is relatively emergent, there are few practical examples of best practice from these strategies. However, looking at how the literature on healthcare IS integration regards organisational and social methods of integration, EHR integration has strong resonance with socio-technical approaches.

CODING AND GROUPING THE LITERATURE

Table 7.1 presents 55 papers coded to four main themes:

1 information systems integration
2 healthcare IS systems and applications review, history and development
3 healthcare information systems integration; and
4 electronic health record systems, integration and use.

It displays the separate articles, texts and sources into main and sub-themes.

TABLE 7.1 Literature organised into main theme groups

Ref.	Author (Year)	Focus and main theme code	Sub-focus and sub-theme code	Ref.	Author (Year)	Focus and main theme code	Sub-focus and sub-theme code
1	Kim and Michelman (1990)	HIS		29	Anyanwu, et al. (2003)	HIS	
2	Hughes and Bayes (1991)	HAPP		30	Hartswood (2003)	EHR	
3	Wyse and Higgins (1993)	IS		31	Cross (2004)	EHR	
4	Conrad and Shortell (1996)	HIS		32	Landry, et al. (2004)	HIS	
5	Fiedler, et al. (1996)	IS		33	Wainright and Waring (2004)	IS	
6	Weber and Pliskin (1996)	IS		34	Weiner, et al. (2004)	HIS	
7	Johns (1997)	HIS		35	Carcinero, et al. (2005)	EHR	
8	McDonald (1997)	EHR		36	Ciccarese, et al. (2005)	HIS	EHR

Ref.	Author (Year)	Focus and main theme code	Sub-focus and sub-theme code
9	Rigby and Robins (1997)	HIS	EHR
10	Rivers and Bae (1999)	HAPP	
11	Grimson, et al. (2000)	HIS	EHR
12	Gulledge (2006)	IS	
13	Hasselbring (2000)	IS	
14	Southard, et al. (2000)	HAPP	
15	Stead, et al. (2000)	HIS	
16	Wainwright and Waring (2000)	HAPP	EHR
17	Waring and Wainwright (2000)	IS	
18	Berg (2001)	EHR	HIS
19	Grimson (2001)	EHR	
20	Makoul, et al. (2001)	EHR	
21	Bates (2002)	HAPP	
22	Burns and Pauly (2002)	HIS	
37	Davidson and Chiasson (2005)	EHR	
38	Hillestad, et al. (2005)	EHR	
39	Shortliffe (2005)	HAPP	
40	Wang, et al. (2005)	HIS	
41	Winthereik and Vikkelso (2005)	HIS	
42	Caccia-Bava, et al. (2006)	HIS	
43	Ellingsen and Monteiro (2006)	HIS	EHR
44	Khatri (2006)	HIS	
45	Khoumbati, et al. (2006)	HIS	EHR
46	Khoumbati and Themistocleous (2006)	HIS	
47	Mendoza, et al. (2006)	IS	
48	Thrasher, et al. (2006)	HIS	
49	Avison and Young (2007)	HIS	
50	Berstein, et al. (2007)	HAPP	

(continued)

Ref.	Author (Year)	Focus and main theme code	Sub-focus and sub-theme code	Ref.	Author (Year)	Focus and main theme code	Sub-focus and sub-theme code
23	Evgeniou (2002)	IS		51	Connell and Young (2007)	HIS	
24	Hersh (2002)	EHR		52	Davidson and Heslinga (2007)	EHR	
25	Tsiknakis, *et al.* (2002)	EHR		53	Hennington and Janz (2007)	EHR	
26	Raghupathi (2002)	HAPP		54	Jensen and Aanestad (2007)	EHR	
27	Raghupathi and Tan (2002)	HAPP		55	Rigby, *et al.* (2007)	EHR	
28	Stuewe (2002)	HAPP					

Literature coding key:
IS – Information systems integration (general)
HAPP – Healthcare IS systems and applications review, history and development
HIS – Healthcare information systems integration
EHR – Electronic health record systems, integration and use

INFORMATION SYSTEMS INTEGRATION DEFINITIONS AND APPROACHES

Table 7.2 captures IS systems integration definitions and approaches mapped to several common themes (shaded cell indicates coverage of topic). Table 7.3 further synthesises the organisation and data extraction from the IS systems integration literature showing main themes grouped around technical, strategic and organisational dimensions.

Table 7.3 findings show common elements of definitions, characteristics and concepts attributed to IS integration in organisations.

TABLE 7.2 IS integration literature concept matrix from content analysis

Reference Number	A9	A8	A7	A6	A5	A4	A3	A2	A1
Article/Text by Author (Year)	Mendoza, et al. (2006)	Gulledge (2006)	Wainright and Waring (2004)	Evgeniou (2002)	Waring and Wainwright (2000)	Hasselbring (2000)	Weber and Pliskin (1996)	Fiedler, et al. (1996)	Wyse and Higgins (1993)
Main concepts, themes and topics									
Enterprise systems/architecture									
Systems integration									
Enterprise application integration (EAI)									
Technical interfacing (e.g. message-based)									
Best-of-breed									

(continued)

Reference Number / Article/Text by Author (Year)	A1 Wyse and Higgins (1993)	A2 Fiedler, et al. (1996)	A3 Weber and Pliskin (1996)	A4 Hasselbring (2000)	A5 Waring and Wainwright (2000)	A6 Evgeniou (2002)	A7 Wainright and Waring (2004)	A8 Gulledge (2006)	A9 Mendoza, et al. (2006)
Legacy systems				■	■		■	■	■
Data/information communication; technical							■	■	■
Standardisation				■	■	■	■		■
Business process re-engineering				■			■		■
Federated systems; data warehouses				■	■	■	■	■	■
Organisational structure (e.g. centralisation)	■	■			■	■	■	■	■
Organisational learning, knowledge				■	■	■	■	■	
Leadership					■	■	■	■	■
Culture			■	■					■
Social communication				■	■			■	■

A9	A8	A7	A6	A5	A4	A3	A2	A1	Reference Number
Mendoza, et al. (2006)	Gulledge (2006)	Wainright and Waring (2004)	Evgeniou (2002)	Waring and Wainwright (2000)	Hasselbring (2000)	Weber and Pliskin (1996)	Fiedler, et al. (1996)	Wyse and Higgins (1993)	Article/Text by Author (Year)
									Strategy; strategic management; competitive advantage; planning
									IT–Business strategic fit

TABLE 7.3 Viewpoints on the approaches and characteristics of the integration of information systems

Dimension of integration	Wyse and Higgins (1993)	Fiedler, et al. (1996)	Weber and Pliskin (1996)	Hasselbring (2000)	Waring and Wainwright (2000; 2004)	Evgeniou (2002)	Gulledge (2006)		Mendoza, et al. (2006)		Relevant concepts and strategies
Technical and systems dimensions		Centralised cooperative computing			Integrated IS (as a product)	Standardised enterprise (ERP)	Enterprise systems ("Big I")		Enterprise systems (ERP)		Enterprise systems; single database; standardisation; single architecture
	Technical integration through interconnectivity	Distributed computing (enabled by networking technologies)		Systems integration techniques	Integrating or interfacing IS components and artefacts (as an activity or discipline)	Decentralised enterprise (federated systems)	Interfacing ("Little i")	Point-to-point	Point-to-point	Point-to-point	Best of breed; interfacing; technical communication; federation; standardisation; legacy systems; heterogeneous systems
						Adaptive enterprise (conceptual approach harnessing EAI technologies and flexible organisational forms)		DB-to-DB			
								Data warehouse	Data warehouse	
								EAI	Internal structural and process integration	
								Application server integration		
								B2B	External integration	

Dimension of integration	Wyse and Higgins (1993)	Fiedler, et al. (1996)	Weber and Pliskin (1996)	Hasselbring (2000)	Waring and Wainwright (2000; 2004)	Evgeniou (2002)	Gulledge (2006)	Mendoza, et al. (2006)	Relevant concepts and strategies
Organisational and social dimensions	Data integration defined by utility of technical integration for organisational members	Integration defined by data and resource sharing across organisational units	Integration as cultural synergy	Coupling and integrating interorganisational processes; organisational boundary spanning	Structural view: integration as automation, informatisation; communication across organisational units	Adaptive enterprise (conceptual approach harnessing EAI technologies and flexible organisational forms)		Effective org. change mgmt. for process and structural change	Business process re-engineering; horizontal, vertical integration; organisational forms; delayering, downsizing, organisational boundary spanning
					Social and historical factors			User involved	Organisational learning; knowledge; social communication; communities of practice; leadership
					Power and politics			Effective leadership	
					Culture				

(continued)

Dimension of integration	Wyse and Higgins (1993)	Fiedler, et al. (1996)	Weber and Pliskin (1996)	Hasselbring (2000)	Waring and Wainwright (2000; 2004)	Evgeniou (2002)	Gulledge (2006)	Mendoza, et al. (2006)	Relevant concepts and strategies
Strategic dimension	Data integration defined by systems alignment with business strategy; planning methods				IS integration as facilitator of competitive business strategies: e-business; technology-business alignment; best practices	Adaptive enterprise concept as an integration approach for rapid business strategy realignments			Business process re-engineering; horizontal and vertical integration; competitive strategy

THE EVOLUTION OF HEALTHCARE INFORMATION SYSTEMS AND APPLICATIONS

Table 7.4 displays the main concepts and themes that are mapped to instances of the literature grouped under the healthcare IS systems and applications history and development texts (shaded cell indicates coverage of topic, concept or theme). Figure 7.1 is a timeline that helps visualise the milestones and motives behind healthcare IS developments.

TABLE 7.4 Healthcare IS applications, history and development concept matrix from content analysis

Reference Number	Article/Text by author (Year)	Concepts, themes and topics			
		History of healthcare IS applications and systems adoption	Drivers for healthcare IS adoption and integration	Barriers to healthcare IS adoption and integration	Healthcare IS applications
B1	Hughes and Bayes (1991)				
B2	Rivers and Bae (1999)				
B3	Southard, et al. (2000)				
B4	Wainwright and Waring (2000)				
B5	Bates (2002)				
B6	Raghupathi (2002)				
B7	Raghupathi and Tan (2002)				
B8	Stuewe (2002)				
B9	Shortliffe (2005)				
B10	Bernstein, et al. (2007)				

(continued)

Reference Number	Article/Text by author (Year)	Healthcare delivery process	Healthcare service quality	Seamless/ integrated care	Healthcare strategy	Decision support systems	Electronic healthcare records	Best-of-breed
B1	Hughes and Bayes (1991)							
B2	Rivers and Bae (1999)	▓	▓					
B3	Southard, et al. (2000)			▓	▓			
B4	Wainwright and Waring (2000)					▓		
B5	Bates (2002)	▓	▓				▓	
B6	Raghupathi (2002)			▓	▓			
B7	Raghupathi and Tan (2002)			▓				
B8	Stuewe (2002)				▓			▓
B9	Shortliffe (2005)		▓			▓		
B10	Bernstein, et al. (2007)			▓		▓		

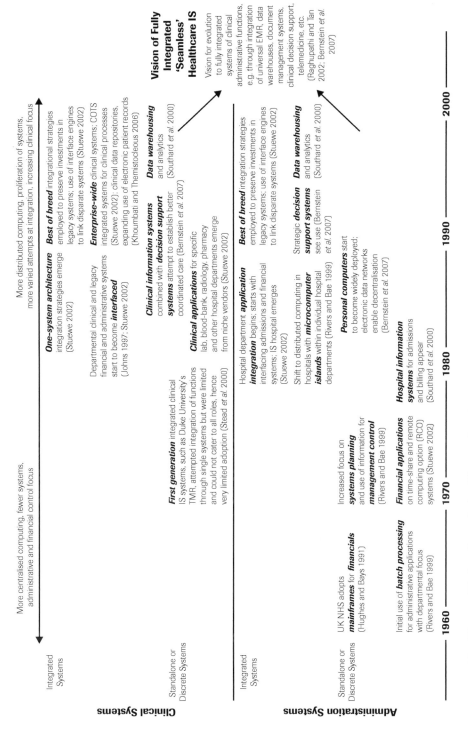

FIGURE 7.1 Healthcare IS timeline of significant developments

TECHNICAL, ORGANISATIONAL, SOCIAL AND STRATEGIC APPROACHES TO INFORMATION SYSTEMS INTEGRATION IN HEALTHCARE

Table 7.5 illustrates the findings from the literature study concerning the strategies and approaches that are advocated by various authors from the healthcare IS literature that was reviewed (shaded cell indicates coverage of topic, concept or theme).

TABLE 7.5 Technical, organisational, social and strategic approaches to electronic health records integration

Reference Number	Article/Text by Author (Year)	Organisational main focus			Technical main focus						
		C11	C10	C9	C8	C7	C6	C5	C4	C3	C2	C1
		Winthereik and Vikkelso (2005)	Weiner, et al. (2004)	Landry, et al. (2004)	Burns and Pauly (2002)	Berg (2001)	Khoumbati and Themistocleous (2006)	Khoumbati, et al. (2006)	Ciccarese, et al. (2005)	Anyanwu, et al. (2003)	Grimson, et al. (2000)	Stead, et al. (2000)

Technical and systems dimension
- Common architecture
- Systems integration
- Inter-systems communication
- Technical standardisation
- Legacy systems integration
- Federation

Organisational and social dimension
- Organisational structural management approaches (supportive structures)

	Organisational main focus						Technical main focus					Reference Number
	C11	C10	C9	C8	C7	C6	C5	C4	C3	C2	C1	Article/Text by Author (Year)
	Winthereik and Vikkelso (2005)	Weiner, et al. (2004)	Landry, et al. (2004)	Burns and Pauly (2002)	Berg (2001)	Khoumbati and Themistocleous (2006)	Khoumbati, et al. (2006)	Ciccarese, et al. (2005)	Anyanwu, et al. (2003)	Grimson, et al. (2000)	Stead, et al. (2000)	**Strategic dimension**
Organisational cultural management approaches		■										
Organisational knowledge and learning management approaches												
Organisational IS/IT capabilities development and management approaches				■								
User participation; user-led evolution; social communication and collaboration; socio-technical approaches								■				
Business process re-engineering approaches											■	
Competitive strategy approaches (IS integration as competitive weapon)												

(continued)

Organisational main focus / **Technical main focus**

Reference Number	Article/Text by Author (Year)
C11	Winthereik and Vikkelso (2005)
C10	Weiner, et al. (2004)
C9	Landry, et al. (2004)
C8	Burns and Pauly (2002)
C7	Berg (2001)
C6	Khoumbati and Themistocleous (2006)
C5	Khoumbati, et al. (2006)
C4	Ciccarese, et al. (2005)
C3	Anyanwu, et al. (2003)
C2	Grimson, et al. (2000)
C1	Stead, et al. (2000)

Quality management and improvement approaches

Patient-centricity approaches

Strategic fit and organisational alignment of IS approaches

Organisational main focus

Reference Number	Article/Text by Author (Year)
C12	Caccia-Bava, et al. (2006)
C13	Ellingsen and Monteiro (2006)
C14	Khatri (2006)
C15	Kim and Michelman (1990)
C16	Conrad and Shortell (1996)
C17	Johns (1997)
C18	Rigby and Robins (1997)
C19	Wang, et al. (2005)
C20	Thrashers (2006)
C21	Avison and young (2007)

Strategic main focus

C22	Connell and Young (2007)

Common architecture

Technical and systems dimension

	Strategic main focus								Organisational main focus			
Reference Number / Article/Text by Author (Year)	C22 Connell and Young (2007)	C21 Avison and young (2007)	C20 Thrashers (2006)	C19 Wang, et al. (2005)	C18 Rigby and Robins (1997)	C17 Johns (1997)	C16 Conrad and Shortell (1996)	C15 Kim and Michelman (1990)	C14 Khatri (2006)	C13 Ellingsen and Monteiro (2006)	C12 Caccia-Bava, et al. (2006)	**Organisational and social dimension**
Inter-systems communication												
Technical standardisation												
Legacy systems integration												
Federation												
Organisational structural management approaches (supportive structures)												
Organisational cultural management approaches												

(continued)

	Strategic main focus								Organisational main focus			
Reference Number	C22	C21	C20	C19	C18	C17	C16	C15	C14	C13	C12	**Strategic dimension**
Article/Text by Author (Year)	Connell and Young (2007)	Avison and young (2007)	Thrashers (2006)	Wang, et al. (2005)	Rigby and Robins (1997)	Johns (1997)	Conrad and Shortell (1996)	Kim and Michelman (1990)	Khatri (2006)	Ellingsen and Monteiro (2006)	Caccia-Bava, et al. (2006)	
									▪	▪	▪	Organisational knowledge and learning management approaches
							▪		▪		▪	Organisational IS/IT capabilities development and management approaches
	▪	▪				▪	▪		▪	▪	▪	User participation; user-led evolution; social communication and collaboration; socio-technical approaches
	▪	▪	▪									Business process re-engineering approaches

Strategic main focus					Organisational main focus						
C22	**C21**	**C20**	**C19**	**C18**	**C17**	**C16**	**C15**	**C14**	**C13**	**C12**	**Reference Number**
Connell and Young (2007)	Avison and young (2007)	Thrashers (2006)	Wang, *et al.* (2005)	Rigby and Robins (1997)	Johns (1997)	Conrad and Shortell (1996)	Kim and Michelman (1990)	Khatri (2006)	Ellingsen and Monteiro (2006)	Caccia-Bava, *et al.* (2006)	Article/Text by Author (Year)
											Competitive strategy approaches (IS integration as competitive weapon)
											Quality management and improvement approaches
											Patient-centricity
											Strategic fit and organisational alignment of IS approaches

Table 7.6 illustrates the findings from the literature study concerning the strategies and approaches that are advocated by various authors from the healthcare IS literature (shaded cell indicates coverage of topic, concept or theme).

TABLE 7.6 Strategies for EHR integration in the literature

	Strategic main focus				Organisational main focus					Reference Number
	D21	D20	D19	D18	D17	D16	D15	D14	D13	Article/Text by Author (Year)
	Hillestad, et al. (2005)	Cross (2004)	Wainwright and Waring (2000)	Rigby and Robins (1997)	Davidson and Heslinga (2007)	Jensen and Aanestad (2007)	Hennington and Janz (2007)	Ellingsen and Monteiro (2006)	Davidson and Chiasson (2005)	
Technical and systems dimension										
Common architecture										
Federated systems integration										
Inter-systems communication										
Organisational and social dimension										
User-led; user participation										
User acceptance										
Social communication and collaboration										
Organisational structural management										

Strategic main focus			Organisational main focus						Reference Number
D21	D20	D19	D18	D17	D16	D15	D14	D13	Article/Text by Author (Year)
Hillestad, et al. (2005)	Cross (2004)	Wainwright and Waring (2000)	Rigby and Robins (1997)	Davidson and Heslinga (2007)	Jensen and Aanestad (2007)	Hennington and Janz (2007)	Ellingsen and Monteiro (2006)	Davidson and Chiasson (2005)	**Strategic dimension**
				■	■		■	■	Organisational knowledge, learning and cultural management
			■						Patient-centricity
■	■								Strategic fit and alignment of IS

DISCUSSION AND ANALYSIS

The proposition that IS has become increasingly important to the delivery of health-care services in highly distributed, complex and information intensive activities is self-evident. However, the link between strategy and implementation in IS integration is not well developed, which means that potential benefits from technology investment are often elusive in healthcare. This has been demonstrated by the proliferation of various isolated systems to meet diverse clinical and administrative needs, which makes the challenge of systems integration ever more difficult.

While we have acknowledged that integration, as a concern, is complex and multifaceted, it can also be shown that the concept may be deconstructed, organised and classified to improve our theoretical and practical understanding. In this section, we attempt to synthesise the different strands of the preceding discussion to clarify our understanding of the approaches towards healthcare information systems integration. This process of drawing the various research threads is depicted in Figure 7.2.

Singularly defining IS integration as an all-encompassing operational term is problematic. The literature reveals that there are numerous and sometimes conflicting interpretations of the concept. Yet achieving clarity of definition for integration, as the subject of analysis, is an important first step in beginning to categorise and evaluate the competing and complementary approaches towards attaining it. To achieve this aim, integration was looked at along three characteristic dimensions

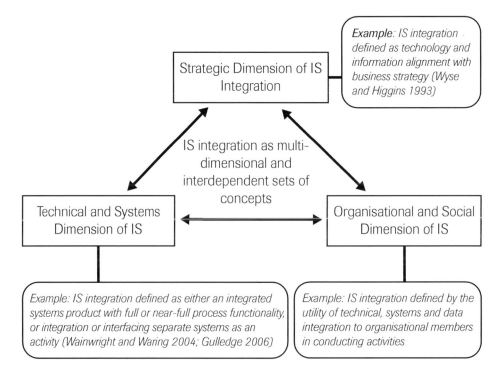

FIGURE 7.2 IS integration conceptualised in multi-dimensions with co-dependent aspects

that were recurrent themes in the IS literature. Observers would describe and define integration in terms of these dimensions: the technical and systems, the strategic, and the organisational and social aspects. This classification not only provides a suitable manner to deconstruct the meanings of integration but it also reveals the co-dependence that different aspects of integration have upon each other. Integration at the macro level, for example, is regarded in a strategic sense, and is often depicted as the linkages between the organisational and inter-organisational value chains that are the focus of strategic management and planning concerns; concepts such as horizontal and vertical integration, and the achievement of strategically competitive efficiencies are the most prevalent here.

As information pervades and links every part of organisational activity in the value chain, the drive towards strategic integration becomes synonymous with integrated IS (entity or product) and where disparate IS are implemented already, it becomes synonymous with the integration of IS (actions and techniques). Where the chain of processes and activities of the organisation and their informational inputs and outputs are required to be modelled, the approaches manifest themselves in technical and systems integration terms, whether these take the shape of technical solutions such as ERP systems or technical interfacing that align and fit to strategic imperatives.

However, integration cannot be useful in terms of these two themes alone and organisational factors must be considered. The implementation of a technical system does not automatically confer the intended benefits of a strategic plan. The role of organisational members in utilising integrated IS for collaborating horizontally across organisational units and functional departments requires that IS integration be seen through a social and organisational lens as well. Integration may mean gaining the acceptance of users for the systems or designing the systems in ways that match actual organisational practices.

Organisational processes in the value chain rely upon people as much as they do on technology and strategic planning. Depending on how integration is conceived as a package of definitions, there is potential for conflict. In these ways integration is not only multidimensional, but these dimensions are co-dependent and also characterised by the tensions between them. This idea is conceptualised in Figure 7.2 and embodies a closer step towards a definition that, though imperfect, improves clarity and is more amenable in structuring the various approaches towards IS integration. The IS integration literature looks at this concept quite generically and even though many organisations would need to alter working practices radically to benefit from the changes brought about by integration, this type of desired organisational change is regarded as a positive outcome.

In healthcare settings, a range of factors complicate IS integration. Generic strategic and technical integration and adoption models that are already challenging to implement in most other industry sectors present added complexities to healthcare. Healthcare is characterised by idiosyncratic, often ambiguous, diverse and structurally unique work activities. It is highly regulated, requires large numbers of people to deliver medical services, is broken up by dual managerial and clinical structures, has institutional characteristics that feature powerful professional groupings, and has a high number of stakeholders ranging from clinicians, to patients, to governments and supporting industries such as insurance companies. IS integration archetypes, having largely been developed as technical solutions for automation within manufacturing environments, have had problems in translation to medical settings.

Furthermore, it has been shown that the historical evolution of healthcare IS has not only contributed to a legacy of fragmented and autonomous infrastructure and practices, but it demonstrated that healthcare organisations have also failed to capitalise on past opportunities to provide information services to multiple stakeholders in an integrated manner. Institutional, professional, regulatory and economic factors have all contributed to this state of affairs, but what ultimately results are highly constrained environmental conditions that hamper current efforts to integrate.

Early financial and management control emphases on IS systems and applications that at first improved efficiencies through automation would later became more strategic as financial management was elevated in status as a result of fiercer competition or regulatory oversight in the case of public healthcare systems. This not only influences future patterns of adoption in which the industry context here is very strong but it fosters the overall need for integration; strategically, in the face of changing care paradigms such as quality, integrated and patient-centred care processes, IS integration is an inherent requisite. Therefore our understanding of the meaning of integration in healthcare must not only account for the collective tensions and dependence of various strategic, technical and organisational definitions but must also be tempered by an appreciation that these dimensions are bound and encapsulated by the various packaged meanings, assumptions and conditions of integration in healthcare. Figure 7.3 presents a visualisation of this framework. Integration is therefore highly reliant on very complex interrelations and typical IS integration models are modified in context to the unique features of healthcare organisations and activities. This contributes to summing up not only what the different views and definitions of health IS integration are, but that this summation cannot be a direct and absolute one. The definitions are relative to one another.

HEALTHCARE IS INTEGRATION STRATEGIES: TYPOLOGICAL CONSTRUCTION

The results from the literature review provide a useful framework for organising the various healthcare IS integration approaches, which have been studied and proposed by a number of different authors, into a more streamlined and consolidated view. This model depicts a typology of the main approaches, classified under their respective dimensions for which justification in formulation has been made, as an aggregation and categorisation of various views in the literature. Not many authors have sought to lay out and structure the various integration strategies for healthcare IS and this effort attempts to synthesise and consolidate the knowledge from the literature in the field in this manner, and therefore this approach, as far as can be deducted from the literature, is quite novel.

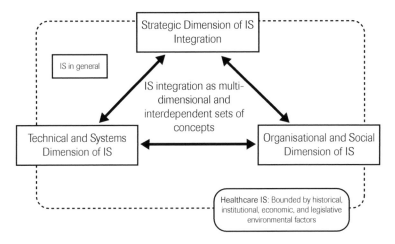

FIGURE 7.3 IS integration in healthcare is influenced by various factors

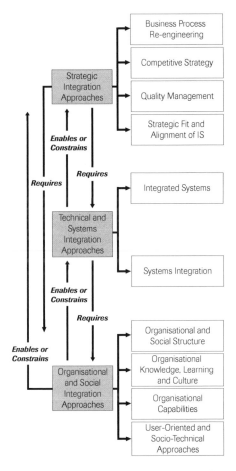

FIGURE 7.4 Healthcare IS approaches from a consolidated review of the literature

Regardless of the main umbrella approach that an author advocates, there is the recognition that the integration strategies comprising a single domain cannot exist in isolation and their interrelationships must be acknowledged as part of a cohesive solution to integration. For example, Grimson, *et al.* (2000) may regard healthcare IS integration from a systems integration viewpoint but they do not deny that their preferred federated common infrastructure approach will likely require complementary business process re-engineering measures to capitalise on the organisational changes wrought by increased integration. In a similar vein, observers such as Johns (1997) may campaign for quality improvement initiatives and competitive approaches as part of an IS integration strategy, but still maintain that these objectives can only be accomplished alongside methodologies conscious of cultural sensitivities that advocate leadership, cultural management and the navigation through often politicised organisational change. In this manner, if we consider the reviewed healthcare IS integration literature in its entirety, the consensus view is that no single dimension should completely dominate.

What is not generally agreed upon is what proportion of the overall emphasis should be devoted to these respective concerns. Organisational issues, for example, receive less attention compared with technical issues. While those arguing for certain technological innovations only superficially touch upon organisational and social changes, all factors are relevant. Equally, different strategic approaches are often in direct conflict, making organisational comparisons useful. For example, a systems approach to consolidate organisational IS into a commercial off-the-shelf enterprise type system may assist in providing greater process efficiencies and tighter inter-organisational coupling. However, where these technologies cannot fit adequately within work practices, organisational level approaches that entail user-led customisation and metastructuring of the technology, popularised for example by expert groups and communities of practice, may be constrained because these monolithic technical approaches afford very few opportunities for adaptation. The framework depicted in Figure 7.4 recognises these dependencies and shows how the respective dimensions may depend, enable and constrain one another.

HEALTHCARE IS INTEGRATION PATHWAYS

The typology shown by Figure 7.4, at its current level of detail, is not immediately useful in providing an integrative view of the strategies mentioned in the literature. Figure 7.5 expands on the high level overview of the typology and shows how elements of each approach, synthesised from contributions of the healthcare IS literature, may be constructed into specific sets of methodological pathways to attain particular integration goals. This schema arranges the individual elements that construct a given route towards a solution for an IS integration goal.

For example, taking the strategic integration dimension and the strategic fit approach, tracing the path of this strategy shows a call for an alignment of IS capabilities to the business concerns of the healthcare organisation. Kim and Michelman (1990) demonstrate how this approach might be undertaken through a strategic

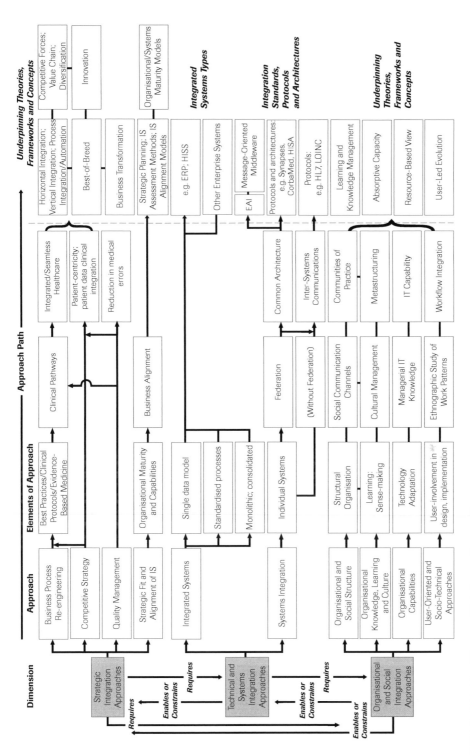

FIGURE 7.5 Healthcare IS integration pathways

capabilities assessment analysis of existing isolated clinical and administrative systems that can be developed into competitive weapons by moving them from purely operational automation-oriented systems to integrated strategic systems. Thrasher, *et al.* (2006), on the other hand, show that organisational and information systems maturity models can also be leveraged to assess the level of strategic fit and where appropriate inform managers where corrections are needed. This pathway is an example of one that utilises the tools of the strategic management discipline and can reinforce an informed decision-making process.

Where relevant, this expanded typology gives three dimensions to healthcare IS integration pathways: strategic, technical and systems integration, and organisational and social integration. It further gives the approach pathways leading to the underpinning theories, frameworks and concepts. For example, we can consider an earlier example of the strategic objective of integrated seamless care. Tracing the BPR route in the schema, we are reminded of the healthcare analogue of clinical care pathways and their relation to business process re-engineering principles based on the concept of the value chain and horizontal integration of medical activities. The typological pathways are a useful instrument for understanding how healthcare IS integration is approached in a consolidated and integrative fashion. The systems pathways can be perceived as a form of standardisation.

We recognise, however, the limitations of this model. The primary source of its validity is the evidence from the literature upon which it is grounded. The strategic domain pathways are generally accepted as they mirror much of the current thought of strategic interventions in healthcare IS, including those initiatives that intend to integrate overall information and care processes while guaranteeing high data and service quality with the patient as the focus of attention. Likewise, strong evidence and perhaps the best-known approaches fall under the technical and systems categorisation. The technical and systems typological pathways represented by the model embody typical healthcare IS technological solutions that have a constellation of practitioner and vendor experiences that are well documented. Systems integration protocols and standards such as HL7, DCOM and Synapses are highly represented in the systems-oriented literature as well as the concept of federation.

Where the model can only provide less definite assurance of the approach pathways are in parts of the organisational and social integration domain. While macro-level strategies of structural interventions such as working groups and communities are well known in practice, there has been less evidence in the literature concerning the softer social approaches in relation to implementing healthcare IS integration. Even though socio-technical proponents such as Berg (2001), Winthereik and Vikkelso (2005) and Ellingsen and Monteiro (2006) have conducted qualitative research within a range of healthcare settings from physician practices to clinical laboratories and hospital wards at local and regional scales, their conclusions tend to focus on 'what should not be done' rather than on 'what should be done' when it comes to integration.

This lack of direction can, in part, be placed on the more recently emergent attention to the interests of a social nature in the integration of IS into clinical practice from which a technical focus has previously predominated. However, most of the recommendations made by these observers are generally an attack on the limitations of technical and systems design in relation to organisational members' ways of working and there are fewer practical contributions of how organisational and social integration approaches can be made operational as part of a set of best practices or a framework for implementation. User involvement is far more ambiguous than the ideas related to technology acceptance and use that has long been a main research stream in the field of IS. In addition, the model does not vouch to be fully comprehensive of all the approaches studied in the field; such a claim must be backed up by a fully extensive systematic review of all literature sources.

Even with these extant vulnerabilities, the typological model achieves what it sets out to do. For one, it highlights where the research community should address gaps in knowledge where it is shown that organisational and social interventions on the subject of healthcare IS integration are sorely needed. Second, on a more practical basis it can help inform a reliance on the dominant positions of strategic and technical systems integration methodologies that can potentially create an imbalanced and non-holistic overall approach to what are essentially organisational concerns for integration. Third, it informs on the theoretical and conceptual basis upon which many of the advocated integration pathways are grounded. For example, concepts and theories related to knowledge and learning are relevant capabilities in attaining organisational integration. This provides an avenue to relate integration approaches to wider management interests and perhaps more interestingly how these management interests can in turn be applied to clinical concerns and stakeholder affairs. Therefore, to be absolutely clear, the development of the model is not our end purpose here – it is a necessary objective milestone for analysis – but what and how it can tell and inform us about integration practices.

APPLYING THE TYPOLOGY CONCEPT: EHR INTEGRATION AND PATHWAYS

The discussion thus far follows a structured analytical journey in which the literature has been used not only as a source of direct data to be analysed, but as the starting point in the construction of a template against which specific examples in the literature can be referenced and analysed. Hence the typological representation of healthcare IS integration strategies and methodological pathways was formulated not only as a useful exercise and conceptual framework in its own right, but also as a starting point from which subsequent analysis of integration strategies could be conducted for specific types of IS.

It is within this frame of mind that the application of the typology can be adapted to schematise a consolidated view for a better understanding of how approaches towards electronic healthcare records integration are advocated in the literature. Figure 7.6 depicts the typological representation of the EHR integration pathways built from the literature analysis. It is not feasible to examine all the possible streams and paths of EHR integration and therefore certain examples will be selected to illustrate what we can learn from the analysis. The integration of EHRs have closely followed the solution patterns and recommendations made within generic health-care IS and general IS strategies. We might dismiss this as a lack of innovation on the part of healthcare organisations. In fact it might be said that EHRs as an emergent form of healthcare IS are being approached more conservatively than the average integrated application. For instance, the pathway for the technical systems approach in the EHR schema (Figure 7.6) depicts as only viable the federated common archi-tecture systems integration methodology, which narrows the approach to certain standard protocols and architectures developed for the healthcare sector. Although isolated instances in the literature may present rival methods such as inter-systems communications for integration (e.g. McDonald 1997; Rigby, *et al.* 2007), these are in the minority and often cited for niche or specialised purposes and therefore the model represents federated common architectures as the main technical approach.

However, to infer this cause as the explanation of the phenomenon would be premature and we must appraise any generalisations made in terms of the valid explanations contributed by the literature overall. This line of reasoning may appear tangential to the actual point being made but we will complete the argument for the sake of clarity and show its relevance. EHRs are constrained in terms of technical and systems approaches for the sole reason that the great majority of patient and clinical data reside in numerous heterogeneous, autonomous and distributed legacy systems that have been heavily invested by healthcare organisations. Historical, economic and institutional factors make other systems integration or enterprise systems alter-natives unfeasible or at least less tenable for immediate needs; common architecture federation present healthcare organisations with a good compromise between tight systems coupling and the maintenance of autonomy.

Returning to the main point, we see this as structured evidence that EHR integ-ration cannot necessarily utilise all the approaches available for the reasons already mentioned. What can be more easily communicated visually here is that technical and systems EHR strategies are more limited and constrained in comparison to the wider portfolio of approaches (as seen in comparison to the general healthcare IS typology and pathway shown by Figure 7.5). To furnish another example for EHR, consider the strategic integration dimension and the approach pathway of strategic fit and alignment. The same contextual factors that affect systems integration choices affect the path towards clinical alignment with EHRs with clinical processes, the med-ical analogue to business processes.

Where, previously, strategic planning and fit methods were in general terms lev-eraged towards more immediate 'business' transformation as in the general schema, the EHR case in contrast recommends an evolutionary approach (Wainwright and Waring 2000; Tsiknakis, *et al.* 2002). Wainwright and Waring (2000) provide a partic-ularly interesting analysis of the NHS Information for Health 1998 policy mandating the provision of healthcare provider-independent EHRs. Utilising Nolan's (1979) systems maturity framework alongside Galliers and Sutherland's (1991) adaptation of Nolan's framework, Wainwright and Waring (2000) show how the NHS's rela-tively low IT/IS maturity and capabilities as well as its high levels of fragmentation

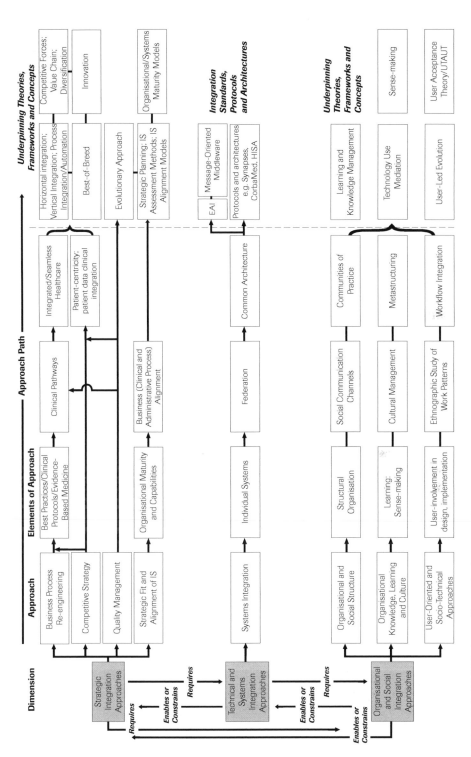

FIGURE 7.6 EHR integration strategy pathways

are incongruent with its strategic mission of providing integrated EHRs. This means that smaller steps need to be taken towards a fully integrated record to allow for the organisation to keep up with the pace of change. For many healthcare organisations this situation is the norm, so it follows that an evolutionary rather than revolutionary change is inevitable.

Considering the organisational and social pathways, we can see that much the same methods for achieving integration are present. However, from our discussion of EHRs, we note that many of these approaches have not been studied in depth in a systematic manner and therefore we can accept these as only tentative contributions to the literature. Indeed, many of the approaches of EHR integration do not deviate widely from typical IS or healthcare IS pathways. One explanation for this might be that different approaches are not needed, or more plausibly that existing approaches have not been fully realised as EHRs are only recently emerging on a wide level of adoption. Therefore our attention now turns to how these insights contribute to our understanding of how the integration of complex healthcare IS/IT in the form of electronic healthcare records are practically integrated. However, within this area it must be conceded that the typology is less conclusive. Organisational issues appear to be the most complex especially in their intricate interrelationships. While we may strive to make organisational and social elements discretely, schematically and neatly arranged, as has been attempted here, some observers demonstrate just how problematic this is. For example, Davidson and Chiasson's (2005) study of formalised, organisationally sanctioned adaptations of technology in healthcare organisations through technology-use mediation theory encompasses a broad range of organisational and social concerns. As an approach that calls for the adaptation of technical artefacts and working practices to fit working patterns, this includes sophisticated interplays between organisational structures, individual learning, social communications and organisational knowledge. This presents not only a highly intricate set of co-dependent elements but also the institutional contexts in which these interactions occur.

Although it might be interpreted as a shortcoming, this section of the investigation with the test and critique of its typological schema highlights that the organisational and social approaches towards EHR integration still require more interdisciplinary study and research. The current gaps in knowledge in this area need to be addressed to be able to better understand what types of practical interventions and mediations are needed to formulate and improve EHR integration practice in healthcare organisations.

CONCLUSION

Several views and approaches regarding the successful integration of healthcare information systems have been collected and analysed from the existing literature base. These have been organised and arranged to show that many of these approaches conform to the categorical dimensions that have been established as the research exercise has progressed. It has also been revealed that there are tensions and co-dependencies between these integration strategies and that the contextualising factors of healthcare organisations, the nature of their work, institutional characteristics, history and environment have influenced the trajectory of the development and implementation of these approaches.

The healthcare IS literature has shown that a range of strategies are available but that these often take the form of certain prescribed pathways that are used to achieve specific organisational goals. Of these, the most well understood and developed are the technical and systems pathways to integration, but these are acknowledged to only be effective as a holistic systems approach with complementary organisational and social integration strategies. It has also been noted that the knowledge and capabilities to operationalise these organisational and social mediations in integration practices are less well established, although their importance and influence are not in doubt. It is evident that integration is still very much a technical and systems concern borne from generic strategic management objectives that have been transplanted into the healthcare setting. Business process re-engineering and quality management for instance have found their clinical analogues in integrated seamless care and patient-centricity concerns.

Applying what has been constructed from the separate pieces of healthcare IS integration literature to the concerns of EHR integration has highlighted certain similarities and differences. EHR integration strategies are less well developed and, in many cases, constrained by the moderating factors that are characteristic of the healthcare sector, although the solution patterns are very much the same even for generic IS integration. This raises some questions in light of the unique challenges in healthcare whether more innovative solutions are needed. Certainly, the organisational changes necessary for the integration of EHRs will require effective organisational and social solutions to be applied, but a lack of substantive findings in the literature do not make this proposition very clear at this juncture.

REFERENCES

Ahgren B, Axelsson R. Determinants of integrated health care development: chains of care in Sweden. *Int J Health Plann Manage*. 2007. 22(2): 145–57.

Anyanwu K, Sheth A, Cardoso J, *et al*. Healthcare enterprise process development and integration. *J Res Prac IT*. 2003; 35(2): 83–98.

Aveyard H. *Doing a Literature Review in Health and Social Care*. Maidenhead: Open University Press; 2007.

Avison D, Young T. Time to rethink health care and ICT? *Commun ACM*. 2007; 50(6): 69–74.

Banker RD, Kauffman RJ. The evolution of research on information systems: a fiftieth-year survey of the literature in management science. *Manage Sci*. 2004; 50(3): 281–98.

Bates DW. The quality case of information technology in healthcare. *BMC Med Inform Decis Mak*. 2002; 2(7): 1–9.

Berg M. Implementing information systems in health care organisations: myths and challenges. *Int J Med Inform*. 2001; 64(2–3): 143–56.

Bernstein ML, McCreless T, Cote MJ. Five constants of information technology adoption in healthcare. *Hosp Top*. 2007; 85(1): 17–25.

Bloomfield BP. The role of information systems in the UK National Health Service: action at a distance and the fetish of calculation. *Soc Stud Sci.* 1991; 21(4): 701–34.

Boulton M, Fitzpatrick R, Swinburn C. Qualitative research in healthcare: II. A structured review and evaluation of studies. *J Eval Clin Pract.* 1996; 2(2): 171–9.

Brazhnik O, Jones JF. Anatomy of data integration. *J Biomed Inform.* 2007; 40(3): 252–69.

Brown PJB, Warmington V. Data quality probes: exploiting and improving the quality of electronic patient record data and patient care. *Int J Med Inform.* 2002; 68(3): 91–8.

Burns LR, Pauly MV. Integrated delivery networks: a detour on the road to integrated health care? *Health Aff.* 2002; 21(4): 128–43.

Caccia-Bava MDC, Guimaraes T, Harrington SJ. Hospital organization culture, capacity to innovate and success in technology adoption. *J Health Organ Manag.* 2006; 20(3): 194–217.

Carnicero J, Blanco O, Mateos M. The application of information and communication technologies to clinical activity: electronic health and clinical records. *Pharm Pol Law.* 2005; 8: 69–82.

Ciccarese P, Caffi E, Quaglini S, *et al.* Architectures and tools for innovative health information systems: the Guide Project. *Int J Med Inform.* 2005; 74(7–8): 553–62.

Connell NAD, Young TP. Evaluating healthcare information systems through an 'enterprise' perspective. *Inf Manage.* 2007; 44(4): 433–40.

Conrad DA, Shortell SM. Integrated health systems: promise and performance. *Front of Health Serv Manage.* 1996; 13(1): 3–40.

Cross M. In sickness or in health? *IEE Review.* 2004; 50(10): 38–41.

Currie G, Brown AD. Implementation of an IT system in a hospital trust. *Public Money Manage.* 1997; 17(4): 69–76.

Currie WL, Guah MW. IT-enabled healthcare delivery: the UK National Health Service. *Inf Syst Manage.* 2006; 23(2): 7–22.

Currie WL, Guah MW. Conflicting institutional logics: a national programme for IT in the organisational field of healthcare. *J Inf Technol.* 2007; 22(3): 235–47.

Davidson E, Chiasson M. Contextual influences on technology use mediation: a comparative analysis of electronic medical record systems. *Eur J Inf Syst.* 2005; 14(2): 6–18.

Davidson E, Heslinga D. Bridging the IT adoption gap for small physician practices: an action research study on electronic health records. *Inf Syst Manage.* 2007; 24(1): 15–28.

Department of Health. *Delivering the NHS Plan.* CM 5503. London: HMSO; 2002.

Devaraj S, Kohli R. Information technology payoff in the healthcare industry: a longitudinal study. *J Manage Inf Syst.* 2000; 16(4): 41–67.

Dixon BE. A roadmap for the adoption of e-Health. *e-Service J.* 2007; 5(3): 3–13.

Ellingsen G, Monteiro E. Seamless integration: standardisation across multiple local settings. *Comp Support Coop Work.* 2006; 15(5–6): 443–66.

Evgeniou T. Information integration and information strategies for adaptive enterprises. *Eur Manage J.* 2002; 20(5): 486–94.

Fiedler KD, Grover V, Teng JTC. An empirically derived taxonomy of information technology structure and its relationship to organizational structure. *J Manage Inf Syst.* 1996; 13(1): 9–34.

Finnegan DJ, Currie WL. A centrist approach to introducing ICT in healthcare: policies, practices and pitfalls. *J Cases Inf Technol.* 2008; 10(4): 1–16.

Finnegan D, Willcocks L. *Implementing CRM: from technology to knowledge.* Chichester: Wiley; 2007.

Grimson J. Delivering the electronic healthcare record for the 21st century. *Int J Med Inform.* 2001; 64(2): 111–27.

Grimson J, Grimson W, Hasselbring W. The systems integration challenge in health care. *Commun ACM.* 2000, 43(6): 49–55.

Gulledge T. What is integration? *Ind Manage Data Syst.* 2006; 106(1): 5–20.

Hart C. *Doing Your Masters Dissertation.* London: Sage Publications; 2005.

Hartswood M, Procter R, Rouncefield M, *et al.* Making a case in medical work: implications for the electronic medical record. *Comp Support Coop Work.* 2003; 12(3): 241–66.

Hasselbring W. Information system integration. *Commun ACM.* 2000; 43(6): 33–8.

Haux R. Health information systems – past, present, future. *Int J Med Inform.* 2006; 75(3–4): 268–81.

Hayrinen K, Saranto K, Nykanen P. Definition, structure, content, use and impacts of electronic health records: a review of the research literature. *Int J Med Inform.* 2008; 77(5): 291–304.

Hendy J, Fulop N, Reeves BC, *et al.* Implementing the NHS information technology programme: qualitative study of progress in acute trusts. *BMJ.* 2007; 334: 1360–7.

Hennington AH, Janz BD. Information systems and healthcare. XVI: physician adoption of electronic medical records: applying the UTAUT model in a healthcare context. *Commun AIS.* 2007; 19: 60–80.

Hersh WR. Medical informatics: improving health care through information. *JAMA.* 2002; 288(16): 1955–8.

Herzlinger RE. Why innovation in health care is so hard. *Har Bus Rev.* 2006; 84(5): 58–66.

Hillestad R, Bigelow J, Bower A, *et al.* Can electronic medical record systems transform health care? Potential health benefits, savings and costs. *Health Aff.* 2005; 24(5): 1103–17.

Hsu MH, Chiu CM. Predicting electronic service continuance with a decomposed theory of planned behaviour. *Behav Inf Technol.* 2004; 23(5): 359–73.

Hughes JT, Bayes J. Managing IT: the introduction and adoption of new systems. *Public Money Manage.* 1991; 11(3): 31–6.

Jensen TB, Aanestad M. How healthcare professionals make sense of an electronic patient record adoption. *Inf Syst Manage.* 2007; 24(1): 29–42.

Johns PM. Integrating information systems and health care. *Logistics Inf Manage.* 1997; 10(4): 140–5.

Kaplan B. Addressing organisational issues into the evaluation of medical systems. *J Am Med Inform Assoc.* 1997; 4(2): 94–101.

Kaplan B, Duchon D. Combining qualitative and quantitative methods in information systems research: a case study. *MIS Quarterly.* 1988; 12(4): 571–86.

Kaplan B, Farzanfar R, Friedman RH. Personal relationships with an intelligent interactive telephone health behaviour advisor system: a multimethod study using surveys and ethnographic interviews. *Int J Med Inform.* 2003; 71(1): 33–41.

Khatri N. Building IT capability in healthcare organisations. *Health Serv Manage Res.* 2006; 19(2): 73–9.

Khoumbati K, Themistocleous M. Evaluating integration approaches adopted by healthcare organisations. *J Comput Inf Syst*. 2006; 47(2): 20–7.

Khoumbati K, Themistocleous M, Irani Z. Evaluating the adoption of enterprise application integration in healthcare organisations. *J Manage Inf Syst*. 2006; 22(4): 69–108.

Kim KK, Michelman JE. An examination of factors for the strategic use of information systems in the healthcare industry. *MIS Quarterly*. 1990; 14(2): 201–15.

Kuziemsky CE, Jahnke JH. Information systems and healthcare. V: a multi-modal approach to health care decision support systems. *Commun AIS*. 2005; 16(9): 407–20.

Landry BJL, Mahesh S, Hartman SJ. The impact of the pervasive information age on healthcare organisations. *J Health Hum Serv Adm*. 2004; 27(3–4): 444–64.

Lee AS, Baskerville RL. Generalising generalisability in information systems research. *Inf Syst Res*. 2003; 14(3): 221–43.

Lemmer B, Grellier R, Steven J. Systematic review of non-random and qualitative research literature: exploring and uncovering an evidence base for health visiting and decision making. *Qual Health Res*. 1999; 9(3): 315–28.

Lenz R, Beyer M, Kuhn KA. Semantic integration in healthcare networks. *Int J Med Inform*. 2007; 76(2–3): 201–7.

Levy Y, Ellis TJ. A systems approach to conduct an effective literature review in support of information systems research. *Inform Sci J*. 2006; 9: 181–212.

Lutchen M, Collins A. IT governance in a health care setting: reinventing the health care industry. *J Health Compl*. 2005; 7(6): 27–30.

McDonald CJ. The barriers to electronic medical record systems and how to overcome them. *J Am Med Inform Assoc*. 1997; 4(3): 213–21.

Makoul G, Curry RH, Tang PC. The use of electronic medical records: communication patterns in outpatient encounters. *J Am Med Inform Assoc*. 2001; 8(6): 610–15.

Mark AL. Modernising healthcare – is the NPfIT for purpose? *J Inf Technol*. 2007; 22(3): 248–56.

Mendoza LE, Perez M, Griman A. Critical success factors for managing systems integration. *Inf Syst Manage*. 2006; 23(2): 56–75.

Newell S, Swan JA, Galliers RD. A knowledge-focused perspective on the diffusion and adoption of complex information technologies: the BPR example. *Inf Syst*. 2000; 10(3): 239–59.

NHS Executive. *Information for Health*. A1103. Wetherby: Department of Health Publications; 1998.

Nolan RL. Managing the crises in data processing. *Har Bus Rev*. 1979; 57(2): 115–26.

Ram MB, Campling N, Grocott P, Weir H. A methodology for a structured survey of the healthcare literature related to medical device users. *Evaluation*. 2008; 14(1): 49–73.

Raghupathi W. Information technology in healthcare: a review of key applications. In: Beaver K, editor. *Healthcare Information Systems*. Boca Raton, FL: Auerbach Publishers; 2002.

Raghupathi W, Tan J. Strategic IT applications in health care. *Commun ACM*. 2002; 45(12): 56–61.

Rahimi B, Vimarlund V. Methods to evaluate health information systems in healthcare settings: a literature review. *J Med Syst*. 2007; 31(5): 397–432.

Rigby MJ, Robins SC. Building healthcare delivery and management systems centred on information about the human aspects. *Comput Methods Programs Biomed*. 1997; 54(1–2): 93–9.

Rigby M. Applying emergent ubiquitous technologies in health: the need to respond to new challenges of opportunity, expectation, and responsibility. *Int J Med Inform.* 2007; 76(Suppl.): S349–52.

Rigby M, Budgen D, Turner M, *et al.* A data-gathering broker as a future-orientated approach to supporting EPR users. *Int J Med Inform.* 2007; 76(2–3): 137–44.

Rivers PA, Bae S. Aligning information systems for effective total quality management implementation in healthcare organizations. *Total Qual Manage.* 1999; 10(2): 281–9.

Shortliffe EH. Strategic action in health information technology: why the obvious has taken so long. *Health Aff.* 2005; 24(5): 1222–31.

Southard PB, Hong S, Siau K. Information technology in the health care industry: a primer. *Proceedings of the 33rd Hawaii International Conference on System Sciences.* Maui, Hawaii, 2000 Jan 4–7.

Stead WW, Miller RA, Musen MA, *et al.* Integration and beyond: linking information from disparate sources into workflow. *J Am Med Inform Assoc.* 2000; 7(2): 135–45.

Stuewe S. Interface tools for healthcare information technology. In: Beaver K, editor. *Healthcare Information Systems.* Boca Raton, FL: Auerbach Publishers; 2002.

Tange HJ. The paper-based patient record: is it really so bad? *Comput Methods Programs Biomed.* 1995; 48(1–2): 127–31.

Thrasher EH, Byrd TA, Hall D. Information systems and healthcare. XV: strategic fit in healthcare integrated delivery systems: an empirical investigation. *Commun AIS.* 2006; 18: 692–709.

Tsiknakis M, Katehakis DG, Orphanoudakis SC. An open, component-based information infrastructure for integrated health information networks. *Int J Med Inform.* 2002; 68(3): 3–26.

Turban E, Sharda R, Aronson JE, *et al. Business Intelligence: a managerial approach.* New Jersey: Pearson Education; 2008.

Wainwright D, Waring T. The information management and technology strategy of the UK National Health Service. *Int J Public Sector Manage.* 2000; 13(2–3): 241–59.

Wainwright D, Waring T. Three domains for implementing integrated information systems: redressing the balance between technology, strategic and organisational analysis. *Int J Inf Manage.* 2004; 24(4): 329–46.

Wainwright D, Waring TS. The application and adaptation of a diffusion of innovation framework for information systems research in NHS general medical practice. *J Inf Technol.* 2007; 22(1): 44–58.

Wallace M, Wray A. *Critical Reading and Writing for Postgraduates.* London: Sage Publications; 2006.

Walsham G. Learning about being critical. *Inf Syst.* 2005; 15(2): 111–17.

Wang BB, Wan TTH, Burke DE, *et al.* Factors influencing health information system adoption in American hospitals. *Health Care Manage Rev.* 2005; 30(1): 44–51.

Ward J, Peppard J. *Strategic Planning for Information Systems,* 3rd ed. Chichester: John Wiley and Sons; 2002.

Waring T, Wainwright D. Interpreting integration with respect to information systems in organisations: image, theory and reality. *J Inf Technol.* 2000; 15(2): 131–48.

Weber Y, Pliskin N. The effects of information systems integration and organisational culture on a firm's effectiveness. *Inf Manage.* 1996; 30(2): 81–90.

Webster J, Watson R. Analyzing the past to prepare for the future: writing a literature review. *MIS Quarterly.* 2002; 26(2): xiii–xxiii.

Weiner BJ, Savitz LA, Bernard S, *et al.* How do integrated delivery systems adopt and implement clinical information systems? *Health Care Manage Rev.* 2004; 29(1): 51–66.

Winthereik BR, Vikkelso S. ICT and integrated care: some dilemmas of standardising inter-organisational communication. *Comp Support Coop Work.* 2005; 14(1): 43–67.

Wyse JE, Higgins CA. MIS integration: a framework for management. *J Syst Manage.* 1993; 44(2): 32–7.

CHAPTER 8

The NHS National Programme for Information Technology: a socio-technical systems perspective

Ken Eason

INTRODUCTION

The National Programme for Information Technology (NPfIT) was planned as a 10-year programme to transform the way patient records were handled in nearly 400 trusts and over 8000 General Practice surgeries of the National Health Service in England (Brennan 2005). The aim was to move from vaults full of paper records to electronic care records that could be shared across all of the trusts. To achieve this goal a few large information technology consortia were contracted to deliver common technical solutions across the trusts in England. Contracts worth £6.2 billion were awarded in 2003. It is clear from these beginnings that the main driver for the programme was the implementation of technical solutions. However, it is also clear from the objectives of the programme that the goal was to transform the working practices of all healthcare teams from the use of paper-based records to the sharing of electronic records. This constitutes a major organisational change programme that impacts on the working practices of thousands of clinicians, nurses, paramedics, administrators and others. If the programme is to be successful it has to address both technical and organisational change and, as such, can be considered a programme for very large socio-technical systems change. This chapter reviews the progress of the national programme after five years from a socio-technical perspective. How has a programme based on the centralised delivery of common technical systems managed the organisational changes that are necessary for the objectives of the programme to be achieved?

SOCIO-TECHNICAL SYSTEMS THINKING

Socio-technical systems thinking provides a perspective on the operational reality of delivering work on a daily basis in organisations that emphasises the need for close integration of the human and technical resources that gets the work done. Understanding organisational behaviour as a socio-technical system began in earnest at the Tavistock Institute of Human Relations in London in the 1950s. The initial studies were about technical change in weaving mills in India (Rice 1958) and coal mining in England (Trist and Bamforth 1951). These studies found that the new technologies that were introduced to increase work productivity disrupted the social system of the workplace. The staff in work roles who relied on one another to get the overall task done found that the new technology was making it more difficult for them to work together. The result was that the overall performance of the work system deteriorated. The researchers recognised that the technical and social systems were interdependent at many levels and they coined the principle of co-optimisation as a statement of a fundamental aim when designing a work system: the technical and social systems have to be integrated at every level. The socio-technical systems theory that came out of these studies was also an open systems theory. It recognises that the environment in which a work system exists can be turbulent and that this can affect the inputs to the work process, the outputs it has to produce and the conditions under which the work is done. As a consequence an operational socio-technical system has to be one that can adapt and adjust to change in both the short term and the long term.

This frame of reference has been widely used to study the impact of ICT on organisations, for example, Mumford (1993) and Eason (1996). The majority of studies investigated what happened when a new ICT system was implemented in an already operational socio-technical system. The results demonstrate the mechanisms by which the existing socio-technical system adjusts to the new technical system. In some instances the adjustment might be full adoption to achieve the planned purposes. However, other outcomes are more likely: the new system may be rejected or it may cause stresses and strains in the operation of the work system that render it less productive. Other common outcomes are that only parts of the functionality of the new systems are adopted or that users devise elaborate 'workarounds' to cope with the differences between what the system offers and what is required to get the job done. All of these outcomes point to a process whereby the linkages between the new technical system and the working practices of the existing socio-technical system are being explored and new practices emerge as opportunities and problems are encountered. The results suggest that overall 'co-optimisation' can be difficult to achieve.

After five years of 'rolling out' the NPfIT to the NHS trusts we should be in a position to gauge what kind of process of assimilating the new technical systems into existing healthcare practices is occurring. The national programme has an array of targets for the deployment of its systems to the trusts, that is, the dates by which technical systems should be installed and operational. However, deployment is not the same as the adoption of the technical system into the working practices of the existing socio-technical system. The analysis below reports on both the achievements in technical system deployment and on the adoption of the systems into healthcare practice.

PROGRESS OF THE NATIONAL PROGRAMME

As a major source of government expenditure, the NPfIT has been subject to very close scrutiny and, in May 2008, an official review of the progress of the programme was published by the National Audit Office (NAO 2008a, 2008b). Despite the fact that there has been widespread agreement in the NHS that the general use of electronic patient records could bring many benefits, the programme has been beset by problems from the outset and the overall NAO judgement is that it is four years behind in its 10-year plan. However, although it was devised as one large integrated IT programme, in reality the programme is a suite of many different computer applications and some of them have fared better than others. In Table 8.1 the progress of nine of these developments is summarised using the data from the NAO reports. Three of the developments are IT infrastructure projects, to create an IT structure to enable communication across the NHS, three are specific user applications and three are more general purpose, that is, they are to create full electronic care record systems to support all the different healthcare activities that take place in the trusts.

There are major differences in the achievements of the different projects in the programme. The three infrastructure projects have achieved their technical delivery targets on or before the target dates. These are enabling projects and as such there is no process by which they directly impact the working practices of healthcare teams. They may have been large and complex technical tasks but, since they did not have to engage with user issues directly, there is not a separate process by which they are adopted by healthcare professionals. They are the basis upon which the applications below enable electronic records to be shared and it is in these other projects where the socio-technical issues come into play. NHSmail is slightly different because it does enable staff to send and receive e-mails. The NAO report states that, although it was deployed in 2004, 'take-up has been slow' (NAO 2008b: 33).

At the end of May 2008 43% of the NHS users with e-mail addresses were using NHSmail. NHS staff have existing e-mail accounts on other systems and, although NHSmail offers a secure way of sending information, its widespread adoption by staff is a relatively slow process. This is an indication of a common adoption issue; if there is already a similar system in use, what advantages does the new system offer that would cause it to be adopted?

TABLE 8.1 Progress of the NPfIT Programme May 2008 (based on NAO 2008a, 2008b)

Project	Purpose	Progress
ICT Infrastructure		
N3 – The National Network	To provide fast, broadband connections between all trusts.	Target: connect all sites by March 2007. Achievement: two months before schedule.
NHSmail	To provide a secure e-mail service for all trusts.	Achievement: delivered on time in October 2004.
The National Data Spine	To provide the architecture for the national databases.	Technical delivery achieved on time in a number of releases from May 2006.
Specific applications		
The Summary Care Record	To mount limited care records of all patients in England on the Spine.	Deferred for two years. Early adopter pilots in March 2007.
Choose and Book	To enable GPs to help patients choose referrals and to make electronic bookings.	Target: 90% of referrals by March 2007. Achievement: 31% referrals by March 2008.
Picture Archiving and Communications System	To store and share electronic images.	Brought into the NPfIT in 2004. Fully deployed by December 2007, three months ahead of schedule.
The full electronic care record systems		
The London Programme for IT	To deliver common and full electronic care records to all trusts in the London area.	Programme proved impracticable. Revised plan from 2007.
The Southern Programme for IT	To deliver common and full electronic care records to all trusts in the South of England.	Programme proved impracticable. The main contractor left the programme in June 2008.
North, Midlands and East Programme for IT	To deliver common and full electronic care records to all trusts in the North, Midlands and East of England.	This was originally three separate 'clusters'. The programmes in each case proved impracticable. The main contractor for two of the clusters withdrew from the programme in September 2006 and the three areas were merged. The main IT system is still under development and other systems are being implemented.

The specific applications and the full electronic care records systems listed in Table 8.1 all involve major take-up processes by healthcare teams and many of them have run into serious problems. In the next section below, the three specific user applications are examined more closely and this is followed by an examination of the implementation of the full electronic care record systems.

THE ADOPTION OF SPECIFIC APPLICATIONS

The Summary Care Record (SCR)

One of the major objectives of the NPfIT programme is that clinicians anywhere in the country should be able to access a summary electronic record of every patient in England that provides not only demographic information but clinical information on allergies and current medication. The plan is that this information will be uploaded to the Spine from the records of GPs. The NAO report that 'in 2005 the implementation of the Summary Care Record was deferred by two years on the grounds of complexity and the need for wider consultation, for example, on patient confidentiality issues' (NAO 2008b: 20). From the beginning of NPfIT there had been a public debate about the Summary Care Record because it meant that confidential information about patients previously only available in systems held within GP clinics were now to be held on very large databases. There have been questions about the security of the information, who would have access to it and the rights of patients to check the accuracy of information held or even to withhold it from the system. The process was delayed while these issues and technical issues were addressed.

In March 2007 summary care record trials were undertaken at five early adopter sites and the NAO reported that by March 2008 over 153 000 care records had been established (NAO 2008b). Greenhalgh, *et al.* (2008) undertook a year-long evaluation of the early adopter pilots and concluded that there were many social and organisational issues to be addressed before there could be widespread adoption of the summary care record.

1 Many GPs remained anxious about the confidentiality and security of the patient records and were protective of 'their' patients' data.
2 The system raised issues about patients' rights with respect to their healthcare record and whether they would have to be asked to 'opt in' to the system or whether consent would be assumed unless they 'opted out'. Regardless of the procedure, it would take time and effort to consult patients and many GP clinics were concerned about the effort involved.
3 The uploading of information to the database ran into technical difficulties in some of the pilots because of problems linking the Spine software to the systems which GPs held their patient records. In some cases the GP clinics held the clinical and demographic information about patients on separate systems and this increased the effort involved.
4 The views of GPs about the SCR were influenced by the fact that uploading the information was effortful and time consuming for them and their staff but yielded no specific benefit to them. GPs who had roles where the SCR could be of value,

e.g. they also provided an out-of-hours GP service, took a more positive view in adopting the system.

The Picture Archiving and Communications System (PACS)

The PACS collects, stores and communicates electronic X-ray and other forms of medical images. It replaces the previous film technology for X-rays. PACS has been under development for many years in the NHS and was not originally part of the NPfIT programme. It became part of the programme in 2004 and was fully deployed in hospital trusts by 2007, three months ahead of schedule. Although substantive studies of its usage are not available, many reports speak of its rapid take-up across the country. The NAO team visited 15 trusts and report that radiologists and radiographers felt it aided diagnosis through the flexibility of being able to manipulate images easily. They noted in particular a change in working practices whereby doctors were using mobile display devices to discuss scans with patients at their bedside (NAO 2008a). The widespread adoption of PACS makes it an exception in the suite of NPfIT applications that have direct impact on the working practices of healthcare teams. It is the only one to have been readily accepted and to have been rapidly assimilated into healthcare practice. One reason for this is that the user community sees direct benefits arising from this application. It cuts out a lot of messy and time-consuming film development. It provides good quality images that can facilitate accurate diagnosis.

As a study before the NPfIT programme revealed (Cox and Dawe 2002), electronic images can be processed faster, it is easier to find them in a store and they can be shared easily with colleagues. There have, in the past, been doubts and questions about it, for example, whether the display quality is adequate, and its use does have implications for staff workload and for the allocation of duties, but the long period of development and exploration of its use before its adoption in the NPfIT means that these issues are now widely understood. There remain further developments that may pose new organisational issues, for example, how to share images with a wider population of clinicians, but the process of assimilating this technology into the practices of specialists such as radiologists and radiographers is well under way.

Choose and Book

Choose and Book is a system that enables general practitioners to offer patients a choice of where specialist treatment might be undertaken and it then facilitates making a booking. The system was launched in 2004 and links GP clinics and the appointment processes in acute trusts. It has been slowly deployed but in March 2008 was available to 95% of GP clinics across England and 84% of acute trusts had access to a compatible system. However, the rate of take-up has been slower than planned and patchy. The target was that 90% of GP referrals would be made via Choose and Book by March 2007. In practice 38% of referrals were made by March 2008 and there was a very large variation across primary care trusts, three achieved more than 90% but four achieved less than 20% (NAO 2008b). Behind these figures is a complex process in which GP clinics have worked out whether to use Choose and Book and, if so, how to do so most effectively. The original scenario for Choose and Book was that during the consultation the GP would show the patient the alternatives on the system and, after the discussion, the GP would book the appointment. In practice, when Choose and Book is used, the NAO report identifies five different processes that have been developed in order to book an appointment. Of these only 9% are bookings made by the GP. In 22% of cases GP staff made the booking, particularly where the clinic had a practice manager. In 33% of cases the patient made the booking either via the Internet or an appointments line. However, in many cases hospitals have been unable to provide an online booking service and indirect booking services have been developed in which the patient telephones the selected hospital to make an appointment.

The history of Choose and Book demonstrates quite starkly the difference between deployment of a system and its adoption as normal working practice. GPs had a lot of reservations about the system and had alternative ways in which they could make referrals and these factors have delayed adoption. The process has also been delayed by the search for appropriate organisational processes to support Choose and Book and a range of different solutions have been found. The expectation that this was a technical system to be used by a patient and their GP has proved ill-founded and adoption has become a hunt for more complex socio-technical solutions.

Full electronic healthcare record systems

The implementation of full electronic healthcare records is a central objective of the national programme. The original aim was that the country would be divided into five areas and, in each one, a local service provider (LSP) would deliver a single 'best of breed' system to all trusts. This would facilitate the exchange of a full range of electronic healthcare data and would bring all the trusts in the area up to a common standard of electronic record provision. The majority of the original funding (80% of £6.2 billion) was targeted for this objective. It is this objective that has been most difficult to achieve – in most cases it was not just a case of missed deadlines, but of 'a plan that proved impractical' and had to be scrapped.

It is useful to begin the analysis of what happened from the perspective of the suppliers. They were first required to modify existing 'best of breed' healthcare systems for NHS use and then to roll them out to all the trusts in their area. The contracts agreed with the NHS stipulated that the suppliers would be paid when systems were installed and working in trusts, so they had a strong incentive to get the systems in and move on to the next trust to meet the targets of the roll-out plan. Each supplier serviced many trusts and a complex roll-out plan was published which provided a limited 'window' for the installation of a system in each trust. The suppliers had more difficulty preparing the systems for NHS use than expected and one of the major systems, iSoft's Lorenzo, is still not ready five years into the roll-out timetable. They also found that different trusts represented different challenges and required different kinds of support. In order to install a new healthcare system it was necessary to migrate data from existing systems (which were then intended to cease operation). In the implementation of these systems, therefore, there is an immediate and direct impact on the working practices of those needing access to patient records. The process of working with each trust at this level proved complex and challenging and, as a result, all of the local service providers fell behind their planned schedule. As difficulties and delays mounted, the main suppliers and the NHS attempted to renegotiate the contracts, but two of the main contractors have now left the programme: Accenture in September 2006 and Fujitsu in May 2008.

In evaluating why it has been so difficult to make progress with full electronic healthcare records it is possible to point to technical difficulties, but by far the biggest issues have been the difficulties of (1) delivering a common technical solution to a very diverse set of trusts and (2) integrating the new e-health system into the complex healthcare practices that exist for every medical specialism and which are already mature socio-technical systems delivering healthcare on a daily basis. These two factors are explored in more detail below.

THE DIVERSITY OF TRUSTS

In each of the areas covered by a local service provider there is a wide variety of trusts including acute trusts delivering hospital care, primary care trusts and general practitioner (GP) clinics, ambulance and emergency trusts, and mental health trusts. Trusts vary in size and specialism, from large city hospitals with teaching and research programmes to small country hospitals and specialist hospitals for cancer, orthopaedics, children etc. They vary in the services they supply, the links they have with other agencies, including private suppliers of healthcare and, of course, with the sophistication of the electronic patient record systems they already operate. They also show a lot of internal variation because the records needed for cancer patients are different from orthopaedic patients and these are very different from those for patients with depression or for elderly people who may suffer from many conditions at the same time.

The trusts were expected to stop using their existing systems and to migrate their patient records to the new common solution. There were strong incentives to do so, including the fact that they were being offered the best systems available for nothing. However, when they looked at what was on offer, many trusts found that it was not a good fit with their requirements. Table 8.2 lists a few of the problems that were encountered.

Table 8.2 illustrates only a few of the trusts that found that the system offered was not appropriate to their needs. The diversity of the trusts meant that the system selected was a misfit for many of them. Michael, the chief executive of Guys and St Thomas' NHS Foundation Trust and a supporter of the programme, declared that 'the flaw of the national programme is the belief that "One-Size Fits All"' (Collins 2006). A particular difficulty was encountered when a trust was already advanced in the use of electronic healthcare records and had installed a system specific to its needs. To be part of the national programme the trust might have to take a step backwards and be downgraded to the common standard of all. As a result of representations from many trusts, Connecting for Health, the agency delivering the NPfIT,

TABLE 8.2 The diverse requirements of trusts

NHS Trust/Healthcare provider	Issue	Outcome
St Mary Sidcup	An earlier adopter site that found the new system 'not fit for purpose'.	System removed and the LSP adopted a different common solution (Clark 2006).
Royal Marsden Cancer Hospital	As an international centre for cancer research, the electronic records needed are very specialised.	The system offered would have much poorer records than those already in place. The hospital continued with its existing system (Milan 2005).
GP surgeries	The majority of GP surgeries had already implemented a successful system that was not the solution offered in the programme.	Many GPs refused the new system and, after extensive negotiations, the supplier of the current GP systems was admitted to the NPfIT.
London Mental Health Trusts	The system offered had no facilities for significant parts of mental health records, especially those that were statutory requirements under the Mental Health Act.	The trusts were allowed to adopt a system specifically designed for Mental Health as an 'interim solution' (NAO 2008b).
The Wirral Hospital Trust	The Wirral had already implemented systems for sharing data with local healthcare agencies.	The new system would be a significant step backwards. They have continued with their existing system (Merrick 2007).

and the LSPs changed their approach and admitted new suppliers of 'interim' solutions better fitted to particular needs into the programme.

THE ADOPTION OF FULL ELECTRONIC HEALTHCARE RECORDS

Although many trusts concluded that the electronic record system they were offered would not meet their needs, many others went ahead with the implementation of the system provided by their local service provider. Within the roll-out programme implementation was in many cases undertaken in a relatively short period and focused upon the technical installation of system software, the migration of patient data from existing systems to the new system, the training of users and the registration of users so they could make authorised use of patient records. However, if the national programme is to achieve its objective of transforming healthcare through the use of electronic records, this is only the beginning of the process. Installing the system has then to be followed by staff finding ways of using it in relation to the everyday practices by which they deliver healthcare. There has been no comprehensive survey of how trusts have fared in this process. However, as the national programme has developed, anecdotal accounts of the issues associated with the adoption of electronic healthcare practices have emerged and it is apparent that this is often a slow and stressful process. There are now accounts of specific research studies in the literature. We have worked in detail with one mental health trust (Eason 2007) and have had extensive discussions about implementation experiences with the information technology staff of 10 trusts, covering both the primary and secondary sector. Below is a summary of the many issues that are reported. They are presented under five headings, starting with the issues for individual users and moving to broader organisational questions.

1 Inputting data into the electronic patient records

A database is only as good as the data it contains and electronic healthcare records depend on the people who administer, diagnose and treat the patient updating the record as necessary. If data is input at source the possibility of errors is minimised and the source of the input can be registered. However, for many users the inputting of data can be a problematic process.

➤ When and how do you input data? It may be relatively straightforward for administrators in offices or clinicians in consulting rooms to enter data on a desktop computer but if the consultation is in the patient's home, on the ward etc. it may necessitate the use of specialist hand-held and portable devices with attendant issues of security and confidentiality.

➤ What is the effect on the patient? Many clinicians, especially those treating patients with mental illnesses, have expressed anxieties about using a computer when they should be attending to the patient. Some patients could react negatively if they felt the doctor was more interested in the computer than in them.

➤ Being turned into 'data input clerks'. Traditionally, records have been updated by clerical staff on behalf of clinicians. Many clinicians are now concerned about the additional load they may have to take on if they have to do all the work directly. For many it is not a good use of their professional skills to be operating a keyboard.

➤ What goes into the record and for what purposes? By far the biggest concern is about what they have to enter. Typically, the inputs required are pre-structured, their source is logged and, after confirmation, the entry cannot be changed. Many clinicians have voiced concerns about the confidentiality of their entries and the need to ensure their patient's privacy is protected. Since they are identified as the source, they may be also concerned about how the data might be used to assess them.

➤ 'Working notes' or formal records? Clinicians often work with colleagues to check assumptions about diagnoses, to assess whether treatments are effective etc. and, as Hardstone, et al. (2004) have found, they traditionally use patient notes to share these informal working hypotheses with colleagues. Electronic record systems usually only record outcomes and conclusions and, as such, the entries the clinician makes may be of little direct value. This is a classical problem with database systems; the user may be entering data for others to use rather than for their own use. Working for the collective good has less motivating power than recording something that may prove of direct benefit in the completion of the current task.

The consequence of these issues is that many users minimise the data they enter in the official healthcare records. Many databases contain demographic information about patients but relatively little clinical information. Some of the NPfIT care record systems in hospitals are at present only PASs (patient administrative systems) and do not have the capability to store clinical records. However, even when they do, the clinical information is often sparse. Clinicians may put the minimum into the official system, put working information of specific relevance to them into other local systems and they may sustain local paper records in order to share information with colleagues.

2 Accessing and using electronic patient records

If they are to be useful, the records have to be accessible to all staff who are associated with the treatment of a patient. However, the privacy of patient information is very important and the security of the records has been a major national concern ever since the programme was announced. Electronic healthcare record systems have in some way to serve what can be two conflicting objectives: to enable data to be shared and to keep data confidential. In order that only staff who need to access a patient's record can do so, the national programme has introduced a strict role-based access process for determining a user's rights of access. In this process, after training, a member of staff is registered as a user and issued with a smart card and a pin number that specify the degree to which they can access records in accordance with their role with respect to patients; for example, clinical staff may view clinical records, nursing staff may view treatment information, administrative staff may only view administrative information etc. And each member of staff can only view the records of patients for whom they have some responsibility. In theory this process means everybody can access what they need to know and no more. While there is strong support for security safeguards, in practice this process is often too rigid for the changing and unpredictable world of healthcare. The members of a healthcare team, for example, might all need to access a patient's record in order to have a full case conference but in practice some of them may only be able to access partial information.

In a mental hospital trust (Eason 2007) we found that staff turnover was very high and many temporary but qualified staff were needed to sustain patient care. However, organising training and registration could take some time and this meant that the staff were technically excluded from accessing patient information during this period. In these and other circumstances an informal practice has developed whereby the senior member of the team who has full access leaves his or her card in the card reader so that any member of the team can access the necessary information. In the Accident and Emergency Department of South Warwickshire General Hospitals Trust (Collins 2007) the medical staff found that the time it took to enter each of their smart cards was too long when there was a heavy emergency case load and they publicly declared they would operate a procedure whereby shift leaders left their cards in the card reader for the whole shift. A more general problem is the matching of local role responsibilities with the formal role definitions used in the registration process. There are organisational policies being pursued in the NHS that devolve clinical responsibilities, for example, to senior nursing staff. Every time this occurs there is a requirement to override the existing registration of the member of staff to enable them to fulfil their responsibilities.

The response of staff to problems of gaining access to records is to find 'workarounds', ways of using the system that enable work to go on despite any constraints or limitations of the technical system. This is a very common phenomenon in the use of many kinds of systems and displays the ingenuity of human beings when the limitations of systems interfere with the tasks they are trying to complete. It results in a wide array of unanticipated organisational practices, sometimes overt, sometimes covert, emerging around the use of new technical systems. The organisational procedures that have emerged around the use of 'Choose and Book' are similar examples, developed in part because the system could not make direct contact with clinic appointment systems in hospitals. Workarounds can be very effective means by which the socio-technical system adapts to new conditions, but they are often ad hoc individual reactions to local difficulties that may create new problems elsewhere in the system.

3 Supporting healthcare pathways

The patient journey through the NHS often involves different parts of the organisation and frequently involves different specialist services. One of the important potential benefits of electronic care records is that they could mean that, at all points along the healthcare pathway, the relevant member of staff has immediate access to the latest information about the patient's condition. This could dramatically improve the effectiveness of healthcare by eliminating the wait for information, cutting out the need to take the patient history many times, reducing the need to repeat tests and ensuring that a holistic view of the patient's medical circumstances is available. However, to achieve these objectives, the information in the system has to be matched to the healthcare pathway so that relevant information is available as and when needed. This is not easily achieved when there are many different medical conditions and many, many possible pathways. There is also a lot of variation between different NHS trusts in the detailed way in which information is kept about different conditions and the pathways that patients follow. As a result there is a need to configure systems to match what is required locally. The adoption of the system may also change the way the pathway operates; with greater provision of information, for example, it may be easier to treat patients in the community rather than in hospital. Achievements of the benefits of using healthcare records may therefore require local socio-technical design (Eason 2005). It might, for example, involve the healthcare team looking at current obstacles and inefficiencies in the process and working out whether a particular technical configuration of the records and changes in the organisational practices might have the potential to overcome these difficulties. In practice, because this involves detailed collaborative and local work, the provisions of the system often do not match the requirements of the healthcare pathway and existing practices are sustained.

It is possible to go further than the provision of patient data in the use of electronic care records to support of healthcare pathways. The records can also be used to provide protocols of best practice in the treatment of patients in particular circumstances and can perhaps act as expert systems, for example, to guide diagnostic work. The system can also be used to monitor performance and to collect statistics about local practice. Systems tend to be used in these ways, for example, to guide the procedures that nurses follow in treating patients. These ways of using technical systems can work to lift standards and enforce good practice but, again, in their daily use in operational healthcare they can cause problems. They may enforce practice that local staff do not consider appropriate in the context of a particular patient's circumstances. The response of staff might be to follow the procedures and 'tick all the boxes' but this may be to the detriment of the patient. Alternatively, the member of staff may ignore the system and use professional judgement to treat the patient, accepting the risk that they may be called to account for their behaviour subsequently. If the detailed design of the healthcare practices embedded in the system is subject to local configuration and emerge as manifestations of how the local team have decided to treat their patients, there is less likelihood that staff will face this kind of dilemma.

4 Organisational changes

The adoption of e-health systems as an integral part of delivering healthcare could have a wide variety of organisational implications. The most direct implications might be for the staff who were previously involved in creating, storing and retrieving the paper documents in patient records. If clinicians can, for example, update the records directly and retrieve them electronically, there is in theory no requirement for the administrative support that sustains a paper-based record system. However, previous research on the organisational adoption of new ICT systems suggests (*see*, e.g. Eason 1996) that such a straightforward change rarely occurs. Administrative staff will continue to have responsibilities for the administrative data in the system and it is likely, as in the case of the emergent organisational practices for 'Choose and Book', that administrative staff will play more major roles in the execution of patient processes than originally intended. There is also the strong likelihood, as Woolgar (1998) has expressed it, that the new e-health systems will not replace paper records but will complement them; some form of paper record systems will remain and will continue to require administrative support.

The lessons from other organisational contexts where ICT systems have been introduced are that there are no inevitable organisational changes but that the new technology creates conditions in which a variety of changes might become possible and desirable. There are likely to be many subtle and indirect routes to organisational change. Access to better records and support locally can, for example, mean that the healthcare process treats the patient more locally. There may be less need, for example, to treat patients in hospital. This could change the roles and responsibilities of every-body in the healthcare processes; hospital specialists may, for example, devote more time, perhaps via telemedicine, to advising colleagues on the treatment of patients rather than treating the patients themselves. Such changes may affect funding, the distribution of resources, the respective responsibilities of members of the healthcare community etc. and the redesign of the organisational arrangements may need as much time and effort as the design and implementation of the technical system.

But it would be wrong to imply that the organisational implications of e-health systems are only likely to result from the impact of a new technical system on a stable organisational structure. The health service is in a state of continuous organi-sational flux and it is just as likely that issues will arise in reverse: that a particular organisational change may have implications for the technical system. Perhaps one of the most worrying features of introducing a centralised, and in many ways fixed, e-health system is that it may obstruct organisational changes that are required either nationally or locally. Flexibility in the delivery of technical systems so that they can evolve as the organisation changes is at the heart of the open systems approach to socio-technical systems and is a major requirement in a complex and volatile organi-sation such as the NHS.

5 The configuration and evolution of the technical system

The diversity of trusts and the diversity of medical conditions mean that a technical system that serves well in one place may well be inappropriate in another. However, the NPfIT plan was to achieve data sharing by all having the same system. The 'one size fits all' assumption has caused a lot of problems in the programme and has led to a greater number of technical systems being deployed. However, there is another way of solving a potential mismatch between what is required and what a system provides. In socio-technical systems theory the requirement is to design according to the 'principle of minimum critical specification' (Cherns 1987), that is, create flex-ibility in the system so that it can be customised to meet local needs. Many modern technical systems have configuring potential. Eason (2007) found in a study of a system being delivered to a mental health trust that there was considerable potential for local decisions about the clinical information that could be kept in the patient record. However, while there may be some potential, there are many barriers to overcome in the national programme if local staff are to get a technical service that matches their particular needs. One problem is that the rapid roll-out programme leaves little time for staff to understand the flexibility of a system and do the necessary local design to deliver services as needed. To achieve this outcome, local clinicians and other users need to work with local IT staff to define what is needed. There are places where this process is in place but it is a slower, more evolutionary process than the 'big bang' implementation of the roll-out programme. Another problem is that there may be aspects of the systems delivered that cannot be changed locally. If a trust wishes to change these aspects of the system, they have to submit requests to the supplier and all the other trusts that are users of the system have to agree the change. This is a change process that can take a substantial amount of time. Another issue is that a system may serve user's needs at first, but the changing nature of healthcare organisations may require changes in the system. An important test for any technical system is how easily it can be adapted as the organisation evolves. If the user communities encounter mismatches between what they need and what the technical system delivers, and it is time consuming or difficult to change the technical system, it is often easier to treat the system as an immovable object and find ways of working round it by, for example, marginalising its use, retaining other technical systems and devising workarounds.

There are then many issues that emerge as healthcare teams seek to adopt electronic healthcare records into their working practice and there are three important conclusions to draw about how they are being handled in the national programme. First, most of the issues listed above are not on the formal agenda of the suppliers responsible for delivering full electronic healthcare records. As a result, they are dealt with in an ad hoc way by the people who encounter them, and socio-technical systems practices may emerge that were not in any sense 'designed'. Second, this process may serve to marginalise the degree of adoption of the new systems and potential benefits to the healthcare process might be lost. Third, the diversity of local conditions means that although the same issues may be encountered in different trusts, each may need to find its own local solutions.

THE NPfIT AS A SOCIO-TECHNICAL SYSTEMS DESIGN PROJECT

Having reviewed progress with the various aspects of the NPfIT, there is a stark conclusion: it has made great strides in creating the technical infrastructure for the national sharing of electronic healthcare records but, whenever the programme has to deal with the needs of particular user communities, it has run into delays and problems. In short, as a technical programme it is achieving success but as a socio-technical programme that will result in the transformation of e-health working practices, it has been much less successful. There are three main reasons:

1 'One size fits all'. The diversity of trusts and the diversity of medical conditions mean that it was always going to be problematic to enforce the use of common technical systems across the NHS. It has led to many trusts demanding alternatives and to those that do adopt the common systems having to find ways of accommodating to the specific characteristics of the systems.
2 Technical resources not socio-technical resources. The original £6.2 billion budget for the programme was for the suppliers to deliver technical solutions. It did not provide money for the trusts to engage in user training or any of the other activities involved in adopting the new systems within the trusts. As a result the organisational issues associated with the programme have hardly figured on the formal implementation agenda.
3 'Big bang' rather than evolution. The implementation programme has been a rapid roll-out process in which the emphasis has been upon taking out old systems, installing the new, migrating the data and training the users. Although the

trusts could call upon the suppliers for some help after the initial installation period, they have been largely left to find their own way in working out how to use the new systems in relation to their healthcare practices and in changing those practices to exploit the new technical capabilities.

In recognising that the roll-out programme of the full electronic health record in particular has not been going to plan, there is evidence that Connecting for Health has been changing its strategy in the delivery of the programme. This culminated in the publication of the Department of Health 'Health Informatics Report' (Department of Health 2008). The report sets out a plan for trusts to be given more local autonomy with respect to informatics developments. They will, for example, be permitted, within a framework of standards, to seek 'interim' IT solutions that meet their particular requirements. It also recognises that installation of technical systems is not sufficient to achieve real benefits and it stresses that trusts must 'take greater responsibility for implementation and subsequent transformational change' (p. 39) to ensure that benefits are realised. The role of Communicating for Health will also change so that it is a 'source of technical, commercial, service and programme management support expertise to the NHS', as well as being responsible for the implementation of the NPfIT (p. 36). In particular CfH is developing its role in the creation of capacity and competence in NHS trusts to implement e-health systems.

These changes suggest that the second period of the national programme will be characterised by a much more devolved structure that recognises the diversity of requirements across the NHS and a more explicit recognition that the achievement of the expected benefits depend upon socio-technical change rather than technical change. But there is little in the report to indicate how trusts are to discharge their responsibilities for 'transformational change'. Greenhalgh, *et al.* (2008) distinguish between two change models: 'make it happen' and 'let it emerge'. They characterise the current NPfIT model as a 'make it happen' approach in which change in working practice is part of the 'managed roll-out process'. I have elsewhere described it as a 'push' strategy (Eason 2005). The 'let it happen' or 'organic emergence' approach leaves the local community to find their own ways of adopting change at their own pace. As a result of their evaluation of the pilot sites adopting the Summary Care Record, Greenhalgh, *et al.* (2008) conclude that the 'roll-out should be undertaken at a pace and style consistent with the "softer" aspects of social and organisational change rather than as dictated by an over-arching Gantt chart'. However, they also conclude in relation to the 'let it happen' approach that 'we do not have firm evidence that the latter approach would necessarily meet with greater uptake' (p. 85).

Having reviewed progress with the wider programme, and especially the adoption of the full electronic care records, we might characterise what has been happening as an intensive 'make it happen' managed roll-out process for the short period of installation followed by an indeterminate 'let it happen' period. The first period often achieves technical installation, data migration, user registration and training but only limited adoption of the new systems within healthcare practices. The subsequent 'let it happen' stages have not been a funded and organised part of the national programme. On the basis of the limited data available it appears that during the 'let it happen' stage uptake is often marginalised, many aspects of the system are not used and existing ways of working are sustained. These outcomes are more the result of ad hoc responses by busy operational staff than a deliberate attempt by local staff to develop new working practices.

Greenhalgh, *et al.* (2008) suggest that what is needed to ensure effective uptake of the new technical systems and the transformation of working practices is a process that is somewhere between the 'make it happen' and 'let it happen' extremes. There is no evidence that ensuring responsibility for transformational change passes to the trusts will result in a middle approach being adopted; they may feel under pressure to sustain the 'technology push' approach. Socio-technical systems theory has for many years been concerned about the integrated development of technical and social systems and has, in particular, pioneered methods by which IT staff and user communities can work together to achieve this integration. It is 'a middle way' that encourages the local health community to 'make it happen' in ways that give benefit in their particular circumstances. As a report on NPfIT by the British Computer Society's Socio-Technical Systems Specialist Group suggests:

> socio-technical thinking and practice can be of practical benefit within NPfIT – provided the programme adopts a more holistic overall strategy that places social and organisational issues alongside technology concerns at the heart of its work. The methods recommended are based on socio-technical design principles which have been successfully applied in many environments over more than fifty years (Peltu, *et al.* 2008: 2).

The next section outlines the principles of this approach as they might apply in the further deployment of electronic healthcare records in the NHS.

PRINCIPLES OF SOCIO-TECHNICAL DESIGN AND CHANGE

The aims of socio-technical systems design are twofold. First, the requirement is to create a set of work practices in which technical resources support human beings who collaborate together to achieve the operational targets. The important element is the local task; the technical resources and the deployment of human resources have to be in the service of the task. The second requirement is that the socio-technical system is flexible and adaptive. There is need for flexibility because the task may present itself in many different forms. This is especially important in healthcare where highly trained professionals are needed on the front line of daily operational delivery because of the complexity and variability of the healthcare task and the many contexts in which patients need care. There is a need for the socio-technical system to be adaptive because the organisational and political context in which the work is being carried out will be subject to continuous change and the healthcare system will need to respond to these changes. These statements have several implications for socio-technical systems development:

➤ the focus has to be on the local form of the collective task
➤ the contributors have to include those who understand this task and particularly the variable forms that it can take
➤ the 'design' has to include both the technical and the social system
➤ the design has to be revisited on a regular basis and adapted to emerging situations.

In the context of the delivery of NPfIT systems these are challenging implications because, even with the autonomy trusts will now have, there is still a requirement to implement technical systems that adhere to standards that will facilitate data sharing. Following the 'principle of minimum specification' the target might be to design or select technical systems that meet national data exchange standards but still leave flexibility for local teams to customise them to their own requirements. Supposing there is suitable flexibility in the technical systems, what then is the process of socio-technical systems design? There are many possible methods that can be used in this process, but here are five key elements.

Participation through transitional systems

The active participation of all local stakeholders, including IT specialists and healthcare staff, is vital if new working practices are to be identified and implemented that take advantage of the opportunities presented by electronic care records. It is often difficult for busy, operational staff to get involved in ad hoc meetings to plan technical systems implementation. The creation of 'transitional systems' (Klein 2005) can help in this context because they provide an explicit vehicle in which people can meet together to explore the future. A 'transitional system' is a temporary structure that carries the organisation from one state to another and it does its work alongside the current operational system. To be effective it needs to be a place in which people can set aside the normal pressures of work and share, explore and experiment with different ways in which things can be done. It normally manifests itself as a temporary organisation with responsibility for a change process, in this case for exploring how electronic healthcare records can best be used to improve the local healthcare practices, it is open to all stakeholders involved and works mostly through a series of meetings or workshops separated as far as possible from the place of work. A transitional system of this kind does not work to fixed deadlines but explores what is possible and gradually implements and reviews new practices. It becomes the 'container' through which the activities below are conducted.

Working from the healthcare pathways

If the uptake process is to move away from a 'technology push' that drives particular kinds of changes in working practices, a different vision of the role of new technical resources needs to be established. A socio-technical view would be that there is a collective task to be undertaken and new technical systems represent resources that might help improve the performance of the collective task. What is needed is for the local stakeholders to explore the benefits that might be possible. To do this they first need to review their aspirations for the improvement of the collective task by examining the issues associated with the current healthcare pathways from the perspective of the different participants. They might ask, for example, how the experience of patients at the transition points in the pathway can be improved, what bottlenecks and delays need tackling, where information is lost or not shared, where procedures are unnecessarily duplicated and so on. Agreement on the kind of challenges they face can provide a strong basis for reviewing what a new technical system might have to offer.

Vehicles for experimentation and change – scenarios and prototypes

It is often difficult for potential technical system users to understand and contribute to systems design projects and, as people busy with their own operational tasks, they may have little time for what may seem obscure and technical discussions. The socio-technical requirement is to offer them grounded and real examples of what the operational practice of working with a new technical system might be like which they can use to identify the benefits that might be achieved and the issues that would have to be resolved. The process also has to demonstrate that there are socio-technical choices, so that participants can explore the benefits and issues of alternative forms of future practice before establishing the route to take. Many studies have shown that the best way of achieving these goals is to put in place pilot systems that can be the basis of experimentation. Since this can be an expensive and time-consuming process, an alternative approach is to create scenarios of future healthcare pathways in which the e-health systems have been adopted. Stakeholders can systematically work through the process to enable each contributor to the process to both understand what it would mean for them and to evaluate what benefits and issues might result. Klein (2005), for example, reports the use of 'Poor Old Henry' scenarios in Greenwich Hospital to evaluate the implications of a new e-health system. In this scenario 'Poor Old Henry' was a fictitious elderly patient with multiple conditions. Healthcare staff used the scenario to evaluate the possible use of the patient's electronic care record by the many different services he encountered and this helped the creation of integrated working practices when the new system was implemented.

Technical system customisation, work practice changes and organisational design

Local socio-technical systems work is not about championing and introducing a predefined set of new working practices. It is a series of design exercises in which local staff work out the work practices they will employ in the future. Starting with the requirements identified by reviewing the current healthcare pathways, the design exercises examine both the technical and human resources needed to meet these requirements and the outcomes may, for example, be specific customisations of the technical system, changes in work practices and organisational changes such as changes in the responsibilities of members of staff and perhaps a redistribution of roles across the organisational units involved in the healthcare process.

Evolutionary implementation and action research

The process of integrating a new technical system into operational work practices takes place over an extended period of time. A mechanism is needed that monitors the emergent usage of the system, assesses the benefits that are or might be achieved and identifies where problems and bottlenecks are limiting effective usage. The use of an action-research cycle can be an effective way of achieving these goals. Research in this instance involves making periodic evaluations of the use of the system and the issues that users are confronting and the 'action' involves sustaining elements of the 'transitional system', for example, a working group of IT staff and users, to receive the evaluation reports and undertake further socio-technical design work as necessary to maximise the benefits for the healthcare process.

In the discussions with staff from 10 trusts about the implementation of the NPfIT, it has become apparent that many elements of the methods described above have been put in place in different implementation processes. There are, for example, a number of examples of clinicians and IT specialists working together to customise electronic records for local use. However, everybody seems to be discovering these methods for themselves and they are, for the most part, only establishing part of the necessary procedures. At present, the 'middle way' seems to be a patchy, under-funded and often unrecognised bottom-up phenomenon that cannot be expected to help healthcare teams fully realise the benefits of the technical systems that are being deployed.

CONCLUSION

The national programme was created to make significant changes in the way health-care is delivered in England but, like many programmes before it, the focus of its financing and project management practice has been on the installation of technical solutions. Given the complexity and diversity of healthcare practices it is perhaps not surprising that the programme has run into major problems in delivering new forms of healthcare based on electronic working. There are significant indications that the programme is changing direction so that there can be more control of developments by trusts and this creates opportunities for socio-technical change that is geared to the needs of local healthcare. However, the shift of responsibility to a local level is a necessary but not sufficient condition for effective uptake of the potential of new technical systems to be achieved. The thesis of this paper is that the processes of socio-technical change cannot be effectively pursued in a context as operationally challenging as the NHS by either a top-down managed change pro-gramme or by a 'put in the technology and leave it to happen' approach. There is a danger that a review of the programme in five years' time will conclude that, despite the move to more local autonomy, uptake has not improved because no effective methods of supporting the necessary socio-technical systems design work were put in place. The methods evolved by socio-technical systems practitioners offer ways in which local, knowledgeable stakeholders can engage with and manage this process for themselves. Some aspects of these methods are being informally established and they may spread. However, their formal adoption on a large scale will involve confronting a big challenge. There are enormous differences between the formal project management, time and cost controlled methods that have been developed to install technical systems and the more organic, participative, evolutionary and ultimately always unfinished approaches that are necessary for socio-technical systems design. That these are very different would be less significant if the two undertakings could be pursued separately. However, it is an intrinsic feature of socio-technical systems that the technical and social are interdependent at every level, so the struggle must continue to reconcile these two approaches

REFERENCES

Brennan S. *The NHS IT Project: the biggest computer programme in the world . . . ever!* Oxford: Radcliffe Publishing; 2005.

Cherns A. Principles of socio-technical design revisited. *Hum Relat.* 1987; 40(3): 153–62.

Clark L. Trust feels pain of IT roll-out. *Computer Weekly.* 7 November 2006.

Collins T. NHS plan is evolving but one-size-fits-all is a fundamental flaw, says hospital chief. *Computer Weekly.* 14 March 2006.

Collins T. NHS security dilemma as smartcards shared. *Computer Weekly,* 30 January 2007.

Cox B, Dawe N. Evaluation of the impact of a PACS system on an intensive care unit. *J Manag Med.* 2002; 16(2/3): 199–205.

Department of Health. *Health Informatics Review Report 10 July.* London: Department of Health; 2008.

Eason KD. Understanding the organisational ramifications of implementing information technology systems. In: Helander MG, Landauer TK, Prabhu PV, editors. *Handbook of Human-Computer Interaction.* Amsterdam: Elsevier; 1996. pp. 1475–95.

Eason KD. Exploiting the potential of the NPfIT: a local design approach. *Br J Health Comput Inf Manage.* 2005; 22(7): 14–16.

Eason KD. Local socio-technical system development in the NHS National Programme for Information Technology. *J Inf Technol.* 2007; 22: 257–64. Available at: www.palgrave-journals.com/jit/journal/v22/n3/full/2000101a.html

Greenhalgh T, Stramer K, Bratan T, *et al. Summary Care Record Early Adopter Programme: an independent evaluation by University College, London.* London: UCL; 2008.

Hardstone G, Hartswood M, Procter R, *et al.* Supporting informality: team working and integrated care records. *Proceedings of the 2004 ACM conference on computer supported cooperative work.* 2004; 142–51.

Klein L. *Working Across the Gap: the practice of social science in organizations.* London: Karnac Publications; 2005.

Merrick R. NHS chief attacks computer project. *Liverpool Daily Post.* 15 June 2007.

Milan J. The NPfIT in London: a case study. *Br J Health Comput Inf Manage.* 2005; 22(2): 26–9.

Mumford E. *Designing Human Systems for Health Care.* Rotterdam: 4C Corporation; 1993.

National Audit Office. *The National Programme for IT in the NHS: progress since 2006.*

London: National Audit Office, HMSO. 16 May 2008a. Available at: www.nao.org.uk/pn/07-08/0708484.htm

National Audit Office. *The National Programme for IT in the NHS: project progress reports,* London: National Audit Office, HMSO. 16 May 2008b. Available at: www.nao.org.uk/pn/07-08/0708484.htm

Rice A. *Productivity and Social Organisation: the Ahmedabad experiment.* London: Tavistock; 1958.

Peltu M, Eason K, Clegg C. How a socio-technical approach can help NPfIT deliver better NHS patient care. Submitted for publication to *Behav Inf Technol;* 2008. Available at: www.bcs.org/upload/pdf/sociotechnical-approach-npfit.pdf

Trist E, Bamforth W. Some social and psychological consequences of the long wall method of coal-getting. *Hum Relat.* 1951; 4: 3–38.

Woolgar S. A new theory of innovation. *Prometheus.* 1998; 16: 441–53.

PART THREE

Global ICT Adoption and Implementation in Healthcare

New IT and the Kaiser Chiefs: EMR integration in the Aloha State

Tim Scott

INTRODUCTION

Kaiser Permanente is the largest integrated healthcare programme in the USA. It comprises The Kaiser Health Plan (health insurance) and the Permanente Medical Group (healthcare). In early 2003, I was asked to investigate the abortive implementation of an $800 million electronic medical record (EMR) system in the organisation's Hawaii Region. The findings of the study are reviewed in this chapter, which further examines some of the multiple integrative issues raised by the preparation, partial implementation and ultimate withdrawal of the EMR. Respondents' own words are used liberally, to preserve the freshness and authenticity of their narratives.

THE RESEARCH CONTEXT

Adopting new IT is a major challenge to healthcare organisations (Cutting 1984). By 2003, despite frequent calls in the US for greater use of EMRs (Institute of Medicine 1997, 2001, 2003), adoption of such technology had been limited (Miller, Hillman and Given 2004; Miller and Sim 2004). Few large systems had introduced or evaluated an EMR, due to their high cost and unquantifiable benefits. Few EMR studies have found positive evidence of benefits on care processes and health and financial outcomes (Department of Health 2001: Øvretveit 2007a, Øvretveit 2007b). Others had found disappointingly small or no effects (Evans 1998; Fiscella, *et al.* 2000; Gibbs 1997; Kaplan 1998; Littlejohns, Wyatt and Garvica 2003). Such projects face complex organisational challenges to integrate the new technology into workflows and redesign care processes to harness its potential (Miller and Sim 2004; Brynjolfsson and Hitt 2000). Succinct reviews of empirical research up to 2003 on the effectiveness of EMRs on specific functions have been published (Scott, *et al.* 2005; Scott, *et al.* 2007).

A BRIEF HISTORY OF KAISER PERMANENTE

With no national health service, most working Americans and their dependants are insured against ill-health as an employment benefit. Persons aged 65 and older are covered by the federal Medicare health insurance programme. Very low income individuals and families are eligible for health insurance benefits under Medicaid. Sixty-one million (35%) of the total US population are either uninsured (45 million) or underinsured (16 million) (Schoen, *et al.* 2005). Most people without insurance receive medical care from county or city-funded public hospitals and clinics. Even those with adequate insurance can find accessing healthcare in America difficult and expensive. Healthcare in the US is still dominated by the solo provider, fee for service practice model. From its outset in the 1930s, Kaiser Permanente adopted a different model, based on prepaid group practice. Its history was profoundly influenced by two individuals, Sidney Garfield MD and industrialist Henry J Kaiser.

The Mojave Desert

In 1933, at age 27, Garfield completed his training in general surgery at Los Angeles County Hospital (Smillie 1991). He intended to establish himself in a typical fee-for-service practice in Los Angeles. But 1933 was the worst year of the Depression and such opportunities were scarce. The Metropolitan Water District of Los Angeles was building an aqueduct from the Colorado River to Los Angeles and looking for a salaried physician to staff a small medical unit at Indio, on the edge of the Mojave Desert. Garfield was offered the job but thought the salary too low. Instead, he and Gene Morris built the small Contractors General Hospital, at Desert Centre, 60 miles east of Indio. Contractors and insurance companies supported the hospital, offering workers compulsory industrial and voluntary non-industrial coverage, for 10 cents a day.

When, 125 miles long, the aqueduct reached the Parker Dam construction site, Garfield built a second hospital. Then, in 1938 the Henry J Kaiser Company won the contract to build the Coulee Dam in Washington State, so Garfield established a prepaid medical programme for Kaiser employees and their dependants at the construction site. By emphasising preventative care, Garfield and his associates observed reductions in the severity of conditions presented by workers and their dependants.

SECOND WORLD WAR AND THE SHIPYARDS

In 1941, facing the Axis Powers alone, Britain depended on shipping convoys from the United States. The British Admiralty commissioned 60 freighters ('liberty ships') from the Todd-California Shipbuilding Consortium, organised by Henry J Kaiser and the Todd Shipbuilding Company of Seattle. Thirty freighters would be built in Richmond on San Francisco Bay. The Japanese bombing of Pearl Harbour in December 1941 brought the United States into the war, and the US Maritime Commission also became a Kaiser client. To accelerate production, Kaiser and others applied assembly line production methods to shipbuilding. By late 1943, around 90 000 men and women worked in the Kaiser shipyards and Garfield was again called upon to organise their medical care. By the end of the war, Kaiser Permanente was the largest civilian medical programme in American history. Garfield employed 100 physicians and their support staff to care for 200 000 workers and dependants, with 790 beds in four hospitals, in the Richmond yards, the Vancouver-Portland yards on the Columbia River between Washington and Oregon, and the Kaiser steel mill in southern California (Smillie 1991).

THE POST-WAR ERA

When the shipyards closed at the end of the war, the Richmond workforce shrank from 90 000 to 13 000, and the medical group from 75 to 12 physicians. Many doctors left to take up fee-for-service practice. The medical staffs at Vancouver and northern California met with dissolution on the agenda. Instead they voted to open the health plan to local communities.

In the immediate post-war years, Garfield struggled to maintain the programme. Most employers did not then provide health insurance for their employees. In the mid-1940s, Blue Cross and California Physicians Service (Blue Shield) were the two major plans. Some unions were wary of associating with Kaiser the industrialist. Politically conservative unions and employer groups were wary of prepaid group medical care. And many Bay Area residents assumed it was still a company programme. However, universities and civil service organisations were anxious to establish healthcare provision for their employees, and membership rose from a baseline of 10 000 members in mid-1945, to 72 000 by April 1948. Permanente medical care was affordable, consistent and efficient, its facilities integrated at one location.

In 1947, the United Steelworkers of America union chose Permanente as an alternative plan and asked the employers to provide payroll deductions. The companies refused. In arbitration it was determined that the employers must offer health insurance payment by payroll deduction, even when the group health plan was unilaterally selected by the union.

In 1948, civilian workers at Hunters Point Naval Shipyard enrolled in the programme. In 1950, the International Longshoremen and Warehousemen Union and the Retail Clerks union in Los Angeles brought Permanente to southern California. The ILWU membership required the establishment of Health Plan cover along the entire US Pacific coast, so new Permanente Plans were located in Seattle, Los Angeles and San Diego. The Group Health Cooperative of Puget Sound already operated in Seattle, so Garfield arranged for it to take up the ILWU contract. By August 1952 Permanente served 250 000 members, 160 000 of them in northern California.

The struggle for control

But a power struggle was brewing between Kaiser and the doctors (Smillie 1991). Kaiser persuaded the Health Plan and the Hospitals to formally adopt his name: Kaiser Foundation Health Plan and the Kaiser Foundation Hospitals. But the Permanente Medical Group refused to change its name to Kaiser and remained an autonomous medical partnership, to avoid any false imputation of being Kaiser employees.

The biggest issue between Kaiser and the Medical Group was ownership of the programme. While physicians saw Kaiser Health Plan as an agency to enrol their patients and collect dues, Kaiser Industries saw the Foundation and the Health Plan as leading the programme: members belonged to the Plan, not to the Medical Group. By April 1955, dissent between stakeholders had paralysed the organisation (Chall and Cutting 1985). On 21 April, the regional medical groups proposed the formation of a working council to address the impasse: 'We consider the basic problems to be the obtaining of a mutually satisfactory integration of all managerial activities, mutually satisfactory representation at policy-making levels, mutually satisfactory methods of monetary distribution and control, and mutually satisfactory methods of selection of all key personnel.'

The working council met on four occasions to consider the options: theoretically, doctors could take ownership of the Health Plan, but only by acquiring massive tax and other liabilities. The only feasible alternative was to draw clear contractual agreements between Health Plan and Medical Group.

The final session of the council was convened at Henry J Kaiser's Fleur de Lac estate on Lake Tahoe. The 'Tahoe Agreement' created integrated regional executive management teams, comprising the regional Health Plan Manager, the Hospital Manager, and the key physician administrators of each region. These teams would mediate between regional personnel and the national advisory council, and coordinate all activities of the Health Plan, the Hospitals, and Permanente Services within the region. The regional teams were not intended to merge or amalgamate existing administrative structures. Each of the regional Health Plans, Hospitals and Medical Groups retained its authority and responsibilities. The Tahoe Conference also created area management teams, comprising the chief physician of each area and the local hospital administrator. It was agreed that neither party could take any action that might affect the other without prior mutual consultation. Thus, Kaiser Permanente's unique integration of health insurance and care was reaffirmed: each region had its own geographical identity, and each regional Medical Group worked closely with, but remained independent from, the Health Plan.

On 27 March 1958, the Permanente Medical Group approved Medical Service Agreement 1958. This established a policy framework for the Kaiser Foundation Health Plan and the Permanente Medical Group, which has persisted to the present day. The Agreement stipulated that the Health Plan would contract exclusively with the Permanente Medical Group, as long as the group adequately served its needs. In return, the Medical Group would contract exclusively with the Health Plan and not render professional services to anyone else in the area.

Kaiser Permanente in Hawaii

In 1965, at 75, Henry J Kaiser retired from active direction of the Kaiser companies and moved to Hawaii. In Honolulu he saw the potential to develop a major tourism and convention destination. He also decided to create a health plan in Hawaii that could be run without the 'interference' of the Permanente Medical Group. Kaiser personally recruited the medical staff to form a partnership called Pacific Medical Associates (PMA).

PMA enrolment was disappointing. Needing 15 000 to 16 000 members to be financially viable, it opened with only 5000. The PMA partners were shunned by their fee-for-service peers. They and their wives were ostracised and excluded from the social life of the medical community (Smith Hughes and Hancock 1986). The partners became disgruntled. From mid-1959 Lambreth Hancock, the Kaiser Health Plan's regional manager, detailed a progressive deterioration in relations between the PMA partners and the Kaiser organisation. Kaiser had senior staff sent over from the mainland to monitor the situation. Ernest Saward, director of the Kaiser Permanente programme in Portland Oregon, spent the month of April 1960 with PMA. Ostensibly a visiting practitioner at the Honolulu Medical Centre, Saward assessed the medical staff and the situation for himself.

In summer 1960, the five PMA partners broke contract, demanding immediate increases in compensation from the Health Plan. The following day, Kaiser executive Clifford Keene sacked the partners, served them a written notice to vacate the premises by 5.30 pm. The remaining 33 employed physicians were assembled and invited to continue to practise as a medical group. All but two stayed.

It took another five years to get the Hawaii Kaiser Permanente programme on its feet. Its troubled first years reaffirmed Garfield's conviction that not just any competent physician had an aptitude for prepaid group practice. After Hawaii, great care was taken to select the core cadre for any new medical group. And every physician recruited to Hawaii Permanente Medical Group still has to pass an acid test: 'would I want this person to treat a member of my own family?'

1960s – present

In May 1960, the programme's first inter-regional management conference was held in Monterey. There, Sidney Garfield (1) reaffirmed his belief in health maintenance and illness prevention over the traditional treatment model. It should be a health plan, not a sickness plan. This ethos was enshrined in the US Health Maintenance Act 1973. Garfield also advocated (2) the greater use of new technology to record and store medical information; and (3) that non-physician health personnel should be more integrated into the healthcare process, under physician supervision, in order to extend the physician's effectiveness and efficiency. These three ideas still exert a strong, formative influence over the Kaiser Permanente programme.

By September 1962, Kaiser Permanente had become the single largest group-practice health plan in the United States, comprising 12 hospitals and 38 clinics, serving 337 000 subscribers (911 000 family members) in California, Oregon and Hawaii. In January 1969, the board of the Kaiser Permanente Committee elected to expand into Denver Colorado and Cleveland Ohio. A driving force behind Kaiser Permanente's expansion was the growing participation of employees in capitation prepayment. During the 1960s, the percentage of members for whom the employer paid some or all of the dues increased from 68% to 91%. By September 1968, Health Plan enrolment had reached 845 000. The Medical Group had 917 full-time equivalent physicians, which put the physician-member ratio at 1:921, the most favourable in the programme's history. Including family members, however, would presumably have increased the ratio to around 1:2400.

Henry J Kaiser died in 1967 at the age of 85. Sidney Garfield MD died on 29 December 1985. Garfield 'captured the principles and significance of prepayment to a group of physicians as a more efficient and effective mechanism for healthcare. He developed the concept against opposition and obstructions that would have been overwhelming to many without his dedication and courage' (Cutting 1984). Both leaders in their fields, Kaiser and Garfield understood the need to integrate industry and healthcare, comprehensive health insurance, prevention and treatment under one programme.

The structure of Kaiser Permanente has not changed fundamentally following the 1955 Tahoe Agreement, although it has continued to evolve. On 2 January 1984, the Permanente Medical Group ceased to be a partnership and became a professional corporation. Today, Kaiser Permanente is the largest not-for-profit, integrated healthcare delivery system in the United States, serving more than 8 million members in eight regions across the US. The same general organisational model is used in each region. Doctors join regional exclusive partnerships or professional corporations that contract with the Kaiser Foundation Health Plan and assume full responsibility for providing and arranging necessary medical care for members.

CIS IN HAWAII

Hawaii Kaiser Permanente region serves 234 000 members across the three largest islands in the state, with 26 primary healthcare teams in 15 clinics, and one hospital. Nine Kaiser Permanente clinics and the hospital are located on the island of Oahu. Primary care teams include physicians trained in internal medicine and family practice. Members have prepaid health benefits, that is, fully capitated care.

Kaiser Permanente had previously implemented two systems in two other regions: one based on a vendor-created, commercially available system (EpicCare), the other (Clinical Information System, or CIS), jointly developed between Kaiser Permanente and IBM. Hawaii's EMR was the second-generation CIS.

In late 2002, the health system experienced a change in its senior leadership. The new Chief Executive Officer was previously CEO of another US health system, which had successfully implemented EpicCare, the same EMR used by Kaiser Permanente in the Northwest. CIS implementation in Hawaii was promptly halted due to delays in delivering promised capacities, and other problems. Its fate in Hawaii provides an opportunity to examine the process of EMR implementation of a large system in one region and to analyse relevant organisational factors (Aarts, Doorewaard and Berg

2004; Friedman and Wyatt 1997; Halfpenny 1979; Lorenzi and Riley 1995; Lorenzi and Riley 2000; Stiell, *et al.* 2003).

METHODOLOGY

An exploratory approach was taken in the research. Semi-structured audio-recorded interviews were held with a sample of 26 senior clinicians, managers and EMR project team members in Hawaii (Ives 1995; Whyte 1982). An interview prompt sheet gave consistency to the topics covered in the interviews, which lasted from 60 to 90 minutes. Information was elicited about respondents' experiences of the planning, implementation and use of the EMR in clinical practice. The topic guide contained a sequence of open questions relating to organisational factors potentially relevant to EMR implementation and care redesign, including organisational culture, leadership, functionality and use, previous IT implementations, and effects on processes of care. In addition, respondents were encouraged to describe their own experience of their EMR.

Respondents representing a range of occupations and roles – as CIS sponsors, leaders, users and support team members – were recruited. Most had multiple roles. Senior leaders in Hawaii Kaiser Permanente invited volunteers to participate in the research. Volunteers were not screened or briefed to influence sample composition or responses.

Interviews were recorded using digital audio recording equipment. A research assistant independently assessed the accuracy of the transcripts against the recordings. The findings were analysed thematically and inductively (Krippendorff 1980). Additional information was obtained by e-mail. The author conducted all interviews using a constant comparative method: treating each interview as an opportunity to check and corroborate data collected in previous interviews. The research was approved by the Kaiser Permanente Hawaii Region Internal Review Board.

EXPERIENCES OF CIS IMPLEMENTATION

CIS was a controversial choice of EMR, as some Hawaiian doctors preferred the proprietary system used in the Northwest region successfully for five years. When CIS was delivered, 14 months late, its functionality did not meet expectations. By April 2002, one third of clinics and specialties were implemented. The remaining two thirds had read-only access, many also with order entry. Users typically found CIS frustrating to use, as one specialty chief noted:

> Within a few weeks it was apparent that this product was not a state-of-the-art system. The main thing physicians do is document their notes, and it wasn't a very good word processor. It didn't have some of the most basic things, like macros for repetitive tasks, [or] spell checking. It wasn't giving me any information that I didn't have before.

The news that CIS was 'clunky' and improvements slow and costly spread quickly through the region. A support team member noted:

> This product had a lot of problems, from our very first site. Technically, it went up fine. But the tool was not as good as people expected. That spread like wild-fire. We picked very credible people to do the initial install; [they] were saying, 'You know, we can do this but if this is all there is we are in big trouble.'

A senior support team member observed:

> The fact is this application's a turkey. So that's superimposed on all the problems [of] trying to implement this kind of change even with a good product.

Weekly clinical debriefings, and monthly meetings in California, were held to collate and prioritise CIS problems. But after 12 months their clinical recommendations were given secondary importance:

> All that work basically got scrapped. Executive decisions were made to limit the scope to increase revenue, do a better job of coding, and make the system scalable to be used in California – all of which are organisational imperatives, but usability literally got crossed off the page. And that was a very, very difficult thing to deal with because we had been telling people from the beginning, 'We know it's not perfect, but give us your ideas: we will help to make it better.'

Finally, in late 2002, a decision was made by the group executive to halt CIS implementation and adopt EpicCare.

Why did CIS IT fail in Hawaii, when Colorado had been using it successfully? As we shall see there were many reasons. One was a simple difference in consultation times across the regions, as one support team member observed:

> A number of us went to Colorado, where they had CIS for a number of years. Some of us came away thinking: 'That's going to be very difficult to implement here.' Colorado has 20-minute appointments and we have 15. Having 20 minutes gives them the time to do all the necessary documentation, review of labs, and other things associated with the CIS system. Over here, we are already challenged trying to keep up with the schedule.

The same individuals saw EpicCare being used in Northwest region, as one chief recalled:

> We really liked this Northwest system. But Colorado had made CIS work and so we were using some of their tools and methods, but some of them wouldn't work in Hawaii. Like, they had a big phone centre, and our philosophy is: no big phone centre. They had physicians who did not have patients: they would

be roving physicians on the floor to help support. Whereas we grab our docs and say: 'You will see this patient!' because access is a problem for us.

Another physician confirmed that some of CIS's shortcomings were predictable:

> We set up a group called the CIS Workflow Team prior to us even really knowing the system, trying to figure out how we'd have to change our way of thinking and operating. And we pretty much predicted many of the problems we experienced. Because we're going to document more, there's a price for documentation, you can't see as many patients.

Most respondents did not solely blame IBM for CIS's failings. One chief thought the fault lay in its contract with Kaiser Permanente.

> I think that IBM was just responding to what we were telling them to do. And the advice Kaiser Permanente was giving them was what was handcuffing them.

Others opined that improvements to CIS were slow and expensive because IBM had no interest in marketing the application elsewhere. In fact, IBM's efforts to market CIS were unsuccessful because it was too specific to Kaiser Permanente to adapt to other customers economically.

Some respondents thought inadequate attention had been given to the long-term implications of Kaiser Permanente bearing the entire cost of CIS's development and improvement, as another support team member noted:

> We should never have started down this road of trying to build software ourselves. It's extremely expensive – we are the only client funding the entire R&D. It doesn't make any sense.

Time burden

Most interviewees discussed the additional time burden of using CIS.

> The physicians in [one clinic] all work 10–11 hours per day, so there was no capacity for implementing CIS. On the other hand, their attitude was very gung-ho and patriotic. If somebody comes along and says, 'We would like you to do this', they will not say 'No'. [This] puts them under a lot of pressure that would not be seen because it wouldn't be shown. Although with CIS we did try and give some hints, when people got up and said, 'This is going to be a real challenge, but we're going to do this!'

A strong Hawaiian taboo on disagreeableness inhibited physicians from voicing their concerns stridently. And regional leaders appeared not to interpret euphemistic expressions of concern like 'This is going to be a real challenge', correctly. It meant, 'This looks impossible.'

Additional cover provided during the settling-in period only deferred the additional time burden. Some respondents expressed particular concerns that using CIS would reduce access to care, as a clinic chief noted:

> It was not an easy roll-out for any of us and we're still having a lot of difficulty. We all dread April 1, [when] we lose the extra locum provided because of CIS. I would see 24–26 patients in an eight-hour day. Come April 1 we lose that extra help and we're expected to handle the pre-CIS load. At each clinic people are developing contingency plans for 'What if we can't?'

There was a general feeling that the additional time burden of CIS might compromise access and standards of care. And the promise that physicians would return to their previous productivity looked increasingly hollow in the light of experience. One clinic chief remarked:

> We certainly said, 'Well, I'm gonna work harder; we're gonna stay later; we're gonna get over this hump and such,' and we discovered that we really couldn't. We had started out in the high ninetieth percentile in terms of our utilisation, so when we tried to add the constraints of the system, basically it broke.

Opening Pandora's box

Preparing for and implementing CIS had many significant unanticipated consequences. A truism was coined: it has nothing and everything to do with CIS.

According to one support team member, the standardisation of work that was a precondition of automation was novel to many physicians:

> To roll out CIS you have to really study the workflow. We gained a lot of efficiencies in workflow, and the agreements physicians needed to make with each other about how they do their work and how the hand-offs work. We made tremendous improvements, because those things had never been expressed before: 'So, how am I going to get this to you?' And, 'How are we going to work together on this?'

In the process, many hitherto unsuspected problems were uncovered:

> I think the other lesson learned is that CIS is going to magnify any challenges that are non-CIS related. It's a huge magnifier. If you have access issues, we're going to magnify that when we come in and reduce your schedule.

Thus, according to one support team member

Implementing CIS really did open Pandora's box. It caused us to look at every single workflow process within clinic operations, because it touches almost everything. CIS tends to bring your hidden problems to the fore. Things that were there before, but now it's critical that we solve because it has implications for our deployment.

Workflow analysis

Much pre-implementation work was undertaken, especially at the first site. Internal consultants analysed systems and workflows. Moreover, CIS was implemented in a context of quality improvement initiatives, as a clinic manager explained:

> We started our patient flow improvement process in 1999. We began [by map-ping] how a patient moves through our clinic – from the patient's point of view, and then identify the steps, and look for redundancies, inefficiencies, so the patient had a better experience with us.

The patient flow improvement, which predated CIS, was supplemented by a 'patient flow straw man process', shifting the focus to care processes. This helped break down communication barriers, flush out idiosyncratic practices, and foster standardisation:

> We would put up a straw man of every clinic process, and then we would have a team meeting for the physicians, appointment clerks, nurses: everybody got in a room and said 'OK, is this how it goes?' And the receptionist goes, 'I don't do that – this is what I do.' And the doctor would go, 'Well, why do you do that?' Or, 'If you do that I don't need to do that.' Or the RNs would say, 'Well, I'm doing this.' And the physicians go, 'Well, why are you doing that? The MAs can do that.' So it was really a good dialogue.

The potential contribution of these process improvements to support CIS imple-mentation was quickly evident to the support team:

> We started this process at one clinic and we said, 'Wow! We should use this tool as we implement CIS.'

Even under the group practice model a high degree of individualism was observed by some respondents. Preparing for CIS helped to establish a more collective attitude. Sharing information about individual practices was an epiphany for some physicians. And sites with functioning teams were more successful with CIS than those operating as de facto sole-practitioners. One support team member compared a medical centre (except its internists, who refused to implement CIS) and another clinic:

> [The medical centre] already had pretty sophisticated care models. When we

started training them in 1998, they had hand-offs established to all their ancil-
lary providers; they had named teams; they really hung together and huddled.

At [the] clinic there was more of a culture of practising alone together.
You know, they came in, they had their MA, they worked heads down in the
same clinic, but they weren't really doing a lot of collaboration. And so I think
that this is making up for years of that type of practice, which is common in
healthcare.

One clinic chief recalled how its team building strategy had targeted dysfunctional
individualism and supported CIS implementation:

We knew that if we couldn't work as a team there was no way CIS was gonna
fly: we would just fall flat on our faces. So we spent a lot of time talking about
what we do in the clinic, why we are here in the first place, why do we want to
work in this clinic versus other clinics, stuff like that. It's the clinic as a whole
taking care of the patient. Trust and respect for each other and our patients;
work and grow as a team based on honesty, integrity, compassion and dependability; strive for excellence; live by our principles in regards to ourselves, clinic
and region. The whole clinic built those: the housekeeping, the front desk, the
doctors and nurses, the MAs. So I think that gave us a good basis when we had
to make a lot of changes in how we do things. We had some underlying respect
for each other's jobs.

Training and support

Yet the initial emphasis was on integrating CIS into individual practice styles.

One of our principles is that doctors need to be able to practise in a style that
works for them. And so we worked hard to discover ways, workflows, different
ways of clicking, different ways of working from an exam room to a nursing
station, to help them find their stride.

This suggests a divergence of expectations between Program Office and Hawaii. Were
these expectations explicit, or tacit? If the automation of disparate styles was the
Hawaiian aim, the implementation workload for its support teams would be mas-
sively increased – which was exactly the experience reported. This error may have
flowed out of the decision to build a bespoke system. The initial mindset was towards
making CIS work for the physicians, when the physicians should really have been
adapting to a system with an established track record.

Though most informants spoke highly of the training and support team, one
expert user criticised a focus on adapting clinicians to the application, rather than
showing them how to use CIS as a tool to change their practice:

So we had a whole bunch of trainers: very good at what they do; very nice; very easy to work with; doing their very best to teach us something that they actually didn't have to spend a lot of time to teach us, because the program itself was relatively easy. But figuring out how to incorporate it into the actual care we were giving to patients – that was a more difficult task, which our trainers weren't really equipped or prepared for. That wasn't their insight, their focus. In retrospect that was a mistake. We should have recognised that. And it was part of a larger mistake when we think about CIS itself, and why it was not the best solution for us.

In discussing the integration of IT into organisations we risk limiting the analysis unduly. Should we not expect radical advances: new IT and practice transcending their relationship, taking healthcare to a new level? This is precisely what sophisticated users sought:

> We quickly found that what we were trained to do was how to use CIS. But that isn't what we really do. We were trained that 'if you hit this button, this is what happens'. But that's the least of what we're doing when we're taking care of patients. And what we weren't trained to do – and what we really hadn't prepared for as well as I hoped we would, is the thinking that, 'Your goal is to give good healthcare and you're going to use this as a tool to provide good healthcare'. The training was around 'using this tool'.

Yet some support team members attributed a conservative attitude to users, obsessed with pressing the right buttons, instead of considering more radically what CIS might support:

> They were focused on the buttons and translating their paper workflow exactly into an electronic workflow, just to get over that transition; and then finally they discovered that in a lot of the things that they were trying to translate it was not efficient to do it the exact way they did it. They didn't even need to do that sometimes – things they had always done but there was not a lot of value to it.

Support team members observed different speeds and types of adaptation, some beginning with hesitation and creeping forward incrementally, others making sudden leaps forward.

The theme of integration also understates the extent of practical change a health system must undergo to implement a new EMR successfully. If an EMR is developed with multiple clients, it should be functionally superior to an EMR designed for a single organisation. And a convergence in user practices is likely to result. Users and EMR will be mutually adaptive, each new client adapting to a greater degree to the tool than vice versa, as the tool already incorporates the cumulative learning of all previous clients.

Scope of practice

The support team found many nurses and medical assistants routinely undertaking tasks for which they were competent but unlicensed. This was due to local preferences and exigencies and interstate differences. Certain CIS functions originally designed for Colorado could not be implemented without adaptation to the Hawaiian State Licensing Laws. This issue would have arisen in the other regions too. Common examples included Hawaiian nurses ordering urine analyses or altering patients' medication levels without a doctor's order. As a senior administrator put it:

> Scope of practice for a medical assistant or a registered nurse may be different across states. For example, can an MA adequately perform a monofilament sensate testing of a diabetic's foot? Well the answer is yes, absolutely, they can do a great job. Is it in their scope of practice as it relates to State law? No, only a registered nurse is allowed to do that type of diagnostic testing.

Such questionable practices increased vulnerability to litigation, or prosecution by state and federal authorities, as a support team member noted:

> When I was working for [one of Hawaii Kaiser Permanente's competitors], the FBI came in and seized files. Medicare fraud was the charge and you are talking about a meticulous audit of records and charges. So I think the risk is very real. And we are now going into HIPAA* compliance. As an organisation we have to decide what risk we are going to assume. I think that in this age of whistle-blowers, you have to run a pretty tight ship.

Care process innovation

The additional time pressures introduced by CIS prompted some users to revise their usual models of care, and even question the sanctity of the personal visit. This resonated with Institutes of Medicine and Health Improvement reports questioning the need for face-to-face visits in all cases ('The visit is not the visit'). Some clinics experimented with alternatives, including telephone triage, group consultations and improved chronic disease management. One support team member said:

> To me, probably the most exciting thing that happened in CIS is that there are pockets of people who have got it: who've said, 'This is not just a way to document my chart: it's a totally new way of taking care of patients.'

The online patient record helped make alternative appointments viable:

---

* The (US) Health Insurance Portability and Accountability Act (HIPAA), passed in 1996, intended to ensure appropriate protection of confidential healthcare information. Wide-ranging in scope, covering both storage and transmission of this data, as well as stipulating comprehensive compliance requirements, HIPAA is having a substantial impact on the healthcare sector.

We were able to start MD triage: since the charts are available, the patient can call in the morning and, instead of having to be seen, maybe we can take care of it over the phone. It's helped open up appointments, and the patients like it because they don't have to come in.

As one chief explained, the online patient record was pivotal to improving the integration and continuity of care:

It used to be so frustrating that somebody got seen first at an outlying clinic, and now they're seeing you for follow-up, and you have no idea what they did. You'd have to try and piece together from lab and X-ray and medication, and this and that: 'OK, well, he must have done so-and-so' – you're just guessing. Now, all you have to do is pull up the note: you can know what your RN did, or talked about the day before, or a week before, whatever. You can read what your colleague did last month. Everything is documented now and all the information is at your fingertips.

Even the dysfunctional aspects of CIS could be useful when they revealed absurdity enshrined in custom and practice, as another chief observed:

To my mind some things are the fault of the IBM system, but in many ways it's kind of a mixed blessing because it really showed a fault in our system, in which our automatic response was: patient has a problem? The doctor has to see you. If someone called in, I could overhear the medical assistant say, 'Oh no, the doctor will have to see you. I know you've had this sinusitis every year, but the doctor will still have to see you.' You know, we all said, 'Do we have to do this? I mean I know the guy: he knows sinusitis. It's like a lady with UTI (urinary tract infection): once you've had one it's not too tricky to figure out it's come back!'

One chief regarded longer visits as a potential improvement:

Maybe CIS takes longer because we take better care of the patient and we're doing more for the patient. So maybe it should take longer. Maybe we don't want to go back to the number of patients that we were seeing before. We were just running 'em through, putting band-aids on them and not really taking care of them. By [CIS] time-limiting us, so that we can't put all these extra patients on our schedule, it's kind of better actually.

Automation or transformation?

I asked respondents if they thought CIS implementation had just automated, or radically transformed, care processes. Over the course of CIS implementation some clinicians' expectations shifted from one to the other, but for others the experience was mainly disruptive of their usual care:

> What I hear from some providers is: 'I need help in integrating this tool into my practice. I need a coach. Because I was successful, I had my routine; I knew how the visit was going to go. And now this alters the dynamic, the time, whatever. And so I need to go through the visit differently maybe.'

Some respondents envisaged a very different kind of healthcare system. One chief remarked:

> If you look at the Institute of Medicine's report, all that CIS did was to uncover the fact that our system was not able to function and we weren't able to fix it by working harder – because we certainly tried that. [. . .] We tried to say, 'OK, we're gonna just come in earlier, we're gonna go home later' and we still couldn't fix it. In retrospect, what we needed to do is rethink how we practise medicine.

New IT was seen as one important factor in wider health improvement and innovation. Teams were another. For example, preparation for CIS capitalised on the previous introduction of team-based care at some sites. Not only were teams conducive to CIS implementation, teams with CIS could offer group clinics:

> Instead of making one appointment and then another, where you say the same things, you try to get all the team members in one appointment. So you have the dietician, the nutritionist, clinical diabetes educator, clinical pharmacist, physician, nurse, nurse practitioner, so they're all there with the members.

Did CIS spur innovation? There is no simple answer, but it did appear to have jolted the region into action. If the software had been a little better, Kaiser Permanente might have persisted with CIS. Its ultimate rejection permitted the adoption of a superior alternative.

Accountability

CIS obliged clinicians to become more accountable than with paper records. They were required to sign off every decision on a date-stamped record. Attitudes to enhanced accountability varied. As well as bringing more openness to care processes, CIS was perceived by one member of the support team to rationalise roles and responsibilities at the affected sites:

> It forces you to be very explicit about how you do things. I think we've seen more sharing of responsibility: having nurses do follow-up phone calls, and follow-up on certain types of results; and understanding what an MA specifically can and can't do for you; shifting some work off the physician to others.
>
> And improving coverage when people were away: how do you handle results? That used to be informal: somebody would just throw it on a desk. Now you have to be very explicit – if Joe is away, who is going look at his results? The computer's got to know who to send it to.

Other clinicians thought CIS had excessively formalised roles and responsibilities. One specialty chief complained that CIS increased his administrative load:

> CIS has made the most expensive employee a clerk in terms of input of data, orders, and notes. Now we have to input everything. So the verbal order part has disappeared.

The perceived demise of the verbal order can be interpreted as part of a wider transformation of medicine from a verbal to a recorded practice. EMRs are designed to exert more rational control over the classification, treatment and cost of health risks. By virtue of its function as an apparatus of capture, the EMR is a disciplinary technology, helping to transform traditional medicine into a 'modern' profession. Such an infrastructure compromises clinical autonomy – a perennial professional demand and a rearguard action against the erosion of traditional privileges – to which verbal orders bear witness. Some physicians, though not all, resented their increased accountability for clinical decisions.

Physicians used to writing their patient notes mainly for their own reference suddenly acquired a large potential readership. One physician said CIS had forced him to record his actions better. He should have set a higher standard for himself, but had felt no external pressure to do so.

> No question in my mind, it's forced me to be more organised, more accountable – and that's the hard part. We see a lab and we sign off on it. Everyone knows when you looked at it; when, what your plans are. Previously, it was easy to look at a sheet of paper with the lab report and decide what you're going to do, and it [was] a bit nebulous. But now [it] is there for everybody to see. It's forced me to do what I should have been doing all along.

This view was supported by members of the support team, who attributed improvements in clinician accountability both to the bureaucratic demands of the software, and a change in minds.

> Somehow it has changed the psyche of people documenting, and they are much more aware of what they are putting in the chart, something we never really anticipated. When you see the electronic signatures on the charts, people sit up. It's almost like they didn't really care about what they wrote on paper, but now that it's electronic and people can read everything, you can't hide behind, 'Well that scribble says this.' It has really opened people's eyes and made them more careful. It's legible, attributable, accountable.

CIS brought a new visibility into the exam room, and helped integrate healthcare activities. According to a support team member:

> It has sort of opened up the doors to the exam room. I don't think there was

that openness before CIS. Putting in the computer allowed us to talk about the workflow. Before, the physicians wholly defined the workflow. It allowed us to discuss things that we really didn't discuss before. CIS was perceived to empower a transformation of Kaiser Permanente into a virtual panopticon.* The invisible all-seeing eye became generalised into anyone and everyone who could log on to the system. CIS realised Bentham's model by subjecting clinicians to the virtual, unseen and unconfirmed presence of the Other, inducing physicians to keep better records, and to internalise the disciplinary gaze, to become their own overseers. Hence the social impact of CIS, and of new IT in healthcare more widely, is in part a political apparatus to render hitherto discreet behaviour visible and accountable, to the corporation and perhaps even society: to integrate healthcare into a surveillance culture. At the same time, uploading data onto an organisation-wide system enables concrete and beneficial process of integration to occur: instead of many individual practitioners, a collective mind forms by virtue of their contribution and access to an electronic archive.

The panoptic principle is a totalising social fact (Durkheim 1982). Physicians' evasion of its supervisory gaze, to which society has been object for at least two centuries, is remarkable. A feature of American medicine's history is its struggle to retain craft status against precisely such forces of modernisation (Starr 1982). It is reasonable to assume a dawning apprehension of its constraint by Hawaii Permanente physicians, informing resistance.

Communication

CIS implementation also led to the development of collective decision making:

> The chiefs have not been organised around a project like this before. There are projects always happening but usually it's like, 'How's this going to affect my

---

* English social philosopher Jeremy Bentham proposed a technically efficient design for prisons, consisting of a circular arrangement of cells surrounding a high tower. The structure allowed every inmate to be observed by a single person in the tower, who remained invisible to them. Nor could inmates see one another. Being uncertain as to whether they were being observed, inmates would have to assume constant surveillance. Bentham named this design the Panopticon. Michel Foucault (1977) proposes the Panopticon as a model of the disciplinary technologies based on mass-surveillance that grew to dominate Western society from the late 18th century. The penitentiary at Stateville Illinois, for instance, was built on the panoptic model. The Panopticon is really a refinement of earlier systems of visibility, such as simple segregation between sick and healthy in times of plagues, and the rectilinear arrangement of schools, barracks and hospital wards. Computer networks operate in a similar way to the Panopticon by allowing the decisions of dispersed operators to be monitored centrally and remotely. Foucault identified in panopticism a psycho-social principle: one internalises the rule of surveillance to become one's own supervisor or warder – the soul, as Foucault puts it, which is the pilot of the body. In the present context, an EMR permits the remote assessment of inputs by identified operators, who can never be certain whether they are being watched. When Hawaii Kaiser Permanente physicians adapted their note-making to CIS, they began to behave like the inmates of a Panopticon. The fact that some agreed with this increased accountability confirms that their warder-consciences were already aware of their lack of rigour. They were even glad to be coerced in exchange for an easier conscience.

department?' This project made them come together and say, 'OK, we have to make some big decisions; we have to make policy decisions. And we can't make it different for ortho and medicine and paeds: it all has to be the same.' So we put a structure together to meet with them project-wide, for the whole region, and that was something new. Getting them together was challenging but now they have regular meetings and they know the kinds of decisions to be made. So that infrastructure is a lot more organised.

One chief noted that CIS had supported better communication between Hawaii Kaiser Permanente and external bodies:

> I would never really have thought about giving a copy of my note to care homes. I do that routinely now. In the past I would write my own note in the chart and then I would write a very abbreviated note in the care home chart, that they needed to maintain their accreditation. But now I actually just give them the entire note. We do the same thing when we use consultants outside Kaiser. It's a lot easier to give them the documentation, because they don't have to worry about not being able to read it. There aren't pieces attached that may not be appropriate. I actually let the patient carry it with them to see their consultant. All of these things I don't think we would have done earlier. It never dawned on me to do it.

A support team member discussed how CIS, and now EpicCare, might change global perceptions of Kaiser Permanente in the context of US healthcare:

> We used to talk about how this was going to change Kaiser as an organisation in ways that nobody understands yet. Even within Kaiser I think there are still areas that you could probably describe as a collection of private practices. I think now the organisation is actually welcoming conversations about, 'Let's standardise our intake process; let's standardise other processes and procedures.' Because they recognise that it's to our members' benefit not to see large variations in healthcare services. And it's advantageous to [the] organisation because now we can predict and control costs much better if we know how everybody is doing it across the board. But maybe it's just setting a baseline, which should have been there for a long time anyway.

The reference to standardisation in this excerpt carries connotations of 'socialisation'. These are specifically American concerns. It is paradoxical that, in the land of Fordism, standardisation is maligned as an enemy of consumer choice and sovereignty, supposedly exercised through the market. Despite that corporate capitalism's essential aim is to monopolise, suspicion of any state or corporate monopolistic control in the USA is entrenched. Such paradoxes seem to define the culture. In practice a rhetoric of choice glosses over a reality of equivalent alternatives. And the dogma of competition in a free market is contradicted by a reflex preference for American products over imports. Republicans especially are still influenced by Cold War values, fearing in any organised and integrated healthcare system a soviet-style conformity; the individual totally subsumed and subjugated to 'the system', which Americans feel they are not. American individualism remains the national fantasy and, as JB Priestly observed, America is the only national culture founded on a dream.

Another support team member thought that, in view of increasing scrutiny by Federal government, the standardisation wrought by the implementation of CIS was necessary:

> Much of what was previously done was not acceptable. But we got away with it. I don't mean that people were deliberately trying to, but that was how they coped with, 'My panel of patients is getting bigger: I need more time, so I'll do that three line summary.' But it may not pass muster when it comes to what the Federal government is going to require from us. So I see it in a different perspective. CIS requires it, but it's always been required. We got sloppy. I hesitate even to say that word about these hard-working people that have all this heart for their members, but we just didn't do the work we needed to do. Chart audits were potentially very poor.

One chief agreed with this assessment:

> To my mind, it really identified areas where we had been lax, or areas where we hadn't really thought it through. In that sense I think we do a much better job.

Symbolic integration of CIS

CIS was functionally designed to automate and integrate coding, billing, ordering, results management, and other processes. But what were the effects on doctor-patient relationships? The support team concentrated on helping clinicians integrate CIS into their existing practice styles. The implication that CIS could be individualised in this way is surprising, suggesting a weak grasp of its real purpose – to make an organisation-wide system of information, standardisation and economy. The support team encountered wide variations in responses to the arrival of the 'Cisco Kid' in the consulting room:

> There are people who do a lot more sharing of information because the computer is in there. Somehow it's just easier to show people a screen than a paper chart. Then there are people who are struggling so hard to get everything in the computer that their members are telling us: 'They talk to the computer; they don't talk to me anymore.'

CIS was referred to as 'the Cisco Kid' by two pairs of respondents, with interesting connotations. 'Cis-' conceives CIS as another person present at the consultation; '-co' denotes a corporate presence, and the San Francisco Bay Area, where Kaiser

Permanente HQ is located. Thus CIS was viewed ironically as (1) a benevolent digital stranger sent to deliver Hawaiians from an analogical Dark Age, and (2) invasion by the corporate agents of IBM and Program Office. The Cisco Kid label had classical mythic and derisory functions: to render the complexity and contingency of decision processes higher up the organisation comprehensible; to satirise those responsible; and to personify a diffuse and incomprehensible technology. By anthropomorphising CIS, its threat and complexity were symbolically domesticated.

Chronic disease management

Effective chronic disease management (CDM) is arguably a mark of well-integrated care. CIS had little impact on CDM. Some respondents referred to the Population Care Registry (PCR), an existing computer programme providing a limited population focus. One clinic had begun to use PCR and CIS together to improve CDM, though it remained unwieldy, as a clinic chief outlined:

> It's a project that started this year. We meet in this room, we've got two computers going: somebody's laptop with PCR running, and then CIS – so if there's a question we can just pull it up. And we've got our list of CHF (congestive heart failure), or diabetes patients and we just go through them, see what medications they're on and everything like that. We can take care of a lot of patients in a short period of time. I don't think we could have done it with paper charts because we would have had to pull maybe 40, 50 charts.

In contrast, a specialty chief reported that CIS reduced his CDM:

> In the one year that we've used CIS, I'd say that it's had a negative impact, because it diverted so much of my mental capacity towards, 'Get the note done, get the note done. Not enough time, hurry up, get the note done!' I didn't have time to stop and ponder, 'What else needs to be done?' And CIS wasn't advanced enough to provide us with those reminders or those flow charts that would facilitate care. The PCR had chronic disease reminders on it. When CIS came I had my nurse stop printing out the PCR because I would never look at it anyway. I was too busy flipping between CIS screens just trying to make it through the clinic visit.

Several respondents reflected on the global lessons of CIS for Kaiser Permanente. According to one support team member:

> It became apparent how many different attitudes in the organisation had to change. I think we learned a lot organisationally. We learned a lot about what our limitations are; what we do well and what we don't do well as an organisation. I think all the regions learned how to work together much better; less [as] separate little empires and more aware that we needed to act in concert not in dissonance. An awful lot of that came about as a function of attempting to install CIS.

Summary

Implementing an EMR requires a comprehensive analysis and redesign process. CIS touched everything. As a bespoke system, it was designed to replicate and automate Kaiser Permanente's systems. It was a functional failure but still played an important role in Colorado, Hawaii and beyond. Its dysfunctional aspects led physicians to review their procedures in order to cope and maintain access, and it gave a foretaste of what they could do with a good EMR. Although CIS was itself disappointing, the planning and implementation processes were nonetheless conducive to integrating medical and administrative processes. By comparing their individual procedures, physicians and their teams learned from each other and reduced variation and redundancy.

This suggests a strong need to distinguish between implementation processes and outcomes, and between specific and global consequences. It supports other scholars' findings that implementation is a crucial aspect of intervention. CIS showed that even a deficient IT system can yield important unintended benefits by virtue of thorough preparation and implementation processes. CIS represented a total investment of about $800 million; the cost of its replacement, EpicCare, an estimated $2 billion. Spread across around 8 million members, $2.8 billion works out at about $350 per member. Whether the organisation's gains in computer literacy, commitment to an EMR, and enhanced integration of care organisation and delivery systems were justified to prepare Kaiser Permanente for a proper functioning EMR is ultimately a value judgement.

Ultimately, the CIS experience revealed a new vision of care not entirely based on the face-to-face visit, which was revealed as a questionable assumption. Ardent supporters of 'going electronic' saw CIS as a medium to transform their healthcare delivery system. Anything less meant failure. One advantage of a proprietary EMR such as EpicCare is that its constant improvement is in response to a range of customers, instead of only one. Thus, multiple efficiencies can be gained by every user. By contrast, a bespoke system might constantly reaffirm fundamental and possible flawed organisational assumptions. And this is where integrity and integration could conflict. Since integrity is a function of culture, the organisation's culture will offer the greatest sources of resistance to the integration of, or to, new IT.

ORGANISATIONAL CULTURE

This study originated in two hypotheses: (1) that organisational culture mediates between policy and practice, and (2) that a distributed organisation's culture would be heterogeneous, each site exhibiting a unique ethos and style of leadership; factors that would influence how CIS was implemented. These hypotheses were confirmed. Although core values were often invoked by respondents, the culture varied between clinics, specialties, member profiles, personalities, leadership, and team size.

The general ethos harmonised with Hawaiian culture. Traditional values of friendliness, family and care for others were promoted within the organisation,

and in the media in the slogan 'Caring for Hawaii's people like family'. US mainland culture was viewed in contrast as impersonal and unfriendly. Hawaiian culture
celebrates three core values (among others): aloha, love; ohana, family; and hanai,
extended family. It is easy to see how such a set of beliefs could suit a healthcare
organisation. Indeed, it was invoked proudly by most respondents to account for a
wide range of behaviour:

> We are the Aloha State. People are friendly and we extend that to everybody.
> There are lots of extended families. Hawaiians traditionally take care of every-
> body. I lived on the mainland for six years and I found that people are not
> friendly there. Here relationships are important, and it carries into your work.
> The cornerstone of our healthcare is the relationship between the member
> and the physician – that's the most important thing. Everything else needs to
> support that relationship. So when we talk about changes and computerised
> systems that enable us to do things, we never get away from that it's the rela-
> tionship that's the most important thing.

As the fieldwork progressed, a more managed aspect of the organisational culture
emerged. Some years earlier the organisational culture had been rather dysfunctional, and a deliberate effort made to transform it by importing traditional Hawaiian
values.

This raises a question concerning an organisation's integrity with society. Being
usually despotic, management seems immune to democracy. Yet Hawaii Kaiser
Permanente repeated accepted socio-cultural values in the workplace. Certainly, there
was a rhetorical aspect to this cultural congruence, as nurses and others were treated
with less ceremony and consideration than physicians – but it was also real.

Several informants observed differences between regional cultures. One support
team member spoke about how these differences affected the mediation of organisational innovation, including CIS:

> Kaiser Permanente Northern California is a very top-down driven organisa-
> tion. Programs are developed at the top and, 'You shall do them!' There isn't a
> whole lot of input coming from the bottom to say, 'Should we really do this, or
> not?' Here in Hawaii they make a very big push to let everything be controlled
> at the lowest level possible, and to get a lot of input, a lot of buy-in, a lot of
> decision making at the lower levels. If you're trying to push automation and
> efficiency above all else then I think the Northern California approach works
> well. If you're trying to push the more intimate, one-on-one relationship, then
> the Hawaii one works. It's not quite as efficient time- and money-wise, but
> value-wise – I think that's the question. Do the members want a quick service,
> like calling up Hertz – you don't care who you get, you just want a doctor – or
> do you want to call up and talk to your personal physician?

He saw the differences between the two regions epitomised in Hawaii's fidelity to its core principle: the physician–member relationship. The core principle was regarded as a genuine base for decision making:

> And that's one of the things we push here, and I'm sure you've heard it: our core principle is that the physician–member relationship is the number one thing. At no time do we ever compromise the core principle.

Specialty subcultures

Most respondents thought that different specialties presented characteristic challenges and opportunities to CIS implementation (Rogers and Shoemaker 1971). Certain specialties – general surgery, and obstetrics and gynaecology – were amenable to computerisation:

> Specialty care is very problem-oriented. You get presented with a problem and you need to fix it. Once it's fixed, barring ongoing complications or problems, then it's done. So you can develop algorithms for specific problems, like breast problems: how to take care of it, how to approach it, and there's a defined end-point. And that lends itself to computerisation.

Differences between primary and secondary care were also emphasised, and another chief concluded that computerisation would be much harder for primary care:

> [In secondary care] you have a set problem that you have to fix. The history that you have to take is pretty well known. The physical examination you know what to expect. And the studies that you'd need to support or refute those diagnoses are pretty much known, so you already have them set up in the CIS system. So because of that algorithmic style it can be structured in the computer pretty nicely actually – and the procedures. When you pull up your diagnoses, you don't have to go hunting for something weird that often. So there's less ambiguity. Whereas in primary care: oh man, you don't know what's going to walk through the door.

Even more specifically, another chief noted the strong individualism of surgeons compared to other specialties:

> Paediatricians and family practitioners tend to be a little more, 'Let's all get together; let's go forward as a group; let's play together.' Surgeons tend to be a lot more independent. The herding cats analogy is apt. Basically, just by saying that we should all do this, you create poles of people saying, 'Well, if you say that, obviously we should think about it and maybe not do it.'

Culture and implementation

A member of the support team referred to a psychological typing exercise, designed to spread understanding of responses to the CIS:

> We've done these profile studies, and I forget what you call them, but there is the Amiable group, the Driver group, Expressives and then the Analytics. We've all been given this test to show what categories we are in so that we can tell it to each other: 'Well, you're an Amiable and therefore you feel this way, and I'm an Analytic.' Basically we are 70% Amiable! There's a bit of unbalance there.

In the case of CIS, a Western analytical gaze was refracted by a benign Hawaiian duplicity. The sort of feedback welcomed by systems engineers Hawaiians viewed as 'talking stink':

> It's hard getting real constructive criticism out of people because we have such a strong drive for team building, that to be the dissident voice is almost seen to be unpatriotic. A lot of Amiables find it hard to say: 'Wait a minute – I don't think this is going to work.' It's very important that we get along: everybody knows that. It's the culture of Hawaii to be polite. We don't beep our horn; we don't cut our way in line. You never talk stink. That's a phrase that's used here: 'You don't talk stink.' You don't say bad things about other people. If somebody asks for constructive feedback, they are little bit shocked if they actually get it. So culture: big influence here.

Another support team member noted:

> A very noticeable difference between Colorado region and Hawaii: a very different culture. It's very collaborative, very consensus-driven, a sense of ohana, the family. Part of that is driven by the high percentage of Asian culture that we have here. They don't want to conflict with people. People don't want to walk up to you and say, 'Thou shalt do this.' They'd rather come up and say, 'Wouldn't it be a really good idea if we did this?' Just wanting to get a lot of buy-in, a lot of consensus. It's been very successful for the region. They've spent quite a lot of money and time educating folks to instil that kind of thinking.

Another team member described Kaiser Permanente culture as a complex weave of clinical and financial threads, reflecting the programme's closely integrated binary structure:

> The culture is twofold. We have business and clinical leadership cultures, and two leaders who partner at each level. Two threads of culture running through the same building. At a large clinic you've got a physician lead, and an Area Manager. That Area Manager might run the nursing supervisors in a very positive way, but that physician just may cut that process off at the knees. So we tend to do a lot of work with our area managers, trying to bring our chiefs along.

To regard the constant tension between administrator and clinician as a distraction may not be helpful. It might be constructive, keeping both partners on their mettle. If one enemy of quality improvement is complacency, that could be reduced by an ongoing lively debate between managerial and clinical priorities, each moderating the other.

LEADERSHIP

The medical leadership was described as democratic, consultative and consensus-seeking, as one CIS trainer explained:

> One thing coming down from our senior leader: we very rarely mandate anything. His thinking is that if it's a good thing it'll get a critical mass and it will take hold. And if it's not then it won't.

This leadership style harmonised with Hawaiian culture, but did not necessarily support efficient CIS implementation. Several respondents noted that trying to achieve consensus and maintain positive relationships made decision making very slow. Some were bemused and frustrated by this, but thought it integral to Hawaiian culture. The support team was powerless in the face of physician resistance to CIS. And professional etiquette proscribed coercion between physicians. Widespread diffusion, therefore, depended on a power of demonstration by reference group. This produced a circular logic: if CIS was good it would be implemented; if not implemented it was no good. This naïve technological determinism was presented by senior staff as a deliberate strategy, but may have been rationalisation. The latter accords with the ambiguity evinced by some leaders, torn between duty to the company and solidarity with colleagues, against CIS:

> I think in all fairness, our top-level sponsors, they were struggling with, 'This is a turkey and I gotta make people . . .' So he [Chief Physician] waxed and waned and he was in a very, very difficult position to deal with that. And so on down into the higher management levels. Everybody had a real struggle. They knew they had to do a good job as sponsors, and yet you're trying to defend something you don't really believe in.

One support team member noted differences in Hawaiian leadership styles:

> There's a chief at one clinic whose attitude was: implementing CIS was like us taking the beach at Normandy: we're gonna do it. Then there were others who were more, 'Well, let's think about this' and 'Do we really want this? And I want to hear everybody's opinion.' So there was both. I would say more chiefs would be inclined to be of the Amiable type and quietly say, 'Well, if that is where everybody is going and that is what we need to do, we just need to fall in line and show our support for it.' The chief does carry a lot of weight here.

One chief was more explicitly critical of Kaiser Permanente HQ:

> Program Office even criticised our leaders for showing bad leadership because they were not supporting their line, you know, 'CIS will work, CIS will work.' Even our leaders started saying, 'There's better stuff out there.'

The same chief referred to the dilemma in which Hawaii Kaiser Permanente found itself committed to implementing a flawed system:

> In the beginning the [support] team leaders were as militant supporters of CIS as anyone. But then they saw what was happening. It was too clumsy, and they didn't take enough time to get buy-in from docs. They didn't take into account local culture. It got to where Program Office was ignoring the project team leaders, who still very obediently tried their best with their hands tied. And I think people in the front line started seeing that they are not the masterminds of evil here: they are the messengers. We shouldn't be throwing rocks at them. I saw that change at about nine months.

The same respondent interpreted the change of Kaiser Permanente Chief Executive as crucial to a proper evaluation of CIS:

> When [the new senior leaders] came that really restored faith – that, 'Wow, somebody really is listening and they are willing to take a step back.' That didn't come locally. It took the leadership change at the highest levels to do that.

A desire to conform to institutional expectations conflicted with a fear of reducing the quality and efficiency of care.

> So there was that tug-of-war going on. Yes, the leadership did everything they could to empower the physicians. They also wanted to implement it. And therefore a timetable was set which was very aggressive. And they [the physicians] all looked at that timetable and said, 'Well, we have no choice but to go along!' So I think they saw mixed signals. They felt mixed signals I should say.

The mixed signals emitted by some leaders made the task of implementing CIS ever harder, bringing the issue of leadership into sharp focus for support team members:

> The ease or difficulty with which CIS can be implemented depends on the leadership, primarily the physician leadership. If the physician leadership is strong and willing to hold their people accountable to doing the change, we have an easier time. And I think in the long term it's those groups that have been most successful. If the leadership is very wary, then they end up either going or not going, but then you find pieces of their departments falling backwards. And it's

harder to support, because [in] an area that's committed to going in one direction we can help the folks that have difficulty, because there is commitment to the change. As the commitment dwindles, it's much harder to get them to where they want to be as a group.

Another team member endorsed that view:

We've learned that sponsorship and leadership are the most important aspects of the deployment, because without the sponsorship of the areas, without our team leaders working with the chiefs, we really had no authority in going in to do any kind of process improvement.

Leaders' ambivalence, combined with a low risk of censure, encouraged resistance to CIS, as a support team member noted:

There has been some hesitance with CIS at the very highest levels of our organisation. I don't think the physician chiefs or individuals who have not fulfilled their CIS commitment feel any repercussions. In fact they have been told, 'It's OK.' So they don't really have anything to worry about by saying 'No.' From a change management perspective that was the nightmare, because we depended on the chiefs and the supervisors of the clinic to be really clear about what their expectations were in terms of performance in CIS.

Their observations of leaders made some support team members sceptical about the region's ability to implement CIS's successor, EpicCare:

Epic is more accepted by the leadership. So hopefully, if the same issues come up, with, 'Well, I don't care if it's CIS or Epic, I'm not going to play!' then there will be more pressure on them to conform – but I'll believe it when I see it.

Clearly, the fate of CIS was heavily contingent on the professional identity of Permanente physicians, whose clinical autonomy had been preserved in the face of proposals in the 1960s to make them health plan employees. This defence was lodged in the organisation's oral and written history. The doctors are salaried Permanente employees. Despite many declaring allegiance to Kaiser Permanente and its model of prepaid group practice, they also belong to the American Medical Profession, an institution transcending any specific healthcare provider. This informed the open scepticism and resistance of some physicians:

The chiefs knew who we were going to have problems with, and were open about it. Who was going to deal with those problems was the question. We could help with more training, more support, more one-on-one work; but there's always been the question – even from the chiefs themselves. 'Now, after all that, if I still got somebody who can't do it, or won't play, what kind of support will I get from the very highest levels of the physician organisation to deal with this?' And I don't know that they ever really got an answer for that. Whereas with nursing supervisors it's like, 'Do it, or else.' You know, if you don't do it you're out of a job.

While nurse supervisors and clinic managers actively promoted CIS, some clinic chiefs refused to stamp their authority. This was a key determinant according to one chief:

> I think a lot of the differences between teams and clinics, why some were easier than others, had to do with a whole attitude of change. That was the biggest factor. If your leaders weren't really for it that was crucial. Internal medicine at [one clinic] never did go up. They haven't even used partial functionality. It was the leadership [view] in that department that this was not the system.

This is corroborated by observations concerning the autocratic chief of one specialty, as two respondents remarked:

> In OB/GYN the leadership was terrific, so implementing OB here and at [this clinic] went very well. It was more autocratic. A decision was made – 'That is how it is going be' – so that made it easier for the team to roll it out. Because it was real clear for the team, really clear.

Leadership was salient to the implementation of CIS, and leaders' prevarication, hesitation and ambiguity were interpreted to support the status quo. But leadership is only one factor in an organisation's readiness for new IT. Variation in compatibility between specialties was another factor. As was workload: when clinicians felt overburdened the best leadership may be insufficient to support lasting change. We need to distinguish between the leadership to promote implementation and to achieve successful outcomes, which are quite distinct challenges.

CONFLICT

CIS caused conflict at several levels. Clinic chiefs and support team members felt internal conflict between their awareness of CIS's faults and their responsibility to promote its uptake. Regional clinical priorities conflicted with the parent organisation's financial and administrative priorities. Friction was perceived between Kaiser Permanente's customised application and IBM's ability to produce a marketable product. And some behaviour described by respondents can be characterised as conflict avoidance – all in a conflict-averse culture.

Personal conflict

Personal conflict was implied in all the interviews and explicit in some. Some clinic and specialty chiefs felt the organisation had put them in a very difficult position:

There was a faction who felt strongly that the functionality of CIS was not state-of-the-art. So as a clinic chief I'm trying to get my staff ready for this, and I'm being addressed by people who I respect, saying, 'This is a mistake: you should do what you need to do to stop this before it goes on.' And I felt very conflicted then.

Realising that its adoption had been mistaken, one chief felt the dilemma of leading his clinic through CIS implementation acutely:

I felt like an officer asked to take my troops to Vietnam, and people are telling me I should go to Congress about why we are going to Vietnam. But my focus needed to be on making sure that my troops survived and did well. My thinking was, 'Well, so maybe it isn't the most functional system, but we're hooked up with IBM for Christ's sake, and if IBM can't help us, who else can fix this?'

Another chief reported similar misgivings:

It's like working with a bad medical assistant. It's better than not having one, but sometimes it drives you crazy. And I really thought it was going to be a lot easier to chart on the computer than it was. It was really cumbersome and I was really irritated with it. So, on a personal level I had to bite my tongue to try to lead the rest of the clinic through it.

Regional–national conflict

Respondents often referred to the importance of voicing one's concerns and being listened to. But Hawaiians are not aggressive communicators, and their polite protests were not heard by Program Office in California. Besides, as costs mounted, national and regional priorities diverged, as one chief reflected:

With CIS, the highest priority was not 'What's going to make the clinician's day easier, or more efficient?' The highest priority was, 'How can we document as completely as possible and then extract information easily, so that we can get paid?' [It] had very little to do with taking care of the patient who comes to your office.

Another chief pointed to a difficult relationship between Hawaii region and Program Office:

A weak point of CIS was Program Office; and I refer to them almost as an entity out there, like the IRS [Internal Revenue Service], like the Government. I don't think Program Office realises how the average frontline physician is alienated by them. If you add on top of that a heavy-handed mandate from Program Office – that this is coming down, and you will implement it; then ignoring local leadership and their opinions on the culture of the local environment in rolling that out: it's a formula for failure.

One support team member also blamed senior Program officers:

> They had difficulty dealing with being told: 'Hey look, you gotta fix this because it really makes it hard for users.' And to an extent they didn't understand it. And to some extent their hands – the people making the decisions – were tied by people above them, very high in the organisation, that were focused on budget.

Conflict between Kaiser Permanente and IBM

Hawaiian physicians were recruited to specify certain CIS functions, including care templates. They invested many additional hours in this work with no previous experience of software design, or even a functioning version of CIS to work with. They were annoyed when IBM delivered templates that bore little relation to those specified. Nevertheless, respondents tended to blame Kaiser Permanente for this shortcoming:

> CIS was an internal development project for Kaiser. Kaiser [specified] their requirements, and IBM responded. The bottom line is IBM is still a manufacturing company. IBM is not in the healthcare industry. The onus [is] on the customer to decide what they want in a product. It was no different in the CIS project.

Some respondents, however, attributed CIS's problems to a difficult relationship between Kaiser Permanente and IBM:

> I've heard that the relationship with IBM was not very good. We wanted to make a whole lot of changes and they would point out why it would take time and cost money, and the smallest change would be a fight and it would cost tens of thousands of dollars. It seemed a very confrontational relationship.

CONCLUSION

By the withdrawal of CIS, Hawaii Kaiser Permanente had begun to conceive of IT's integration with healthcare as an intermediate phase towards establishing radically new models and standards of care. Integration was no longer their ultimate goal, but part of a necessary process that would open new trajectories of care. One respondent concluded that implementing CIS was not about new IT in the narrow sense of computers and software, but a radically new approach to health technology, in the broadest sense of all the ideas, techniques, interventions and organisation involved in the maintenance of health:

> What we need to focus on is to change our healthcare delivery system, which is very different. That would make Epic a part of what we are doing, rather than the centre. Let's put the patient in the centre.

This perhaps suggests a different meaning to integration, where the EMR becomes part of a new ethos of healthcare, not so much a reconfiguration as a reorientation to a new electronic environment. In this conception, the EMR does not colonise the organisation any more than the organisation populates the system. The purpose of any EMR should be to support further innovations in the organisation and delivery of care. An investment of such magnitude should yield proportionate outcomes. The potential for such change arguably decreases the more exactly the system is tailored to existing administrative and clinical arrangements.

In light of this research, implementing NPfIT into the NHS seemed a task of unimaginable complexity and difficulty. In 2003 I could not imagine its success. Shortly after returning to the UK, I was contacted by a young member of the NPfIT support team. He questioned me for two hours, then left rather depressed saying, 'We're doomed, aren't we?' A few weeks later he resigned from his post. Perhaps I had only confirmed what he already suspected: that NPfIT and the Department of Health and Social Care was a hazardous marriage that might well harm his career.

Many in the DoH knew of my research in Hawaii, and some asked if I would be willing to speak to significant groups, including the NPfIT team, about it. These overtures were not followed up. I surmised that NPfIT leaders were either dimly aware of the hazards of the project they were embarking on, actively did not want to know about negative lessons from elsewhere, or both. Sometime later, the then Chief Executive for Health and Social Care summoned me to Whitehall to hear about the research. After half an hour he commented that the NHS would have no problems of resistance from doctors, as they had been 'tamed'. I left with a remark by Robert Cooper (Lecture, 1989, University of Lancaster) in my mind, 'Organisations love meaning and hate information.'

REFERENCES

Aarts J, Doorewaard H, Berg M. Understanding implementation: the case of a computerized physician order entry system in a large Dutch university medical center. *J AMIA*. 2004; 11: 207–16.

Brynjolfsson E, Hitt L. Beyond computation: information technology, organizational transformation, and business performance. *J Econ Perspect*. 2000; 14(4): 23–48.

Chall M, Cecil C, Cutting MD. History of the Kaiser Permanente Medical Care Program. In: *Regional Oral History Office of the Bancroft Library*. Berkeley; 1985. p. 52.

Cutting C. *Annual Report, Kaiser Medical Care Program*. 1984. p. 39.

Department of Health. *Building the Information Core: implementing the NHS Plan*, London: Department of Health; 2001.

Durkheim E. *The Rules of Sociological Method*, New York: Free Press; 1982.

Evans R, *et al.* A computer-assisted management program for antibiotics and other anti-infective agents. *N Engl J Med.* 1998; 338: 232–8.

Fiscella K, *et al.* Inequality in quality: addressing socioeconomic, racial, and ethnic disparities in health care. *JAMA.* 2000; 283: 2579–84.

Foucault M. *Discipline and Punish.* Harmondsworth: Penguin; 1977 (1975).

Friedman C, Wyatt J. *Evaluation Methods in Medical Informatics.* New York: Springer-Verlag; 1997.

Gibbs W. Taking computers to task. *Sci Am.* 1997; 278: 64–71.

Halfpenny P. The analysis of qualitative data. *Soc Rev.* 1979; 27(4): 779–825.

Institute of Medicine. *The Computer-Based Patient Record: an essential technology for health care.* Washington DC: National Academy Press; 1997.

Institute of Medicine. *Crossing the Quality Chasm: a new health system for the 21st century.* Washington DC: National Academy Press; 2001.

Institute of Medicine. *Priority Areas for National Action: transforming health care quality.* Washington DC: National Academy Press; 2003.

Ives ED. *The Tape-Recorded Interview: a manual for fieldworkers in folklore and oral history,* 2nd ed. Knoxville, TN: The University of Tennessee Press; 1995.

Kaplan B. Development and acceptance of medical information systems: an historical overview. *J Health Hum Res Admin.* 1988; 11: 9–29.

Krippendorff K. *Content Analysis: an introduction to its methodology.* London: Sage Publications; 1980.

Littlejohns P, Wyatt J, Garvica L. Evaluating computerised health information systems: hard lessons still to be learnt. *BMJ.* 2003; 326: 860–3.

Lorenzi N, Riley R. *Organizational Aspects of Health Informatics: managing technological change.* New York: Springer-Verlag; 1995.

Lorenzi N, Riley R. Managing change: an overview. *J AMIS.* 2000; 7(2): 116–24.

Miller R, Hillman J, Given R. Physician use of IT: results from the Deloitte Research Survey. *J Health Inf Manage.* 2004; 18(1): 72–80.

Miller R, Sim I. Physicians' use of electronic medical records: barriers and solutions. *Health Aff.* 2004; 23(2): 116–26.

Øvretveit J, *et al.* Improving quality through effective implementation of information technology in healthcare. *J Qual Health.* 2007a; 19(5): 259–66.

Øvretveit J, *et al.* Implementation of electronic medical records in hospitals: two case studies. *Health Pol.* 2007b; 84(2): 181–90.

Rogers E, Shoemaker F. *Communication of Innovations.* New York: The Free Press; 1971.

Schoen C, *et al.* Insured but not protected: how many adults are underinsured? *Health Aff.* 2005; Web Exclusive, 14 June 2005.

Scott J, *et al.* Learning from Kaiser Permanente's implementation of an electronic medical record in Hawaii: a qualitative study. *BMJ.* 2005; 331: 1313–16.

Scott T, *et al. Implementing an Electronic Medical Record System.* Oxford: Radcliffe Publishing; 2007.

Smillie JG. *Can Physicians Manage the Quality and Costs of Health Care? The story of the Permanente Medical Group.* New York: McGraw-Hill; 1991.

Smith Hughes S, Hancock H. History of the Kaiser-Permanente Medical Care Program. In: *Regional Oral History Office of the Bancroft Library.* Berkeley, CA: University of California; 1986. p. 54.

Starr P. *The Social Transformation of American Medicine.* New York: Basic Books; 1982.

Stiell A, *et al.* Prevalence of information gaps in the emergency department and the effect on patient outcomes. *Can Med Assoc J.* 2003; 169(10): 1023.

Whyte W. Interviewing in field research. In: Burgess R, editor. *Field Research: a sourcebook and field manual,* London: George Allen and Unwin; 1982. pp. 111–22.

.

CHAPTER 10

Some insights into the national healthcare systems of the United Kingdom and the Netherlands

Matthew Waritay Guah

INTRODUCTION

In recent years a considerable degree of concern has been expressed about variations in the standards of healthcare provision based on the distinction between government-centred and private insurance-centred schemes. Fuelled by a spate of healthcare stories in the media (e.g. medical error, patient safety, etc.), the rise of consumerism, a political drive to improve accountability, and a genuine desire to focus on quality rather than costs, there have been calls for systems to be put in place to monitor and ensure the quality of clinical services across a range of healthcare services. Several such mechanisms have recently been introduced into the United Kingdom, including the publication of indicators that aim to describe performance in certain key areas of healthcare. Currently, these performance indicators rely on comparisons of routinely collected outcome data to identify hospitals in which the quality of care might be poor.

In the Netherlands, three approaches to healthcare reform have been adopted in the past few decades: (1) ensuring universal coverage, (2) controlling costs, and (3) creating competition (Schut and Van de Ven 2005). Dutch healthcare has recently initiated a market-oriented healthcare system to enhance bureaucratic efficiency and reduce costs. National healthcare systems have existed in both the UK and the Netherlands for several decades. Over the years voluminous data has been collected on patient admissions and outcomes, changing healthcare services, operational processes and effectiveness, staff administration, national healthcare planning and subcontracting to third party vendors. Comparisons between the two state-run healthcare systems are currently receiving more attention, particularly as governments are keen to evaluate the trajectory of costs to continue to support expanding demand for healthcare services. This chapter is premised on the view that comparative studies on healthcare systems offer a useful guide for evaluating different service offerings and outcomes.

This chapter is structured as follows. First, we look at some of the basic characteristics of the UK and the Netherlands healthcare systems. Second, we consider the policies and plans to develop ICT to enhance the healthcare systems in each country. Finally, we offer some insights into the potential opportunities and threats to ICT development, particularly in the context of offering a national healthcare system in conjunction with increasing commercialisation of the sector.

IT IMPLEMENTATION IN UK HEALTHCARE

The UK National Health Service was set up in 1948 to offer free healthcare at the point of delivery to all citizens. Since then, the NHS has rarely been out of the public eye. The NHS has a budget of over £90 billion per year (Currie and Guah 2007). The annual spend on computer systems and services by the UK Government has doubled since 1999, reaching a figure of around £14 billion, representing the highest in Europe (NAO 2004). This increase has been accompanied by the growing use of large external IT service providers, and smaller, more specialised firms who see great potential in developing skills and capabilities in the healthcare sector. The split between public (in-house) and private (external) markets for IT services now stands at around 55 and 45% respectively.

Healthcare in the UK is a highly complex environment with the NHS providing patient services to around 60 million citizens, free at the point of delivery. The NHS was created by a parliamentary act initiated by the Labour Government following a national healthcare review after the Second World War. The current NHS organisation consists of parliament, a secretary of state for health, strategic health authorities, under which NHS trusts, foundation trusts, primary care trusts, care trusts and non-NHS organisations reside. An independent regulator that monitors these organisations reports to parliament.

Yet the history of introducing ICT into the NHS has produced mixed results. From an information intensive organisation with virtually no computers in the 1960s, the NHS now has tens of thousands (Brennan 2005). One of the first computer systems was the Patient Administration System (PAS) introduced in the 1960s. This was followed by several different systems in the 1970s (laboratory systems), in the 1980s (management systems), in the 1990s (IT strategy such as electronic patient records (EPR), electronic record development and implementation programme (ERDIP) and electronic health records (EHR)).

The past six decades have witnessed the NHS experiencing periods of both stability and change. As a highly institutionalised environment, the NHS has developed a 'public sector ethos' infused with the values of serving the public. Clinicians and healthcare workers have placed these values above issues of finance and cost-effectiveness as treatment has been provided based on medical need rather than ability to pay. Over the years, the NHS has developed many institutionalised mechanisms that make change difficult and often highly controversial, such as the powerful professional bodies that govern the conduct and performance of clinicians. Successive governments have introduced policy documents to modernise the NHS with varying levels of success. One area has been in the use of information and communications technology as a means to enhance efficiency and performance. Healthcare is an information-rich business which consumes vast hospital resources in gathering information. Doctors and nurses spend a large amount of their time collecting and using information.

Against a background of relative underinvestment in ICT over three decades, the government pledged in 2002 to spend around £7 billion on a National Programme for Information Technology (National Programme) – later renamed 'Connecting for Health' – to deliver four critical elements: NHS Care Records Service, Electronic Appointment Booking, Electronic Transmission of Prescriptions, and an IT Infrastructure and Network.

The key objective of the National Programme is to deliver a 21st century health service for patients, citizens, clinicians and people working in the NHS through the increased use of information and communication technology. Table 10.1 presents the range of ICT initiatives developed in the UK since 2002.

TABLE 10.1 ICT Initiatives in UK healthcare

Choose and Book	A national electronic referral service which gives patients a choice of place, date and time for their first outpatient appointment in a hospital or clinic.
	Patients can choose their hospital or clinic and then book their appointment to see a specialist with a member of the practice team, at the GP surgery or at home by telephone or over the Internet, at a time more convenient to them.
Electronic Prescription Service (EPS)	Enables prescribers – such as GPs and practice nurses – to send prescriptions electronically to a dispenser (such as a pharmacy) of a patient's choice. This will make the prescribing and dispensing process safer and more convenient for patients and staff.
GP2GP	Enables patients' electronic health records to be transferred directly and securely between GP practices. It improves patient care as GPs will usually have full and detailed medical records available to them for a new patient's first consultation.
HealthSpace	A secure website where patients can store their personal health information online, such as height, weight and blood pressure. In time, it will give people electronic access to parts of their NHS Care Record.
NHS Care Records Service (NHS CRS)	Improves the safety and quality of patient care. It will give healthcare staff faster, easier access to reliable information about patients to help with their treatment.

(continued)

NHS Number	Fundamental to the National Programme for IT, it is the common unique identifier that makes it possible to share patient information across the whole of the NHS safely, efficiently and accurately.
Patient case studies	These are a helpful way to learn from other patients' experiences of the new technologies that are already in place.
Picture Archiving and Communications System (PACS)	Enables images such as X-rays and scans to be stored electronically and viewed on screens, so that doctors and other health professionals can access the information and compare it with previous images at the touch of a button. It makes X-rays on film a thing of the past, leading to faster and improved diagnosis methods.
Research Capability Programme	The primary objective here is to enable research to achieve its full potential as a 'core' activity for healthcare, alongside other uses of NHS data that lead to improvements in the quality and safety of care.
	There are strict criteria for the uses of patient information for research in that there will be effective mechanisms to protect identifiable personal and confidential information and to seek appropriate consent.
Social Care Integration Project (SCIP)	An NHS Connecting for Health project which aims to enable improved outcomes for people using health and social care services, through enabling better, more seamless service delivery between NHS and adult social services.

CONNECTING FOR HEALTH – PROJECT SETBACKS

Connecting for Health has suffered from massive delays at various stages of the implementation process, mostly due to the scale of this project, the pace of change, and the number of implementation partners involved (Guah and Currie 2005). As a result of significant progress made in the last two years, 2009 is proving to be a year for serious system deployment, with approximately 200 NHS sites having systems upgraded every month under Connecting for Health. Table 10.2 summarises progress in a number of areas against earlier mentioned objectives.

IT IMPLEMENTATION IN THE NETHERLANDS HEALTHCARE SYSTEM

The Dutch Ministry of Health, Well-being and Sports is responsible for healthcare provision for about 60 million people in the Netherlands. The current state of the Dutch healthcare system evolved from the time hospitals were set up for Protestants, Catholics, Socialists and the Liberals – mainly for the purpose of providing healthcare to long-term and chronically sick patients. With growing industrialisation, hospitals treated patients with a range of chronic infectious diseases such as cholera, typhoid and tuberculosis. Those early days saw treatment options limited, particularly for the poor. As a result of the more affluent members of society constantly demanding better treatments and services, a general health insurance policy was introduced (Algemene Ziektekostenverzekering) in 1941, which also extended the availability of medical healthcare to people with low incomes (van der Burg 2007).

As healthcare became available to more people in the aftermath of the Second

TABLE 10.2 Key milestones for the NPfIT

IT system	Milestones achieved
Choose and Book	• A little more than 14 million (14 055 358) bookings made to date achieving roughly 33 000 bookings per day. • Just about 50% of NHS referral activity from GP surgery to first outpatient appointment. • Around 10% of all GP practices in England are yet to use Choose and Book for referring patients to hospital.
Electronic Prescription Service	• Over 175 million (175 895 718) prescription messages have now been transmitted electronically. • While 7958 GP practices have had technical upgrades to the new system, only 6441 of those are actively operating the EPS. • 9523 pharmacy systems have had technical upgrades to the new system and 8393 are actively operating EPS. • Over 75% of daily prescription messages still take place without using EPS.
GP2GP Transfer	• GP2GP has now been used for 504 035 medical record transfers. • 5218 GP practices have had technical upgrades to the new system. • 5086 of these practices are now actively operating GP2GP.
National Network for the NHS (N3)	• Approximately 1.2 million NHS employees now have access to the new broadband network N3, making it one of the largest virtual private networks (VPN) in the world. • By the end of April 2008, there have been over 32 000 connections to N3 including approximately 11 000 delivered through aggregators (mostly pharmacies). • N3 can save the NHS an estimated £900 million over seven years, relative to previous NHSnet contracts. • 100% of existing GP sites who require a connection have had this delivered.
NHS mail	• When migration is complete NHSmail, the national NHS e-mail and directory service, will have over one million users: the largest private, fully featured, secure, single-domain e-mail service in the world. • An average of 983 152 messages are sent/received across the NHSmail platform daily. • The number of users registered for NHSmail is increasing every week. • There are now almost 400 000 registered users. • All NHS 'Connecting for Health' staff have migrated to NHSmail.
Picture Archiving and Communications System (PACS)	• PACS has been fully deployed to all acute hospitals since December 2007 and the focus is now concentrated on image sharing between locations. • There are 127 PACs from NHS Connecting for Health now live across England.
NHS Care Records Service	• 248 542 Summary Care Records have now been uploaded to the Data Spine. • There are 576 328 smart card holders who are registered and approved for access to the Spine.

Source: www.connectingforhealth.nhs.uk

World War, the demand for care increased. Due to government post-war investment priorities (including reconstruction of industry and residential buildings) healthcare experienced under-spending resulting in a shortage of hospital beds and use of old-fashioned medical equipment. Waiting lists had 'exploded' immediately after 1945 and the Dutch government began to make further investments in the healthcare sector. This led to doctors beginning to specialise in different areas of medicine, directly leading to improved services for patients.

Specialisation meant changes to hospital targets from short-term to long-term patient care. The number of beds dramatically increased from 44 000 in 1955 to 74 000 in 1975. In 1964 all healthcare costs were covered by a medical insurance system, regulated by the health insurance act (Ziekenfondswet). This law stipulated that employees with an income beneath a predetermined limit must be insured. Options were further advanced for the care and financing of chronically ill patients requiring long-term care. By 1968 an exceptional medical expenses act (commonly referred to as AWBZ) was introduced to offer a new form of financing hospitals and nursing homes. It also led to an explosive increase in the number of nursing homes.

A significant increase in the demand for healthcare services occurred in 1980 when the number of people over 65 years of age doubled – from 800 000 in 1960 to 1.6 million in 1980. Despite better quality of doctors – using increased knowledge to provide better diagnoses – they were unable to cope with such a high increase in waiting lists. The introduction of ICT in Dutch healthcare by the early 1990s contributed to better management of diseases and other medical improvements.

FINANCING HEALTHCARE IN THE NETHERLANDS

While the Dutch government is responsible for providing healthcare to all, the costs of healthcare are generally paid by the patients through complicated methods, including the following:

➤ insurance premiums: directly and indirectly as a percentage of personal income
➤ AWBZ premium: as a percentage of salary
➤ own contribution: for some medicine such as painkillers, dental fees, and part of the costs of elderly or nursing homes a direct contribution is required
➤ tax: government pays the insurance premium of people under 18, and subsidises the insurance premium for those with low incomes ('zorgtoeslag'). These premiums are distributed between insurance companies, the local government and the patient (who ultimately pays for all bills sent directly to him/her by the healthcare providers)
➤ the government has also mandated that 10% of all healthcare costs covered by insurance are freely negotiated between insurance companies and health suppliers
➤ the remaining 90% of the non-negotiated costs for healthcare consists of fixed prices for each treatment or case, as well as the costs for healthcare with fixed

budgets for the total number of treatments or cases over a fixed period. Because these costs are fixed, transferring money from one healthcare provider to another for specific treatment is unnecessarily complicated.

This new arrangement led to a significant increase in government expenditure to meet the continuous increase in the healthcare demand. The increasing demand was not the only factor causing higher expenditure. Unlike business sectors where productivity may increase as a result of technological progress, healthcare is much more complex. The patient life cycle imposes very high costs, particularly when a person requires long-term care for a chronic condition. With new medicines and more sophisticated treatment options, the financial demands on running a publicly funded healthcare system are increasing, so governments are looking towards technology as a means of rationalising healthcare operations and services.

According to the Dutch Central Bureau for statistics (CBS) the total amount spent on healthcare in 2006 was 72.2 billion euros (consisting of 42.5 billion for GP and hospitalisation, 27.3 billion for mental care and 2.4 billion for policy and management of healthcare institutions). This total represents 13.5% of GDP, demonstrating that the primary need in life is also the most expensive and most valuable. It is anticipated that 2009 to 2020 will see the baby boom generation of post-1945 retire, resulting in fewer people taking care of more people. Thus, healthcare processes must be refined and streamlined in order to handle future demands.

Unlike the UK, the Dutch government is not in charge of the day-to-day management of the healthcare system. Private health suppliers are responsible for the provision of services. The government is, however, responsible for the accessibility and quality of the healthcare. Since 1 January 2006 a new healthcare insurance system has been developed, combining previously separated insurance packages for public and private healthcare in the Netherlands. A basic package has been developed by the government similar to the level of service provision offered under the previous system. All insurance companies are legally obliged to offer this basic health insurance package alongside other more expensive and more sophisticated packages. The basic health insurance package in the Netherlands offers the following:

➤ medical care, including services by GPs, hospitals, medical specialists and obstetricians
➤ hospital stay
➤ dental care (up until the age of 18 years; when 18 years or older you are only covered for specialist dental care and false teeth)
➤ various medical appliances
➤ various medicines
➤ prenatal care
➤ patient transport (e.g. ambulance)
➤ paramedical care.

Additional insurance for circumstances not included in the basic package may be purchased under more expensive options that employees of large organisations usually purchase under a collective health insurance policy. Because contributions to the basic healthcare insurance are determined annually, it proves advantageous for people to change insurers on renewal dates. The regulators decided to make it easier for customers to move between healthcare insurers from 1 January 2007. Now that people can change their insurance more easily, a free market system in the healthcare sector is stimulated. This system ensures competition between insurance companies, allowing patients to benefit from lower prices.

SOME INSIGHTS ON ICT-DRIVEN HEALTHCARE PROVISION IN THE UK AND NETHERLANDS

The aims of a new IT system are to support administration and improve medical decision making. One primary reason for collecting information about patients is for the Dutch government to set budgetary guidelines for insurance companies. The UK government, on the other hand, does not use the insurance system and has focused more attention on developing a national patient database to upload a 'summary care record' of every citizen in England. The priorities and purposes of ICT vary slightly between the Netherlands and UK, but it is important to recognise that investment in technology for specific purposes will result in different outcomes for publicly funded healthcare. So far, it looks as though the UK is attempting to retain its somewhat polarised system that offers healthcare free at the point of delivery, yet is provided by a range of different public and private providers. The Netherlands, conversely, is moving to a more commercialised approach with different providers competing to offer health insurance to Dutch citizens.

The differences between the UK and Dutch systems in terms of data manipulation illustrate the systems' intention and strengths, and can be seen in a number of aspects such as the patient database structure, patient care instruments, disease control, treatments and statistical techniques. In comparison with the Dutch systems, ICT systems developed in the UK include gathering patient data not only from clinical and administrative input but from patients themselves.

Built on different social-cultural backgrounds, each healthcare system contains unique features. Certain aspects, such as the relationship between central and local control of hospitals, show that variation exists. Shared concerns include system functions, data manipulation, standardisation, and medical output reporting. Key issues are the following.

➤ *Accountability*: By tracking patient movement over time and historical trends of a particular treatment pattern or disease observation, applications that are part of the new NHS systems demonstrate an evolutionary way of tracking costs of national healthcare.

➤ *Feasibility and measurability*: Patient data elements can be established and measured to reflect key patient conditions and utilisation of health services. This function demonstrates the need for all healthcare data to offer generalisability.

➤ *Comparability and uniformity*: New comprehensive systems for the NHS can be used within and between hospitals for performance quality control as well as service improvement, and commonly to exchange information. When hospitals achieve greater uniformity of patient data, there will be greater comparability of patient data.

➤ *Reliability and validity*: The national healthcare regulator regularly monitors the accuracy of reported healthcare data.

➤ *Accessibility*: More patient data are available to the public. NHS makes certain types of patient data available through the Web, and Dutch patients are able to access their health records through their insurance providers.

SPECIFIC USE OF ICT IN DUTCH HEALTHCARE

General practitioners have been using computers in their offices for many years. In 1978 the first computer was installed at a Dutch GP's office. Today, 97% of Dutch GPs use a GP information system (HIS). Almost all use their information system to record patients' medical records. The Dutch GPs can choose among eight suppliers offering 11 information systems based on the requirements formulated by the professional organisations of general practitioners (Protti and Smit 2000).

The information systems used by GPs have been designed specifically for use in primary care. They consist of different modules, each performing a specific set of functions: patient administration, drug prescriptions, maintaining a journal and keeping a record of current diagnoses, maintaining a list of important diseases or conditions (problem list), keeping a record of investigations, making risk profiles and detailing family history, choosing patients for preventive programmes, etc. It is important that the GP is using these possibilities correctly in order for the HIS to provide the right information at the right time and to support the GP with his or her primary task: providing care.

The information contained in the medical records include the patient's details, the patient's medical history and any other relevant history, and a complete report of each event with the patient, from signs and symptoms when first presenting, through diagnosis and investigations to treatment and outcome. Paramedics and nurse practitioners are using the HIS to add information about their own encounter with a patient or to add incoming information from third parties like laboratory results and incoming correspondence. It is still in operation today, almost 30 years since it was introduced.

The GPs need to be in mutual communication with care providers at the secondary care level, especially with specialists. As family doctors, GPs need to know what happens to their patients when they go to hospital, especially when they have to continue a therapeutic plan after hospital discharge. In addition, secondary care providers need access to the hospitalised patients' medical records, such as medication data, from primary care in order to provide quality care. Pharmacists also need to be kept in the communication loop.

A number of regional systems have been developed, hosting databases and sharing healthcare information regionally. For example, E-Novation LifeLine started in 1983 providing IT solution for healthcare and became a leading player in the exchange of information within the healthcare sector. With RijnmondNet they created a regional network for the Rijnmond Region. Two decades later, 22 different networks cover most of the Netherlands. A similar development is the emergence of national healthcare networks. There is no national network in the Netherlands at the moment that connects all primary care and secondary care, and eventually third care. The Ministry of Health, Welfare and Sport is working with the National IT Institute for Healthcare (NICTIZ) and the Central Information Point for Healthcare Professions (CIBG) on the development of a nationwide system for the electronic exchange of medical data, the electronic patient dossier (EPD).

At the primary care level, studies show that though 80% of GPs use an electronic prescription system, only 10–35% of prescriptions are transmitted to community pharmacists electronically, and less than 5% of GPs get an up-to-date summary of all medication supplied from the local pharmacy. In the communication between primary and secondary care, the referral letters from GPs do not usually contain the necessary information for specialists, physicians and hospital pharmacists. And less than 1% of the specialists have electronic insight into medication supplied by community pharmacies (NICTIZ 2005a). A hospital pharmacist describes the situation as follows:

> Patients are normally asked about their medication history at the hospital. The information is then registered using paper-based forms and is sent to us to be entered into our information system. Our work and observations are based on this information, which sometimes is not even reliable information at all.

The fact that medication data are not shared among these professionals means many lives are potentially put in danger as a result of avoidable medication errors – avoidable if the patients' medication record had been available to healthcare providers at the right time and the right place (NICTIZ 2005b).

ELECTRONIC MEDICAL RECORDS

Unlike Connecting for Health's N3 component, there is no national network responsible for connecting all primary care and secondary care within a single medical record system. The government, CIBG and NICTIZ are working together to introduce the electronic patient dossier (EPD). NICTIZ (2005a) suggests that an EPD will consist of an individual patient's medical record in digital format with the capacity to coordinate the storage and retrieval of individual records with the aid of computers.

EPD is being developed to include applications used for data exchange on national infrastructure, referred to as 'AORTA'. Two applications that are being introduced as part of the AORTA are:

➤ *Electronic medication dossier (EMD)*: The EMD keeps a record of the patient's medical treatments. The goal is to exchange data between GPs, hospitals and pharmacies. With the EMD, medication errors can be prevented because all the data needed is online, on time and available. This must lead to more secure and improved medical care and prevent avoidable medical errors (Ministry of Health, Welfare and Sport 2008).

➤ *'Waarneem Dossier Huisartsen' (WDH)*: The data elements used in the Dutch systems, as in the UK systems, cover basic patient information (personal details and reasons for hospital visits) and the key services of each insurance policy. The methods of statistical analysis and techniques for comparing details relating to healthcare providers' obligations to the patient is not used to the same extent as in the UK. Some data elements, such as the market concentration of public health insurance, are useful and valuable to show how limited financial resources are allocated. To communicate the efficiency of service providers in the Netherlands, the number of patient complaints against a particular service provider will be one indicator used for decision making about healthcare strategy.

Performance measurement of healthcare providers in both the UK and the Netherlands is an important activity and has increased since the 1980s. In the UK, the National Institute for Health and Clinical Excellence (NICE) plays a role in measuring health-care input and output using uniform measurements developed by experts to promote efficiency, cost-effectiveness and increased comparability in the healthcare sector. Systems designers who developed the national systems used uniform measurements in order to make them a powerful tool for performance measurement in hospitals across the nation. The measurements normally reported by NICE also concentrate on uses and the healthcare services provided to the public. Measures that include 'non-service related information', such as hospital funding and staff salaries, are measured, but the emphasis is placed on the effectiveness and efficiency of use, such as the efficacy of drug treatments.

Like the UK, health spending in the Netherlands is increasing, currently around 5% annually (Westtert, Berg, Koolman, Verkleij 2008). This rate of growth is comparable to that of neighbouring countries. The report claims that, while the quality of many aspects of care is good, the country does not excel at the international level. Concerns exist about the availability of nursing and care personnel and the health-care system in general is not overly concerned with quality as the driving force. The report claims that 98% of GPs use an electronic file and there are around 100 telecare projects ongoing, mostly in the area of e-domestics and personal alarms. Further, five regional hospitals and one medical training centre are connected to the National Exchange Point for the EHRs.

The Dutch Ministry of Health, Welfare and Sport is working with ICT suppliers to build a nationwide system for the electronic exchange of medical data. Like the UK system, it is envisaged that patients will be able to access their own data. Similar to the UK structure, ICT policy is developed by the Ministry of Health, Welfare and Sport, the National IT Institute for Healthcare (NICTIZ) and the Central Information Point for Healthcare Professions (CIBG). Part of the remit to develop EHRs is to improve affordability, access and quality by creating the conditions for an optimum and safe usage of ICT. The EHR with the corresponding infrastructure is expected to be the catalyst for other ICT healthcare initiatives such as telemedicine.

CONCLUSION

This chapter has considered the important and critical roles played by government, despite some of the political, economic, social and technical differences between the UK and Dutch healthcare systems. Our observations suggest that many similarities and differences arise between the two systems, with the UK adopting a highly centrist approach to service provision and the Dutch system introducing an insurance policy scheme. Both systems appear to be moving towards greater commercialisation in their approach to offering citizens healthcare choices, yet the UK system appears to be using ICT as a main driver for transformation in healthcare, perhaps more so than the Dutch example. Both countries recognise the importance of the role of new technology, yet critical issues will need to be resolved around the adoption and implementation of EHRs in an environment that aims to improve quality and service to patients at the same time as reducing the costs of unprofitable healthcare service offerings.

While both countries have decided to take actions within their healthcare sectors to improve the quality of products and services being delivered, the Dutch are clearly attempting to meet goals of higher patient and provider satisfaction, increasing the safety of patient care, and reducing the risk and the cost of liability for medical errors. The UK, on the other hand, is opting for a 'big bang' approach, which is looking more likely to be scaled down as more individual suppliers are being invited to bid for contracts. In short, while the overall aim to develop ICT to improve service delivery in healthcare is shared by both countries, the means of achieving it is different, with each approach offering both advantages and disadvantages.

REFERENCES

Ash JS, Berg M, Coiera E. Some unintended consequences of information technology in healthcare: the nature of patient care information system-related errors. *J Am Med Inform Assoc.* 2004; 11(2): 104–12.

Banker RD, Chang H, Pizzini M. The balanced scorecard: judgmental effects of performance measures linked to strategy. *Account Rev.* 2004; 79(1): 1–23.

Beath CM, Orlikowski WJ. The contradictory structure of systems development methodologies: distracting the IS-user relationship in information engineering. *Inf Syst Res.* 1994; 5(4): 350–77.

Berg M. Patient care information systems and healthcare work: a socio-technical approach. *Int J Med Inform.* 1999; 55: 87–101.

Berg M. Implementing information systems in health care organizations: myths and challenges. *Int J Med Inform.* 2004; 64: 143–56.

Blackler F. Chief executives and the modernization of the English National Health Service. *Leadership.* 2006; 2(1): 5–30.

Boulianne E. Revisiting fit between AIS design and performance with the analyzer strategic-type. *Int J AIS.* 2007; 8: 1–16.

Brennan S. *The NHS IT Project.* Oxford: Radcliffe Publishing; 2005.

Brennan S. The biggest computer programme in the world ever! How's it going? *J Inf Technol.* 2007; 22: 202–11.

Brown T. Modernization or failure? IT development projects in the UK public sector. *Fin Account Manage.* 2001; 17(4): 363–81.

Connecting for Health. *Business Plan.* 2004. Available at: www.connectingforhealth. nhs.uk

Constantinides P, Barrett M. Large scale ICT innovation, power, organizational change: the case of a regional health information network. *J Appl Behav Sci.* 2006; 42: 76–90.

Cordella A. Transaction costs and information systems: does IT add up? *J Inf Technol.* 2006; 21(3): 195–202.

Cox B, Dawe N. Evaluation of the impact of a PACS system on an intensive care unit. *J Manag Med.* 2002; 16(2–3): 199–205.

Currie W, Guah M. IT enabled healthcare delivery: the UK National Health Service. *Inf Syst Manage.* 2006; Spring: 7–22.

Currie WL, Guah MW. Conflicting institutional logics: a national program for IT in the organizational field of healthcare. *J Inf Technol.* 2007; 22(3): 235–47.

Dehning B, Richardson VJ. Returns on investments in information technology: a research synthesis. *Inf Syst.* 2002; 16(1): 7–30.

Doolin B. Power and resistance in the implementation of a medical management information system. *Inf Syst.* 2004; 14: 343–62.

Eason K. Local socio-technical system development in the NHS National Programme for Information Technology. *J Inf Technol.* 2007; 22: 257–64.

Geelhoed J. *Control Deficiencies in the Dutch Health Care Sector.* Enschede: Febodruk; 2005.

Gordon L, Miller D. A contingency framework for the design of accounting information systems. *Account Org Soc.* 1976; 1(1): 59–76.

Government Issue. *Modernizing AWBZ.* Dutch Parliament, 2004–2005. 2006; 26631(138): 3.

Grasbski SV, Leech SA. Complementary controls and ERP implementation success. *Int J Account Inf Syst.* 2007; 8: 17–39.

Guah MW. *Managing Very Large Information Technology Projects.* Hershey, PA: IGI-Global; 2008.

Guah MW, Currie WL. Web services in national healthcare: the impact of public and private collaboration. *Int J Technol Hum Interact.* 2005; 1(2): 48–61.

Heathfield H, Pitty D, Hanka R. (1998). Evaluating information technology in healthcare: barriers and challenges. *BMJ.* 1998; 316: 1959–61.

Hillestad R, Bigelow J, Bower A, *et al.* Can electronic medical record systems transform healthcare? Potential health benefits, savings, and costs. *Health Aff.* 2005; 24(5): 1103–17.

Institute of Management Accountants. *Developing Comprehensive Performance Indicators.* Statement no. 4U; March 1995.

Ishikawa K, Ohmichi H, Umesato Y, *et al.* The guideline of the personal health data structure to secure safety healthcare: the balance between use and protection to satisfy the patients' needs. *Int J Med Inform.* 2007; 76: 412–18.

Izit WM. *Project Electronic Patient Dossier*. November 2004.

Jiang JJ, Klein G. Risks to different aspects of system success. *Inf Manageme*. 1999; 36: 63–72.

Kirsch LJ. Portfolios of control modes and IS project management. *Inf Syst Res*. 1997; 8(3): 215–39.

Mark AL. Modernising healthcare – is the NPfIT for purpose? *J Inf Technol*. 2007; 22: 248–56.

Ministry of Health, Welfare and Sport. *Changes in ICT Requirements*. 2007. Available at: www. dbconderhoud.nl/pool/1/documents/Gebruikersdocument%20uitlevering%20 20071001%20deel%203%20V20071001.pdf

Ministry of Health, Welfare and Sport. 2008. Available at: www.minvws.nl/dossiers/ elektronisch-patienten-dossier/

National Audit Office. *Improving IT Procurement, Report by the Comptroller and Auditor General*. HC 877 Session 2003–4, 5 November. London: HMSO; 2004.

NICTIZ. *Modelrichtlijn en modelvoorlichtingsmateriaal autorisatie voor koplopers Electronisch Medicatie Dossier*. versie 1.0. 2005a.

NICTIZ. *Modelrichtlijn en modelvoorlichtingsmateriaal autorisatie voor koplopers Waarneem Dossier Huisartsen*. versie 1.0. 2005b.

Pollack A. *NHS Plc: the privatisation of our healthcare*. London: Verso Books; 2005.

Porter ME, Teisberg EO. *Redefining Health Care: creating value-based competition on results*. Cambridge, MA: Harvard Business School Press; 2006.

Protti D, Smit C. *The Netherlands: another European country where GPs have been using EMRs for over twenty years*. 2000. Available at: www.hcccinc.com/bcovers/previous/Vol_XX_ No_3/PDFS/TheNetherlands.pdf

Randell B. A computer scientist's reactions to NPfIT. *J Inf Technol*. 2007; 22: 222–34.

Schut FT, Van de Ven WPMM. Rationing and competition in the Dutch health-care system. *Health Econ*. 2005; 14: 59–74.

Soh C, Kien SS, Tay-Yap J. Cultural fits and misfits: is ERP a universal solution? *Commun ACM*. 2000; 43(3): 47–51.

Spainck K. *Information Technology in Health*. Report for University of Twente Faculty of Electrical Engineering, Mathematics and Computer Science; 2005.

van der Burg M. *Making an IT outsourcing decision support system for healthcare organizations using the Analytic Hierarchy Process theory* [unpublished Masters thesis]. Erasmus School of Economics; 2007.

van der Haak M, Wolff AC, Brandner R, *et al*. Data security and protection in cross-institutional electronic patient records. *Int J Med Inform*. 2003; 70: 117–30.

Wanless D. *Securing our Future Health: taking a long-term view*. London: HM Treasury; 2002. Available at: www.hm-treasury.gov.uk/wanless

Westtert GP, Berg MJ, Koolman X, Verkleij H, editors. *Dutch Health Care Performance Report 2008*. 2008. Available at: www.healthcareperformance.nl

CHAPTER 11

Customer value and lean operations in a self-care setting

Jannis Angelis, Cameron Watt and Mairi Macintyre

INTRODUCTION

Today NHS trusts are faced with an increasingly complex list of challenges that range from an ageing population, increased cost pressures and a greater public concern regarding patient involvement and safety. At the same time policy leaders, health professionals and the public's attitude to healthcare is beginning to change due in part to the increased incidence of long-term conditions such as diabetes, asthma and heart disease. This refocusing has resulted in a shift towards greater independence and choice for patients, as politicians push for people to have more information on, involvement in and control over their healthcare.

A central argument for this emphasis on 'self-care' is based on the belief held by healthcare providers that patients can positively affect their condition when placed in a position that facilitates self-management (Odgen 2005). We use the definition of self-care as defined by the Department of Health (DoH 2007) as

> the care taken by individuals towards their own health and well-being. It includes the actions people take for themselves, their children and families to maintain good physical and mental health; meet social and psychological needs; prevent illness or accidents; care for minor ailments and long-term conditions; and maintain health and well-being after an acute illness or discharge from hospital.

As a concept, self-care has been shown to be effective in improving the quality of life of patients and promoting appropriate utilisation of services. It is for this reason that supporting patients to self-manage their conditions and to use health services when appropriate has been identified as an increasingly important element in national health policies and attracted significant support from the staff we have interviewed (Cottam and Leadbeater 2004).

A key issue is how to optimise the advantages of self-care through the implementation of Lean principles while still delivering value to the NHS, individual staff and patients. These principles are a focus on customer value, continuous improvement, inclusion of all employees and managers alike, and waste reduction. Lean also contains several techniques, such as just-in-time, total quality maintenance and error-proofing. These are employed to help realise the principles and in turn improve the product or service provider's value proposition. Central to the NHS challenge is the question of value and the nature of patient as customer. In addition, there is a need for greater agility in the complex self-care environment in order to react quickly and effectively to a changing market (Christopher 2000; Christopher and Towill 2000; van Hoek, *et al.* 2001). Integration through the use of information systems (IS) has been recognised as a key enabler in achieving such agility (Power, *et al.* 2001; Yusuf, *et al.* 2004; White, *et al.* 2005). IS integration within and among organisations enables them to capture data on demand, leading to customer-focused value chains (Christopher 2000). It also allows accessing members to relate information and share their interpretations (Tippins and Sohi 2003), something which in experienced-based operations such as healthcare is essential. An integrated information system is more than just individual component integration. It requires the merger of communication, data and application to enable consistent and real-time connectivity among function units across the value chain (Ross 2003; Muller and Seuring 2007). As shown by Rai, *et al.* (2006), the integration covers data consistency and cross-functional application. The former is the degree to which common data definition and consistency in stored data have been established across a value chain, while the latter is the degree of real-time communication between chain units.

THE QUESTION OF CUSTOMER FOCUS

Lean thinking has wide applicability in many different countries and industries (Womack, *et al.* 1990; Womack and Jones 2003), with demonstrated potential for achieving high productivity and quality (Snell and Dean 1993; Sakakibara, *et al.* 1997; Lowe, *et al.* 1997; Bushell 2002). Empirical evidence by Shah and Ward (2003) and Fullerton, *et al.* (2003) shows that Lean contributes substantially to the operating performance of plants and is increasingly implemented in both private and public services. However, while Lean principles have been identified as appropriate for the public sector in general, implementation and sustainability remain a challenge (Jones 2004; Westwood, *et al.* 2007). In healthcare, this is partly due to the complex dynamics between numerous stakeholders, which may be enabling or inhibiting, depending on their views and agendas (Papadopoulos 2007) as well as their needs.

This role of the customer as value specifier lies at the heart of the Lean philosophy (Womack and Jones 2003). By identifying customer value, Lean operations put pressure on the provider to be efficient and effective in the provision of their services (Drummond-Hay and Bamford 2007). But it may pose a fundamental problem when implementing Lean within the NHS due to the ambiguous notion of the 'patient as customer' (Wright and Taylor 2005). A customer is here defined as an individual or group who has the power to specify and pay for services or products they want and value. Value in Lean operations is defined by what the customer values. Such value is not only seen to exist in the end product but also in the chain of processes that take place for a service to be delivered to the customer. So, for effective Lean operations, there needs to be a clear view of the customer without confusion caused by multiple customers and stakeholders. The argument for many is that customer value in healthcare may mean improvements in areas such as medical mistakes, waiting times and patient satisfaction (Gowen, *et al.* 2006).

Since the early 1980s political pressure has driven the NHS towards a more market-orientated position in a much publicised and debated attempt to cut costs, increase efficiency, effectiveness and accountability as well as improving patient care (DoH 1997, 1998a, 2001a). The focus has been on increasing the degree of patient-centred care through greater customer orientation and partnership working (DoH 1998b, 2001b, 2002). While such a customer orientation in private healthcare is not new in the UK or globally (Weisbart 2002; Whitcomb and Shafa 2001; O'Malley 2004; Stavins 2004), its introduction within the NHS whose culture is more custodial, consensual, equitable and socially driven in nature (Bolton 2002; Antony, *et al.* 2007) has potentially created serious adoption problems (Bolton 2002; McGuire 2003; Wright and Taylor 2005). Many protagonists of such a customer focus argue that the benefits to both patient and organisation are multi-level, including increased flexibility and diversity of staff skills (McBride, *et al.* 2005), cost cutting and overall patient care and positive experiences (Perucca 2001; Whitcomb 2001; Weisbart 2002; Fillingham 2007). Indeed, it would seem obvious that in an organisation whose core values are based on caring for individuals, the adoption of such a customer service orientation would be the logical step. However, while a great deal of benefit could be derived from such a move for the NHS, staff and patients, and it is acknowledged that within a Lean context the customer's specification of value is crucial, a number of fundamental problems do exist in blanket adoption of such a philosophy.

Such a stance may be directly at odds with the fundamental care-driven philosophy of the NHS (Walsh 1994; Beckett 2000; Wright and Taylor 2005), which, while placing the patient at the heart of decision making, recognises the professional autonomy and subsequent responsibility of healthcare professionals to deliver the medical, nursing or recuperative care they judge to be needed and in the best interest of the patient. In other words, power relations, roles, responsibility and accountability are clear and focus is on need-driven care provision rather than meeting or reacting to market-based customer satisfaction performance measures. But such a move could be forcing already limited resources to be focused away from patient care to areas that are perceived to be more orientated towards a public relations agenda, creating unfair and unrealistic expectations of what can be achieved by medical, nursing and social care staff (Drake and Davies 2006). Indeed, Bolton (2002) puts forward the argument that such a situation is damaging to the patient-nurse relationship in that it undermines the professional status of the nurse in the eyes of the patient, and we suggest the patient's intimate social circle, by shifting their role to more of a consumer sector service provider than an expert, professional carer. She concludes that the higher levels of 'emotional labour' (2002: 131) involved in such a relationship will lead to a conflicting tension in the way the nurse behaves: the autonomous professional nurse versus the smiling and closely monitored service provider. This may result in a situation where patients will always be unsatisfied with their care as their expectations are unrealistic due to the want-driven rather than need-driven culture being championed at present. This raises the question whether being a healthcare provider means that one occasionally will upset patients and their intimate social circle in order to deliver quality care. If so, what are the implications of this in a market-led customer-orientated healthcare context?

As a result of these paradigm shifts many staff face increased levels of role ambiguity. This in turn makes a significant contribution to plummeting employee motivation, rising levels of staff stress, burnout and turnover (Ackroyd 1994, 1996; Burnard, *et al.* 2000; McVicar 2003; Gelsema, *et al.* 2006; Hall, *et al.* 2006) all of which negatively impact on the patient's care and experience. It is then not surprising that, in a highly pressurised and scrutinised environment such as the NHS, staff stress levels are high. However, it is crucial that such levels are not increased through the adoption of attractive sounding yet poorly thought out initiatives that will further reduce staff's willingness and ability to engage with day-to-day work as well as commit to innovative initiatives and work practice changes. The question, therefore, is what the potential implications of these paradigm shifts on implementing and integrating changes within the NHS are and whether these will worsen in a Lean context (Conti, *et al.* 2006; Angelis, *et al.* 2007).

THE WANT-NEED DILEMMA

A stakeholder in an organisation is defined as 'any group or individual who can affect or is affected by the achievement of the organisation's objectives' (Pouloudi and Whitley 2000: 46). Within a primary care context these stakeholders are multiple and often geographically as well as socially diverse. As Figure 11.1 shows, at the core lies the patient who, according to the DoH (2001b 2007), should be in a position to specify, if not dictate, the received care. However, there is tension with regard to customer/patient wants and needs. National health provision tends to be a need-driven, resource-limited and socially accountable process delivered free at the point of delivery by autonomous professionals holding expert knowledge. The last point is emphasised by the DoH, noting that it is 'doctors and nurses who are in the best position to know what patients need' (DoH 1997: 11). The patient receives care specified by a tightly bounded care package formed in the main by the analysis and opinions of said professionals. Although the patient's views and needs are considered, this is done so from a custodial-care perspective rather than from a buyer-supplier one. Through the mechanism of consent (DoH 2001c) a patient

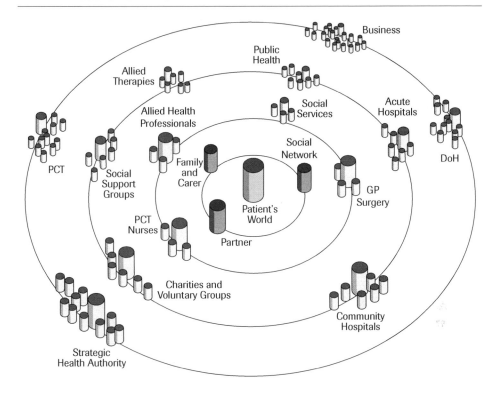

FIGURE 11.1 Patient sphere of immediacy

is able to refuse care, but they cannot dictate the care they receive. In other words, patients are not able to specify or demand what they want. This alone means they are not able to behave as a traditional customer.

Traditional customers are generally seen as autonomous, powerful and knowledgeable people, driven by aspirational wants and actual or perceived needs. They are willing and able to determine what they believe is valuable and assess, across a number of competing suppliers, who will be able to provide them with that value for a price they are happy to pay (Johnston and Clark 2005). Relationships between buyer and supplier are in the main clearly defined and understood, being 'characterised by interdependent, collaborative and long-term relationships' (Wright and Taylor 2005: 206). If a customer is unhappy with a service, refunds and exchanges can quickly occur, or the customer can simply choose to buy from a multitude of different suppliers in the future. However, NHS patients do not easily fit this characterisation. As with any public service with limited and politically distributed resources, the NHS is there to provide services to citizens that are seen to be in the public interest and, as such, it is accountable to the public as a whole not to individual customers. In the case of any public sector service, the interests of individual consumers must constantly be assessed in relation to the interests of the community. Not only is the relationship between the organisation and the community different from the commercial sector, the individuals receiving the service also highlights key differences.

First, patients do not pay for their NHS treatment at point of delivery. They make contributions to the Health Service over their working lives through taxation. Second, even with the market orientation that exists today, choice of service providers is still limited, so market freedom to choose only occurs to a lesser degree. However, these differences pale into insignificance when the nature and disposition of the patient is taken into consideration. Although many people have healthcare experience as a patient, few can be said to be knowledgeable of the stakeholders, operational processes, illnesses, clinical conditions and care options available. Patients are often frightened, unsure and vulnerable rather than powerful, confident and autonomous (Bolton 2002), and often lack the ability to understand their conditions and related care in depth. In addition, many will also find it difficult to understand their felt needs and express them clearly to key stakeholders (Bradshaw 1994) thereby reducing the accuracy of information exchange. This situation may also be compounded in a primary healthcare context by the elderly nature of many patients, geographical dispersal, social isolation and domestic/family-derived pressures.

HEALTHCARE DRIVEN LEAN

This study has involved a number of NHS staff from nurses to managers. The findings illustrate the problems facing them and, in turn, the implementation of Lean in a self-care context. Note, however, that a strategy that focuses on providing a positive experience to users has to be seen as positive in such a people-centred context as healthcare. Instead, it is a question of perspective. It is not the philosophy that is the issue, but how it is being interpreted at a strategic level and implemented at the care frontline. Fundamentally, we argue two key points. First, patients, while having many similar characteristics, are not and should not be viewed as traditional customers. Second, care provision must always be need-driven first and want-driven second.

It is essential that personal non-care-related wants are not allowed to attain a form of expected dominance in the minds of the public where they supersede care-related needs in terms of resource allocation or context. If patient wants are clearly care related then they deserve equal weighting in the minds of policy makers, managers and care providers. This is not to say that non-care-related patient wants should be ignored. Comfortable seating in a waiting room and decent cafeteria food, for example, are all valid issues and should not be ignored just because they are not seen as directly care related. However, they cannot be allowed to divert the limited resources available from direct care provision. Of course there will be grey areas within this concept. A community nurse spending time having a cup of tea with a patient or a consultant communicating in a friendly and open manner may not be seen as directly care related, but no one would argue their potential value in the care experience. The answer lies in collaborative balance. While the patient lies at the heart of this process, it is the healthcare professionals themselves who are in the strongest position to understand the care journey a patient takes and determine the core care needs they have at any point along that path.

This study highlights the point that the question of value within an NHS context is far more multi-dimensional than in a commercial one. This is due to a number of factors. These include the individual nature, wants and needs of patients and their immediate circle, the complex nature of medical and care processes and associated services, society's expectations of the NHS, and the changing political agendas and related conflicting tensions, and indeed even the philosophical and cultural foundations of the NHS itself. The result is a situation where the nature and perception of value is either constantly changing between context to context and stakeholder to stakeholder or is defined in such broad terms as to be meaningless or inapplicable for Lean design. For example, the study results revealed that patients wanted a quality of service that conformed to an expected yet undefined, and by definition multi-dimensional, level of performance. As per Gowen, *et al.* (2006), this was followed by speed in the form of timely and easy access to healthcare services provided geographically and in terms of availability as well as fast throughput time. Interestingly, dependability of service in terms of acquiring accurate information and limited care stoppage was seen as less important, as was quality in terms of fit-for-purpose. Note, however, that it is not clear if this was because patients assumed care was fit-for-purpose by default or they simply could not or did not think to measure the fit. Flexibility was only stated in terms of enhancing service quality and, perhaps not surprisingly, given the context of a nationalised healthcare system, cost had limited impact on patient preferences.

This contrasts with how many senior executives interpret patient needs and wants. As one may expect, there was again an emphasis on quality of service followed by the effectiveness of care in terms of low cost, timely and appropriate information provision as well as external speed in terms of the elapsed time between demanding a service and receiving it in a satisfactory condition. However, flexibility in service delivery time was viewed as less vital, as was service dependability and quality in terms of fit-for-purpose. The latter might be interpreted as an example of the low value given to patient experience throughout the care process, somewhat contrasting the findings of Fillingham (2007), Weisbart (2002) and Whitcomb and Shafa (2001). Naturally, the availability and use of an integrated IS system must take this into account, for instance with less focus on data tracking for enhanced flexibility (Martinez and Perez 2005). Immediacy to the patient of the carer, as shown in Figure 11.1, or position in the care journey, did not yield significant differences in responses. Interestingly, managers believed the patients saw involvement, in terms of improvement suggestions, as a low priority for both themselves as well as their carers. Patients were not perceived to desire involvement in the care provision and similarly the managers did not view such activity desirable for the patients, though it is not clear why. However, managers felt that, in terms of care quality, patient participation and involvement was highly desirable, not for operational learning or innovation reasons, but rather for the benefits obtained through communication and greater opportunity for patient reassurance.

Such findings highlight two key points. First, it can be seen that the above patient-communicated wants are essentially very broad, unspecified and general in nature. This in part could be due to the lack of experience or any reference points patients have in forming judgements or an inability to articulate their wants and needs (Bradshaw 1994). Either way, it illustrates the potential problems associated with limited patient-led informed communication. Second, the differences in perceptions among senior managers of patient wants do illustrate the danger inherent in making judgements that are not based on an agreed set of values or matrices, or are made from a point of distance. In all instances the problem can become one of abstraction and oversimplification that leads to the formation of performance measurements and linked process that do not deliver improved care or patient experiences. In addition, if one is to link perceived patient wants to operational performance dimensions, significant differences are highlighted with the hierarchical Sandcone model associated with Lean operations. The model illustrates that, correctly implemented, Lean within a commercial context leads to eventual cost reduction based on an internal and external cumulative foundation of improvement in other performance objectives. The Lean system transfers improvements in product and service quality, in turn, to improvements in reliability, speed and flexibility, which leads to cost reductions (Ferdows and de Meyer 1990). However, in the care setting this flow of performance benefits is apparently not well understood, or at least not successfully pursued, something which is illustrated by the common view of Lean implementation as a cost-cutting exercise and technique.

How then can meaningful value be specified in an NHS context? Lean techniques such as Value Stream Mapping seek to identify value-creating process and eliminate wasteful activities through the active participation of all appropriate stakeholders. Traditionally, a Lean practitioner would involve staff examining the various steps along the patient journey, getting them to map out how the process currently operates and identify value-creating actions and those that are wasteful. Patient involvement in this process would incorporate the patient perspective throughout the various process steps (Westwood, *et al.* 2007). The employment of connected information systems throughout the value or care chain may well enable necessary data capture. Importantly, it may also help facilitate the knowledge sharing needed for patient and staff involvement that drives Lean continuous improvement initiatives. One commonly used method for mapping value streams has been the Rother and Shook (1998) methodology, which shows customers, suppliers, control functions and key phases of the process, together with key quantitative pieces of information relating to operating process performance. However, one key problem in the NHS context is that the value equation involves multiple stakeholders and yet there is no single metric upon which to measure customer value. Some may argue that patient wants combined with health professionals' definitions of value are all that are needed, but such a simplification is fraught with conceptual and practical problems.

CONCLUSION

Lean principles require that value is specified and that the customer specifies this value. Contrary to the process recommendations, there is no agreement as to who the customer of the NHS environment is. In self-care, patients have a relatively active role which is not necessarily reflected in the value allocated to their preferences by the other stakeholders. The care providers themselves are often better positioned to state what care ought to be given to a particular patient rather than the patient him/ herself. Other care providers may see their primary care trust as the customer or even the relatives of the patient who are essential and unpredictable elements of the care programme. Appleby, *et al.* (2003) argue that promoting patient focus within the NHS may sit uneasily in an institution that traditionally has relied on funding, structure and objectives determined by the government.

Although patients are unable to behave as a traditional customer, which conflicts with both patient-centred care and the value-focused principle of Lean, the reasons are understandable. Hence, contrary to the stated role of patients in self-care, such individuals may not be in the best position to determine their health needs and dictate their care in an authoritative, knowledge-based and clear manner, and while they may be able to articulate 'wants' as a typical customer might, those wants may not have any relevance to their clinical care needs. As such, the question needs to be asked as to whether viewing a patient as a customer who can specify value that will have meaning in a clinical care context is viable. In a Lean and customer-focused perspective the question becomes even more urgent.

REFERENCES

Ackroyd S. Nurses, management and morale: a diagnosis of decline in the NHS hospital service. In: Mackay L, Webb C, editors. *Inter-professional Relations in Health Care*. London: Edward Arnold; 1994. pp. 222–52.

Ackroyd S. Traditional and new management in the NHS hospital service and their effects on nursing. In: Soothill K, Henry C, Kendrick K, editors. *Themes and Perspectives in Nursing*. London: Chapman and Hall; 1996.

Angelis J, Conti R, Cooper C, *et al. Building a High Commitment Lean Culture: the role of shop floor work practices*. Working Paper. Cambridge: University of Cambridge; 2007.

Antony J, Downey-Ennis K, Antony F, *et al.* Can six sigma be the 'cure' for our 'ailing' NHS? *Leadersh Health Care*. 2007; 20(4): 242–53.

Appleby J, Harrison A, Devlin N. *What is the Real Cost of More Patient Choice?* London: King's Fund Publications; 2003.

Beckett J. The government should run like a business. *Am Rev Public Admin*. 2000; 30(2): 185–204.

Bhasin S, Burcher P. Lean viewed as a philosophy. *J Manuf Technol Manage*. 2006; 17(1): 56–72.

Bloomfield B. Power, machines and social relations: delegating to information technology in the National Health Service. *Organization*. 1995; 2(3–4): 489–518.

Bolton S. Consumer as king in the NHS. *Int J Public Sector Manage*. 2002; 15(2): 129–39.

Bradshaw J. The conceptualisation and measurement of need: a social policy perspective. In: Popay J, Williams G, editors. *Researching the People's Health*. London: Routledge; 1994. pp. 45–57.

Burnard P, Edwards D, Fothergill A, *et al.* Community mental health nurses in Wales:

self-reported stressors and coping strategies. *J Psychiatric Mental Health Nurs.* 2000; 7: 523–8.

Bushell S. Discovering lean thinking at progressive healthcare. *J Qual Particip.* 2002; 25(2): 20–5.

Christopher M. The agile supply chain: competing in volatile markets. *Ind Market Manage.* 2000; 29(1): 37–44.

Christopher M, Towill D. Supply chain migration from lean and functional to agile and customised. *Supply Chain Manage Int J.* 2000; 5(4): 206–13.

Conti R, Angelis J, Cooper C, et al. The effects of lean production on worker job stress. *Int J Operations Prod Manage.* 2006; 26: 1013–38.

Cottam H, Leadbeater C. *Red Paper 01 Health: co-creating services.* London: Design Council; 2004.

Department of Health. *The New NHS: modern, dependable.* London: HMSO; 1997.

Department of Health. *The New NHS: a National Framework for Assessing Performance.* London: Department of Health; 1998a.

Department of Health. *Partnership in Action, 38.* Report no. 13684. London: Department of Health; 1998b.

Department of Health. *NHS Performance Ratings, 23.* Report no. 25290. London: Department of Health; 2001a.

Department of Health. *Shifting the Balance of Power, 47.* Report no. 24613. London: Department of Health; 2001b.

Department of Health. *Good Practice in Consent Implementation Guide: consent to examination or treatment.* London: HMSO; 2001c.

Department of Health. *Delivering the NHS Plan.* London: HMSO; 2002.

Department of Health. *Self Care Support Summary of Work in Progress: the evidence pack.* London: Department of Health; 2007.

Drake P, Davies B. Home care outsourcing strategy. *J Health Organ Manag.* 2006; 20(3):175–93.

Drummond-Hay R, Bamford D. An empirical investigation into service strategy within the UK health system. *Conference Proceedings of POMS 18th Annual Conference,* Dallas, TX; 2007 May 4–7.

Ferdows K, de Meyer A. Lasting improvements in manufacturing. *J Operations Manage.* 1990; 9(2): 168–84.

Ferlie E, Fitzgerald L. The sustainability of the new public management in the UK. In: McKaughlin K, Osborne S, Ferlie E, editors. *New Public Management: current trends and future prospects.* London: Routledge; 2002.

Fillingham D. Can lean save lives? *Leadership Health Serv.* 2007; 20(4): 231–41.

Fullerton R, McWatters C, Fawson C. An examination of the relationship between JIT and financial performance. *J Operations Manage.* 2003; 21: 383–404.

Gelsema T, Van der Doeff M, Maes S, et al. A longitudinal study of job stress in the nursing profession: causes and consequences. *J Nurs Manage.* 2006; 14: 289–99.

Gowen C, McFadden K, Hoobler J, et al. Exploring the efficacy of healthcare quality practices, employee commitment, and employee control. *J Operations Manage.* 2006; 24: 754–78.

Hall A, Todd Royle M, Brymer R, et al. Relationships between felt accountability as a stressor and strain reactions: the neutralizing role of autonomy across two studies. *J Occupat Health Psychol.* 2006; 11(1): 87–99.

Jarrett G. An analysis of international health care logistics. *Leadership Health Serv.* 2006; 19(1): i–x.

Johnston R, Clark G. *Service Operations Management.* London: Prentice Hall; 2005.

Jones D. The lean service opportunity. *Lean Service Summit.* Amsterdam; 2004.

Kendall L, Lissauer R. *The Future Health Worker.* London: IPPR; 2003.

Lowe J, Delbridge R, Oliver N. High performance manufacturing: evidence from the automotive components industry. *Org Stud.* 1997; 18: 783–98.

Lucey J, Bateman N, Hines P. Achieving pace and sustainability in a major lean transition. *Inst Manage Serv.* 2004; 48(9): 8.

MacStravic S. Cultivating patient relationships. *Marketing Health Serv.* 2003; Spring: 24–9.

McBride A, Hyde P, Young R, *et al.* How the 'customer' influences the skills of the front-line worker. *Hum Res Manage J.* 2005; 15(2): 35–49.

McDermott C, Stock G. Hospital operations and length of stay performance. *Int J Operations Prod Manage.* 2007; 27(9): 1020–42.

McGuire L. *Transferring Marketing to Professional Public Services: an Australian perspective.* London: Local Governance, Sage Publishing.

McVicar A. Workplace stress in nursing. *J Adv Nurs.* 2003; 44(6): 633–42.

Martinez A, Perez M. Supply chain flexibility and firm performance. *Int J Operations Prod Manage.* 2005; 25(7): 681–700.

Muller M, Seuring S. Reducing information technology-based transaction costs in supply chains. *Ind Manage Data Syst.* 2007; 107: 484–500.

Ogden J. *Health Psychology.* Maidenhead: Open University; 2005.

O'Malley J. Caring before the care. *Marketing Health Serv.* 2004; Summer: 12–13.

Papadopoulos T. *Researching Stakeholder Dynamics towards the Implementation and Sustainability of Lean Process Innovation in Public Healthcare.* Working Paper. Warwick Business School; 2007.

Perucca R. Consumers with options. *Nurs Manage.* 2001; 32: 20–4.

Pouloudi A, Whitley E. Representing human and non-human stakeholders: on speaking with authority. In: Baskerville R, Stage J, DeGross J, editors. *Organizational and Social Perspectives on Information Technology.* Boston, MA: Kluwer Academic; 2000. pp. 339–54.

Power D, Sohal A, Rahman S. Critical success factors in agile supply chain management. *Int J Physical Distrib Logistics Manage.* 2001; 31(4): 247–65.

Rai A, Patnayakuni R, Seth N. Firm performance impacts of digitally enabled supply chain integration capabilities. *MIS Quarterly.* 2006; 30(2): 225–46.

Read S, Lloyd Jones M, Collins K. *Exploring New Roles in Practice.* Sheffield: SCHARR, University of Sheffield; 2002.

Ross J. Creating a strategic IT architecture competency. *MIS Quarterly Exec.* 2003; 2(1): 31–43.

Rother M, Shook J. *Learning to See: value stream mapping to add value and reduce Muda.* Brookline, MA: The Lean Enterprise Institute; 1998.

Sakakibara S, Flynn B, Schroeder R, *et al.* The impact of just-in-time manufacturing and its infrastructure on manufacturing performance. *Manage Sci.* 1997; 43: 1246–57.

Shah R, Ward P. Lean manufacturing: context, practice bundles, and performance. *J Operations Manage.* 2003; 21(2): 129–50.

Shah R, Ward P. Defining and developing measures of lean production. *J Operations Manage.* 2007; 25: 785–805.

Smeds R. Managing change towards lean enterprises. *Int J Operations Prod Manage.* 1994; 14(3): 66–82.

Snell S, Dean J. Integrated manufacturing and human resource management: a human capital perspective. *Acad Manage J.* 1993; 35: 467–504.

Spear S. Fixing health from the inside, today. *Har Bus Rev.* 2005; 83(9): 78–91.

Stavins C. Developing employee participation in the patient–satisfaction process. *J Health Manage.* 2004; Mar/Apr: 135–9.

Taninecz G. *Best Healthcare Getting Better with Lean: Mayo Clinic Division of Cardiovascular Disease improving patient-flow processes.* Brookline, MA: Lean Enterprise Institute; 2007.

Tippins M, Sohi R. IT competency and firm performance. *Strategic Manage J.* 2003; 24: 745–61.

van Hoek R, Harrison A, Christopher M. Measuring agile capabilities in the supply chain. *Int J Operations Prod Manage.* 2001; 21(1–2): 126–47.

Walsh K. Citizens and consumers: marketing and public sector management. *Public Money Manage.* 1991; 11(2): 9–16.

Weisbart E. Patients or customers? *Click.* 2002; Dec: 13–15.

Westwood N, James-Moore M, Cooke M. *Going Lean in NHS.* Warwick: NHS Institute for Innovation and Improvement; 2007.

Whitcomb J, Shafa M. Treating patients like customers: just-in-time inventory control for patient-centered care. *Physician Exec.* 2001; 27(5): 16–21.

White A, Daniel E, Mohdzain M. The role of information technologies and systems in enabling supply chain agility. *Int J Inf Manage.* 2005; 25: 396–410.

Womack J, Byrne A, Fiume O, *et al.* Going lean in health care. In: Miller D, editor. *Innovation Series.* Cambridge: Institute for Healthcare Improvement; 2005.

Womack J, Jones D. *Lean Thinking: banish waste and create wealth in your corporation.* New York: Simon and Schuster; 2003.

Wright G, Taylor A. Strategic partnerships and relationship marketing in healthcare. *Public Manage Rev.* 2005; 7(2): 203–24.

Yusuf Y, Gunasekaran A, Adeleye E, *et al.* Agile supply chain capabilities. *Eur J Operational Res.* 2004; 159: 379–92.

Index

Entries in **bold** denote text in figures or tables.

Accenture 20, 24, 190
action, purposive 69, 75
Actor Network Theory (ANT) 80–1
Additional Supply Capability and Capacity Services (ASCC) 101
ageing population 87–8, 255
appointment booking, electronic 68, 76, 87, 92, 186, 243
architectures
    bespoke 140
    common 51, 53, 138–40, 144, 158, 160, 164, 171, 174–5
    legacy 18, 21, 26, 43–4, 52, 58, 103–4, 136, 138, 140
    proprietary 46
    service-oriented 18, 123
automation 42, 49, 56, 88, 168, 216, 218, 221
autonomy 52–3, 58, 126, 138, 174

behaviour change 28–9
benefits realisation **5**, **15–16**
Bentham, Jeremy 224n
Berners-Lee, Tim 123
Best of Breed model 99, 103, 189
best practice 21, 28, 44–5, 51, 140–1, 143, 145, 173, 195
billing systems 43
BPR, *see* business processes, re-engineering
British Computer Society (BCS) 13, 73, 199
British Medical Association (BMA) 20, 76
brokering engines 139
burnout 73, 258
Burns, Frank 98–9, 103

business processes
    changes in 12–13
    of Choose and Book 28
    re-engineering (BPR) 6, 39–40, 50, 55–6, 141
business strategy 40, 43
buy-in 23, 25, 229, 231, 233

Caché 80
California 78, 209, 211, 214, 229
care
    paradigms of 168
    seamless 44, 46–7, 57, 113, 142, 144
Carruthers, Sir Ian 23
Cayton, Harry 68
CDM (chronic disease management) 220, 227
centralisation 22, 138, 150
change management 89, 100, 202
Choose and Book 14, 20, 24–5, 27–8, 97, 124, 188–9, 194–5, **243**, **245**
chronic illness 87–8
CIS (Clinical Information System) 212–37
Clayton, Harry 11–12
Climbie, Victoria 99
clinical decisions 4, 9–10, 46, 116, 120, 126, 129, 140, 223
Clinical Five 106
clinical integration 51, 54, 140
clinical pathways 43, 49–50
clinical systems 42–4, 47, 52, 58, 99, 103–4, 107, 137–8, 145
cognitive theory 80
Colorado 212, 214, 220, 228, 231

commercial off-the-shelf systems (COTS)
43, 57, 170
Common Assessment Framework 123
communication
barriers 217
between professionals 123
effective 55
electronic 121
informed 262
inter-organisational 56
social 46, 176
standardisation of 46
in value chains 256
communities
of practice (COPs) 55, 79, 143, 175
virtual 88
Comprehensive Health Enhancement
Support System (CHESS) 125
computer literacy 19, 90, 228
computerised physician order entry (CPOE)
90
confidentiality 11, 90, 107, 136, 220n
Connecting for Health (CfH)
and centralisation 77
change in leadership 66
and change management 89
and confidentiality 90
and e-health 87
Evaluation Programme 67
expenditure of 74–5
future of 73
and ICT tenders 27
Local Implementation agenda 75
and NPfIT 20, 23, 98, 101, 190, 198,
243
obstacles to 89, 244
procurement of ICT 20–1
consent 9, 19, 75–6, 89–90, 99, 187, 244, 258
consumerism 88, 241
contingency theory 39
continuous quality improvement (CQI) 51
contracts, psychological 73
coordination theory 39
corruption 77
culture
change in 28–9, 40, 124
classification of 55
ethnographic approach to 55
of Hawaii 228, 231–2
and integrity 228
management of 58, 170
of medical specialties 230
of NHS 257
organisational 7, 55
of professional groups 53
synergy 37, 40, 55

data
collection of 123, 138
formats 138
losses 11
manipulation 248
multimedia 137
security, *see* security, of information
Data Protection Act 19, 128
Data Spine 96–7, 99, 107, 187, **245**
decentralisation 22–3
delayering 39
deregulation 77
detailed care record (DCR) 9, 17–19,
75
diabetes 85–6, 255
diagnostics systems 46
DICOM 139, 172
discharge letters, electronic 57
Dossia 119
dual structure 47, 49

e-health 5, 85–93, 190, 195–8, 201
e-mail 116, 124–5, 185, 213
E-Novation LifeLine 249–50
EAI (enterprise application integration) 40,
51, 61, 140–1, 152–3, 180
EHRs (electronic health records) 3, 5, 9, 12,
81, 92, 135–44, 174, 176–7, 197, 251–2
definition of 9
access to 120
adoption of 36, 58, 136–7, 141, 144,
197
assimilation of 143
benefits of 27, 92, 126–7
categories of **115**
in CIS system 220–1
and consumer-driven approach 3
data in 118
development of 17
future of 85–6
implementation of 189–92, 198
in integrated care 137
integration of 135–45, **164–5**, 173–7,
175
and medical errors 10
national 90, 97, 106
objectives of 193
and patient-centred care 113–14,
119–22, 125–6
professional resistance to 136
role and purpose of 67
in United States 78
eiPHR (electronic integrated personal health
records) 116, 118
electronic images 186, 188
Electronic Prescription Service, *see* EPS

electronic prescription system, in
  Netherlands 250
electronic records
    designing 11
    literature on 10
EMD (electronic medication dossier) 250–1
emergence 42, 55, 198, 250
emotion 80, 114, 125
emotional labour 258
EMR (electronic medical records)
    confusion about term 9
    early 42
    effectiveness of 207–8
    and ethos of healthcare 238
    implementation of 207, 212–13, 219
    in Netherlands 250–2
    proprietary 228
    purpose of 223
Engineering and Physical Sciences Research
  Council 67
enterprise data warehousing (EDWs) 138,
  144
enterprise resource planning (ERP) 51, 138,
  152, 167
enterprise systems 41, 46, 51–3, 58, 138,
  174
enterprise wide arrangements (EWA) 102
EPD (electronic patient dossier) 250
ePHR (electronic patient-held records)
  115–19, **117**, 121, 124–9
EpicCare 212, 214, 225, 228, 234
EPR (electronic patient records), *see*
  personal health records (PHRs)
EPS (Electronic Prescription Service) 17, 20,
  24, 27, 96–7, **243**, **245**
ERDIP (electronic record development and
  implementation programme) 242
ERP (enterprise resource planning) 51, 59,
  138, 167
eSAP (electronic single assessment process)
  123
ETP (Electronic Transfer of Prescriptions)
  96–7
European Convention on Human Rights 19
evaluation
    definitions of 13
    socio-technical approach to 5
evolution, user-led 57

'five forces framework' 50
flexibility 119, 123, 128, 136, 188, 196,
  199–200, 257, 261–2
Foucault, Michel 224n
foundation trusts 21, 71, 190, 242
fragmentation 7, 42–3, 45–7, 51–2, 70–1,
  136, 139, 174

France 68, 70
Fujitsu 20, 24, 26, 102, 190

Garfield, Sidney 208–9, 211–12
Google Health 119, 121, 129
governance, systems of 72, 90
GP Summary Record 99
GP2GP **243**, **245**
GPs (general practitioners)
    and Choose and Book 26–7, 97
    knowledge of IT 11
    in Netherlands 249–50
    resistance to CfH 89
    and SCRs 187–8
Granger, Richard 66
Greenwich Hospital 201

Hancock, Lambreth 211
Hardey, Michael 88
Hawaii 211–15, 218, 220, 224–5, 227–9,
  231, 233, 236, 238–9
health informatics 4–6, 9, 13, 36, 45, 86, 98
Health Informatics Review 104–6
health insurance 207–10, 212, 244, 246–8,
  251–2
health professionals
    attitudes to technological change
      234–5, 238
    attitudes towards patients 128
    management practices of 7
    using EHRs 142
health records 18, 78, 80, 135–6
    convergence in systems 118
    distinctions between types of 119
    evolution of 135–6
    fragmentation of 70
    ownership of 68–70, 78
    paper-based 135, 137, 183, 195
    paradigms of 114–15
healthcare
    affordability of 71
    coordination of 121
    customer orientation in 257
    evidence-based 92
    financing in Netherlands 246–7
    fragmentation of provision 71–2
    'fuzziness' in 46
    in Hawaii 229
    information systems in 44–5, 48, 157,
      169
    institutions in 78–9
    and Lean principles 256
    modernisation of 65
    nature of organisations 4, 49, 58
    nature of work 57
    pathways of 194–5, 200–1

healthcare (*continued*)
    performance measurement 241, 251
    practices 3, 44, 46, 49, 184–5, 188, 195,
        198, 202
    public and private providers 81
    public attitude to 255
    regulation of 89, 91–2
    role of innovation and technology in 6
    strategic consolidation in 50
    and surveillance 224
    in US, *see* United States
    wants and needs 258–63
healthcare professionals
    access to records 120
    and change 4, 9, 18
    and Choose and Book 28
    and EHRs 144
    and PHRs 116
    power of 86
    role ambiguity 258
    sharing information 99
healthcare professions, allied 101
HealthSpace 17, 76, 124, **243**
HealthVault 119, 121, 129
HIPAA (Health Insurance Portability and
    Accountability Act) 220
HISS (hospital information support
    systems) 18, 43, 51–3, 108, 144
HL7 121, 139, 172
hospitals
    absorptive capacity of 55
    PFI 74
    teaching 7, 71

IBM 215, 221, 227, 235–7
ICT (information and communications
    technologies)
    accelerated obsolescence of 18
    access to facilities 91
    adoption and implementation of 4–5,
        7, 11, 22, 24, 26, 28, 195–6, 207,
        242
    benefits and risks of 13, 38
    as change agent 6–7, **8–9**, 252
    disciplines which study 4
    in Dutch healthcare 246, 248–9, 252
    and e-health 87
    evaluation of 8, 13–14, 66–7, 70
    impact of 184, 224
    institutionalisation of 71, 219
    literature on 5–7, 9
    managerial knowledge 55
    and market-driven healthcare 3
    and performance management 6–7
    and politicians 27
    potential of 89

    procurement of 28
    strategies for 25
    suppliers 9, 25, 28, 251
    and systems integration **12**
    in UK healthcare **243–4**, 248, 252
identities 79
iEHRs (integrated electronic health records)
    36, 117–18
IMaGE project 70
individualism 217, 226, 230
Indivo 119, 129
information
    accessibility of 88
    exchange of 50, 250, 260
    health 88, 125
    management 17–18, 70
    quality of 91, 125
    security of 11, **15**, 21–2, 68, 71, 89–90,
        99, 107
    shared 99, 107, 217, 249
    tacit 49
Information Commissioner's Office 20
Information for Health (IfH) 17, 19, 43, 98,
    104–6
information systems
    academic field of 4, 9, 13
    characterisation of 36
    clinical, *see* clinical systems
    and communication 37
    consolidation 54
    dependability of 56
    fragmentation of 42–3, 45–7, 51–2,
        139–40
    investment in 46
    literature on **146–56**, 177
    maturity models 172
    standardisation of 51
infrastructure, fragmentation of 168
innovation
    and CIS system 222
    in healthcare 6
    in ICT 50, 54, 89
    and NPfIT 65
    process of 31, 54, 57, 79
    and social entrepreneurship 77
instantiation 72, 81
Institutes of Medicine and Health
    Improvement 220, 222
institutional entrepreneurship 76–7
institutional logics 53, 68, 70–2, 75–6, 78,
    81
institutional persistence 78–9
institutional theory 67, 72, 74–5, 77
institutions
    and action 69
    change in 77, 103

and NPfIT 69
reproduction of 69, 72–3
integration **5**
    definition of 35–7, 40–1, 166
    and agility 256
    of CIS system 226
    difficulties in 53
    dimensions of 38, 166–7, **166**
    drivers for 37, 45
    factors influencing **169**
    of health records 118
    horizontal 172
    humanistic aspects of 142
    implications of 46
    in Kaiser Permanente 228, 237–8
    link between strategy and
        implementation 166
    literature on 4, 36, 41, 47, 58, 135,
        158–63, 167, 170, 177
    methods 37, 43, 56
    models of 46, 55, 57, 168
    need for 41–2, 45
    organisational 39, 57, 142, 173
    pathways to 170–3, **171**
    seamless 56, 123
    social 56, 172
    strategic 137, 167
    strategies for 38, 40, 44, 49, 57–8, 141,
        144, 168, 170, 173, 177
    technical 52, 58, 167
    of workflow 53
inter-organisational processes 37–8, 45,
    57
interactions, interpersonal 46, 49
interdependence 54
interfacing 37, 39, 43, 46, 52
interoperability 38, 52, 129, 137, 139
ISVs (independent software vendors) 24
IT, see ICT
'IT-readiness' 24
Italy 79–80

Kaiser, Henry J 208–12
Kaiser Permanente 207–13, 215, 220, 222,
    224–9, 231–5, 237
key performance indicators (KPIs) 13
knowledge, orphan 73
knowledge management 55, 88
knowledge workers 143

leadership
    charismatic 66
    effective 40, 66
    styles 228, 232–4
    transformational 66
Lean philosophy 256–8, 260–3

learning
    as embodied capability 56
    'on the job' 25
legacy systems, see architectures, legacy
local implementation strategies (LISs) 105
Local Informatics Plans (LIPs) 106
long-term conditions 120–1, 127–9, 255
Lorenzo 189
LSPs (local service providers) 20, 22, 24,
    95–6, 99–102, 104, 106–7, 189–90

management
    integrated 49
    strategies 46
markets
    as drivers of healthcare 3
    internal 74
Medicaid 208
medical informatics, see health informatics
medical information 7, 47, 78–9, 144, 211
medical records, see health records
medical specialisations 45, 49
Medicare 208, 220
mental health **191**
Microsoft 87, 119
modernisation 53, 65–6, 108, 224
modernity 70
monopolies 25, 28, 75
motivation 66, 74–5, **74**, 77, 80, 124, 258
MRI scanning 71, 137

N3 (New NHS Network) 24, 97, **245**, 250
NASPs (national application service
    providers) 24, 95
National Clinical Leads 21
national infrastructure services providers
    (NISPs) 95
National Institute for Health and Clinical
    Excellence (NICE) 251
NCRS (National Care Record System)
    10–11, 14, 17–22, 24–5, 27–8, 96–7, 104
needs assessment 14
Netherlands 4, 36, 241–2, 244, 246–52
new institutionalists 69
New Public Management 6
NHS (National Health Service)
    administration costs in 17–18
    benefits from NPfIT 102–3
    Care Records Service 19, 32, 68, **243**
    clusters in 96, 100, 107, **186**
    Confidentiality Campaign 11
    correspondence policy 124
    customer orientation in 257–60, 263
    Direct 76
    diversity in 198
    and flexibility 196

NHS (*continued*)
    fragmentation of 7
    future of 77
    HISS in 53
    ICT in 18, 22, 26–7, 29, 42, 98
    and institutions 69, 243
    leadership of 66
    Lean philosophy in 257
    modernisation of 3, 25, 73
    Number 11, **244**
    online resources 125–6
    organisational policies in 194
    overview of 242
    philosophy of 257
    policy purpose of 78
    procurement models 100–1
    Service Delivery and Organisation
      Programme 67, 86
    'spine' of 11
    staff stress levels 258
    Strategic Tracing Service 97
    tracking costs in 248–9
    trusts **191**
    value in 261–2
NHS CFHEP, *see* Connecting for Health
  (CfH), Evaluation Programme
NHSmail 185, **245**
NLOP (National Local Ownership
  Programme) 23, 26, 28, 107
NPfIT (National Programme for IT)
    activities of 71, 76
    aims of 14, 17, 21, 65, 73, 183, 187,
      196, 243
    and centralisation 22–3, 99–100
    clinical involvement in 23
    criticisms of 95, 102, 107
    evaluation of 26, 66–70, 197–8
    expenditure of 24
    future of 25–7, 29, 107–9, 198–9
    implementation of 69, 202
    Local Ownership Programme 73
    milestones for **245**
    mythology of 74
    objective of 106
    obstacles to 20–2, 71–2, 80
    and patient interests 81
    progress of 98, 184–5, **186**
    resistance to 29, 238
    and socio-technical systems 200

Office for Strategic Coordination of Health
  Research 87
Office of the National Co-ordinator for
  Health Information Technology 36
online patient record, *see* EHRs (electronic
  health records), in CIS system

Oracle 80
Oregon 209, 211
organisations
    analysis of 39
    change in 141, 195
    citizenship behaviour 73
    culture of 6, 45, 55, 89, 213, 228–9
    knowledge in 56, 73, 176
    life cycles of 73
    networks in 49
    processes of 37, 41, 136, 167, 189
    resistance in 143
    rules of 73
    structures of 7, 39, 54, 72, 79, 143, 176
outsourcing 24, 70

Pacific Medical Associates (PMA) 211
PACS system 100
Panopticon 224n
PAS (patient administration systems) 11, 18,
  53, 92, 103–4, 106–8, 193, 242
paternalism 128
patient-centred healthcare 47, 51, 58, 72,
  114, 119–20, **127**, 129, 144, 171, 175, 177
Patient Recorded Outcome Measurements
  104–5
patients
    access to health records 19–20, 120–1
    and choice **5**, 28
    cognitive processes of 80
    as customers 257
    data on 11, 16, 20, 28, 75, 79, 89, 96,
      99, 144, 171, 175, 191, 195, 248–9
    empowerment of 86, 88–9, 126
    management plans 122, 128
    rights over health records 75–6, 78
    safety of 4, **5**, 27–8, 80, 88, 241, 252
    sphere of immediacy **259**
    tailored care pathways for 122
Pattison, Sir John 100
PCR (Population Care Registry) 227
performance
    management 6, 92
    measurement 6, 13, **15–16**, 251, 262
    targets 10
personal health records (PHRs)
    definition of 9
    access to 193–4
    business case for 126–7
    data in 118, 121–2, 129, 192–3
    description of 116
    in GP surgeries 26
    ideal 118
    introduction of 20, 67, 75–6, 185
    in Italy 79–80
    motivation and 127–8

paradigm of 115
previous plans for 106
purchasing products 103
research on 70
responses to 80
role and purpose of 81
sharing 124
types of 77
Picture Archiving and Communications
System (PAC) 17, 27, 188, 244, **245**
planning, approaches to 40
Poor Old Henry 201
power
distribution of 72
moving between actants 77
pragmatism 70, 79, 104
Prentis, Dave 70
Prescribing Pricing Authority (PPA) 97
prescriptions
data flows and 97
electronic 68, 97, 122, 137, 243
transmission of 76
private sector
performance management tools 7
practices of 3
probity **74**, 75, 77
productivity 54, 142, 216, 247, 256
professional groups 5, 53, 68, 72, 79, 91,
168, 243
professional guidelines 114
programme theory 14
psychiatry 46
public sector ethos 242

QinetiQ 69–70
Quality Management and Analysis Service
(QMAS) 98
Queen's Hospital, Burton 104

radiology 18, 43, 104, 188
rationality, post-hoc 72
Regional Service Card (Italy) 80
reminders 80, 85, 116, 124, 227
Research Capability Programme **244**
resource endowments 56
risk assessment **15–16**

Sandcone model 262
scheduling 106, 119, 124
Scotland 72, 78
secondary care 11
security, of information 4, 11, 20, 22, 28,
128, 193
self-assessment 122–3
self-care 255–6, 263
self-help groups 126

Separation of Concerns 140
service oriented integration (SOI) 142
shared knowledge structures 55
SHAs 22–3, 105, 107
silos 4, 37, 58
smoking 91
SOA (service orientated architecture) **5**, 99,
101–2
Social Care Integration Project (SCIP)
244
social entrepreneurship 77
socio-technical systems 183–5, 190, 194,
196–7, 199–203
software
development of 22, 108
as service 4
SROs (Senior Responsible Officers) 23
stakeholders
definition of 258
engagement of 29, 66
standardisation
American attitude to 225–6
of care 114
and CIS system 216
of information systems 51, 172
process 53
technical 22, 56–7, 142
strategic fit 51, 58, 172, 174
strategic health authorities 21–2, 73, 96,
242
structural archetypes 55
structuration theory 72
summary care record (SCR)
adoption of 99, 187, 198
consent for sharing 19, 75–6
creation of 75
models of 68
and national patient database 248
in NCRS 10, 17
Summary Care Records Taskforce 67–8
SUS (Secondary Users Service) 98
Synapses 172
systems integration
capabilities for 52–3
description of 51–2
and EHRs 138–9
in healthcare 166, 172
literature on 9
methods 54, 144
as technical approach 53–4
systems maturity models 51, 55

Tahoe Agreement 210, 212
Tavistock Institute of Human Relations
184
technological determinism 232

technology
    impact of new 12, 93, 184
    implications of 54
    innovations in 54, 128, 170
    metastructuring of 143
    role of 6
Technology Acceptance Model (TAM) 144
technology use mediation (TUM) 143,
    176
telemedicine 5, 97, 196, 252
temporality, *see* timeliness
timeliness 15, 40
top-down approach 22, 66
total quality management (TQM) 6, 9, 51
'transformational change' 25, 105, 198–9
*Transformational Government Enabled by
    Technology* 65
transitional systems 200, 202

UK (United Kingdom), devolution in 72,
    78
UK government
    policy agenda of 3, 7, 17, 66, 75
    political language of 65–6

United States
    culture of 226, 229
    healthcare in 10, 43, 208
    in World War II 208–9
user involvement 40, 46, 54, 57, 173, 175
user-oriented approaches 58, 143

value chains 13, 49, 167, 172, 256
Value Stream Mapping 262
virtual private networks (VPN) **245**

Wales 72, 78
waste 35, 103
Wirral NHS Trust 104
Witness Accenture 102
work, types of 79
work practices 57, 202
    changes to 14, 89–90
    idiosyncratic 143, 217
work processes 46
workarounds 184, 194, 197
workflow 28, 44, 53–4, 107–8, 121–2,
    216–19, 224
workplaces, social systems of 184